GUY

Q

GUY Q

1,305 TOTALLY ESSENTIAL SECRETS
YOU EITHER KNOW, OR YOU DON'T

JOE KITA *and the Editors of* **Men'sHealth**

RODALE

© 2003 by Rodale Inc.

All rights reserved. No part of this publication may be reproduced or transmitted in any form or by any means, electronic or mechanical, including photocopying, recording, or any other information storage and retrieval system, without the written permission of the publisher.

Men's Health is a registered trademark of Rodale Inc.

Printed in the United States of America
Rodale Inc. makes every effort to use acid-free ∞, recycled paper ♻ .

Book design by Chris Rhoads

Library of Congress Cataloging-in-Publication Data

Kita, Joe.
    Guy Q : 1,305 totally essential secrets you either know, or you don't
/ Joe Kita and the editors of Men's health.
       p.   cm.
    Includes index.
    ISBN 1–57954–859–8 hardcover
    ISBN 1–57954–860–1 paperback
    1. Men—Health and hygiene. I. Men's health (Magazine) II. Title.
RA777.8.K54 2003
613'.04234—dc21   2003013583

Distributed to the book trade by St. Martin's Press

2 4 6 8 10 9 7 5 3 1 hardcover
2 4 6 8 10 9 7 5 3 1 paperback

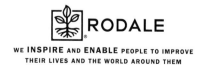

RODALE

WE **INSPIRE** AND **ENABLE** PEOPLE TO IMPROVE
THEIR LIVES AND THE WORLD AROUND THEM

FOR MORE OF OUR PRODUCTS
WWW.**RODALESTORE**.COM
(800) 848-4735

Authors are always dedicating books to parents, husbands, wives, kids, editors. Such sappiness is okay for memoirs, novels, and other earnest endeavors, but this book is essentially about taking control of your life. I don't know about you, but parents, mates, kids, and editors never helped me do that. In fact, they had the opposite effect. So they don't deserve any credit. In fact, it's because of them that I needed to create a book like this to put myself back together.

Instead, I'd like to dedicate this book to you. That's right, *you*. To make it official, just neatly fill your name in here:

This book is dedicated to _____.

If you flip open to this page real quick and show it to friends, they'll be suitably impressed. They'll think you're important. But you won't really be stretching the truth that much. This book *was* created for you. And now that it's been dedicated to you, my wish is that you'll be dedicated to it.

Joe Kita

CONTENTS

ACKNOWLEDGMENTS

I would like to acknowledge all the editors, writers, researchers, photographers, designers, sales-people, and support personnel (unfortunately too numerous to name) who have worked at *Men's Health* during the last 15 years.

This book is not mine. It is ours.

INTRODUCTION

You're about to enter a drivel-free zone. Once past this intro, you will be free of fluff and detail. You will be backed against a leather sofa (or perhaps a porcelain lid) and mercilessly machine-gunned with tip after tip until your sensibility is riddled with new possibilities for life improvement.

This is the *Men's Health* way. The editors, of which I am one, specialize in what's known (rather ingloriously) as "chunk journalism." Pick up a copy of *The New Yorker, Harper's* or any other "serious" magazine, and you'll find bazillion-word essays running for gray page after gray page. Regardless of how well-written or important these pieces are, to finish them requires the endurance of a Kenyan marathoner. Few people have that kind of literary stamina anymore. The time, unfortunately, just can't be spared.

So enter chunk journalism. Like its name suggests, information is delivered in easily digestible bits. We take the raw beef that's slapped on our desks, trim away the gristle and fat (notice I didn't say "butcher"), and deliver only the fillet. It's the print equivalent of, say, *Headline News*. Their anchors break down the world. Our editors demystify the arenas of health, fitness, nutrition, sex, and style. In an age when the quest for new information is insatiable, such an approach eliminates the panning

and quickly supplies the all-important nugget. When we've done our job right, the reader will say "Eureka!"

No doubt, you've already had this experience a few times in your life. When Big Uncle Tony poked his sausage finger into your 13-year-old ribs after that unfortunate incident with the Romano sisters, he said: "Don't let your little head do the thinking for your big head." And that stuck with you, didn't it? Likewise, when Boss Leo asked you to teach your pal Joey a "lesson" and you balked, he said: "Never let friendship interfere with business." And that stuck with you, too. Complex situations reduced to essential lessons. That's what we do.

Although each of the 1,305 tips in this book may look small and inconsequential, they are the painstaking distillation of entire articles, studies, interviews, and even books. In other words, they are the gist. What a great word that is: *gist*. It connotes such value that it should be the name of a currency. Forget dollars and pesos. Those with the most gist are, by far, the wisest and wealthiest.

I've been a writer and editor with *Men's Health* for almost a decade. I've seen it grow from a tiny quarterly ridiculed for publishing articles about cholesterol and prostate cancer (what guy wants to read about *that*?) to the largest men's magazine franchise on the planet with editions in 30 countries and a worldwide circulation of 8 million. I've seen men themselves evolve from being hesitant to talk about a suspicious shoulder mole to openly discussing the merits of Viagra. And in 1994, Congress further validated it all by naming National Men's Health Week as an annual awareness-raising event in mid-June. Although women in this country still outlive men by an average of 7 years, it won't be too long before education and prevention start narrowing the gap.

Because of what we stand for and the progress we've made, people often ask to visit our editorial headquarters in Emmaus, Pennsylvania. They want to get a behind-the-scenes glimpse at such an influential magazine. But I always discourage them from coming because they're bound to be disappointed. (In fact, both my kids prefer school to Take Our Daughters and Sons To Work Day.) There aren't any glamorous models strutting about, the coffee isn't lightened with mandatory soy milk, and there are no circus strongmen testing the latest fitness equipment. I'm sorry to admit that none of the editors work with their shirts off, displaying abs that resemble computer keyboards. Nor do we all have full heads of hair, impeccable wardrobes, or above-average testosterone levels. We're regular guys, just like you, with families and worries and dreams. But, ironically, that's probably been the key to our success. We connect.

You want a peek behind the scenes? I'll give you one. Most of us spend our days hunkered over desks perusing the latest scientific research, talking to experts by phone, or tapping out articles long past deadline. The *Men's Health* editorial office is a central command station from which we monitor the state of health, fitness, and manliness throughout the world. From time to time, we're handed documents called "Sieves," which are compiled by our library and research staffs after scanning hundreds of periodicals. Essentially, these are story leads. They contain information about new studies, programs, and products that might be worth investigating. What gets acted upon is largely determined at staff meetings. These can be raucous affairs at which topics are resolutely defended or collectively doused. The most entertaining ones always involve sex. If you think some of the stories and photography in *Men's Health* are racy, you should see the ideas that never make it into print. (One example: How to Have Sex So Good Even the Cops Will Come.)

After an article is approved, scheduled, and assigned it can take anywhere from a couple of weeks to half a year to write. When it's finally done, the "source packet" that accompanies it is thick with transcribed interviews, studies, journal articles, books, and other supporting material. All this is turned over to the fact-checking department, which recontacts sources and double-checks advice to assure the accuracy of what's about to be published. And just so you have an appreciation for the level at which we're operating, consider that our information comes from nationally recognized doctors and organizations. We're talking the absolute top experts in their respective fields—the equivalent of *Sports Illustrated* chatting up star players, head coaches, and the commissioner for an exposé on the NFL.

What you see in the magazine then is the culmination of a Herculean information-gathering effort. What you read is only the most practical, useable stuff. It's your personal Sieve, delivered 10 times per year. Even more amazing is the fact that this Herculean effort has been going on since the magazine was founded in 1988. The amount of info that's been collected and disseminated during that time is enough to fill a sizable library. To our knowledge, no one has ever been hurt through our erroneous advice. Instead, we regularly get letters like this from grateful readers:

Dear *Men's Health*,

The article you ran last month saved my husband from dying this week. It was entitled "Let My Heart Attack Save Your Life." He read the article a few weeks ago and on Wednesday, when he was home alone for lunch, he started experiencing constrictive-type sensations in his chest—not pain, just odd feelings. He then began feeling some pain in his left arm. Smart guy that he is, he took an aspirin and drove himself to the hospital. (Okay, he's not *that* smart.) He was indeed having a heart attack, and he had another more massive one 15 minutes after arriving at the ER. On Thursday he had triple bypass surgery and is making great progress. At age 44, coronary artery disease finally caught up with him despite his having a pretty healthful lifestyle. He told me he would not have gone to the hospital if he hadn't read all the various and peculiar symptoms listed in your article. Thanks for saving my husband's life.

By the way, could you please renew his subscription? Check enclosed.

Pretty heady stuff, huh? Get a letter like that, even once in a career, and you can rest assured it's all been worth it.

Yet we get them after just about every issue.

What you're holding in your hands right now can save you, too. Maybe not as dramatically as that fellow, but honestly who needs the theatrics? Whether you're overweight, out-of-shape, career-stuck, in poor health, stressed out, looking for love, in the midst of a midlife crisis, or just a spotty dresser, this book has something for you. It represents the accumulated knowledge of 15 years worth of reporting—the absolute best of what *Men's Health* has published. It has the power to change, enhance, and extend your life. Somewhere on the following pages is at least one tip that will be your eureka moment, one tip that will suddenly crystallize the problem, solve the dilemma, or point you in a new direction. Not many books can make that boast. Not many books harbor such potential energy. But this one does. In fact, if it doesn't live up to my hype, send it back and your money will be refunded no questions asked. Here at *Men's Health,* we believe that strongly in what we do *and* how this information can affect you.

Indeed, each of the writers and editors here has their own story of personal redemption. I've lost 35 pounds and run a marathon. Our fitness editor added 3 inches to his chest and 40 pounds to his bench press. Our nutrition editor uses the latest dietary information to better manage his diabetes. After passing a kidney stone, our health editor stays well-hydrated to be sure such a god awful thing never happens again. Our international editor fought back osteoarthritis and returned to the basketball court by taking the supplements glucosamine and chondroitin. Our managing editor lowered his LDL (bad) cholesterol by 71 points through diet, exercise, and the most up-to-date medical advice. And our sex editor, well, let's just say he's usually smiling.

I could go on. The staff is a thriving example of regeneration. And we did it with tips—bits of information picked up here and there. It's hard to make big changes in life. The energy and time commitment that's required are often too great. That's why so many Americans still struggle with their health. The problem isn't knowing what to do, it's doing it. The master plan, even when we hold it in our hands, is often too intimidating or unrealistic.

So why not take the opposite approach? Why not pick a tip, any tip, and begin there. Forget about such grand, amorphous goals as losing weight or getting in shape. They're too ill-defined for you to ever get there. Instead, aim to drink the leftover milk in your cereal bowl each morning to get more vitamins (see page 14), or use smaller, patternless dishes to reduce the amount you eat (see page 55), or "forget" your glasses the next time you're at the gym so you won't get distracted (see page 161). Quirky little tips like these, which on the surface seem almost comical, can make a big difference over time. After all, the statue of Adonis wasn't cast from a mold; it was chiseled. Make things more manageable.

So that's my pep talk. The drivel faucet is being turned off. This is your chance to get the body, the woman, the job, the look, the respect, the *life* you always wanted. From chunk to hunk. Begin the process.

Joe Kita
Executive Writer
Men's Health *Magazine*
August 2003

1

NUTRITION
and
WEIGHT LOSS

Sixty-one percent of Americans are now overweight, compared with 47 percent in 1980. In fact, obesity is about to surmount smoking as the number one health problem in the country, responsible for 300,000 deaths and $100 billion in medical expenses annually. While many people in the world are still scrabbling for rice kernels, we Americans are literally eating ourselves to death.

Whose fault is this? You can point the greasy finger at fast-food restaurants, food manufacturers, an increasingly sedentary workplace, a gluttonous society, or even mom's home cooking and the example your parents set. But you'll be most accurate if you turn that finger 180 degrees and point it directly at yourself. You are the ultimate arbiter of what gets put in your mouth. Every day you make dozens of little decisions that eventually determine your overall composition. Making excuses and apportioning blame is how you got that gut in the first place. It's time to change.

Believe it or not, whenever *Men's Health* asks its readers what they want to see more of in the magazine, they consistently answer "nutrition"—not building washboard abs or having rock star sex, but educating themselves about what they eat and drink on a daily basis. There's a widespread hunger for this information. Most Americans were never taught anything about food, except perhaps how to cook it or, in the case of grocery clerks, how to arrange it in paper sacks. We take food for granted, not only its safety but also its healthfulness. And therein lies our primary mistake. You must be just as discerning a consumer of food as you are of electronics, automobiles, or anything else. Taste is just one of many factors to consider. There's also total calories, percentage of calories from fat, grams of fiber, amounts of saturated and trans-fat, RDAs, etc. It's a bona fide science. In fact, it would probably be more beneficial to the welfare of our country if schools swapped out trigonometry for a class in it.

What you're about to digest is not an all-encompassing diet plan, but rather a piecemeal one—a collection of the best 259 tips *Men's Health* editors have gathered on the subject of nutrition and weight loss. Approach it like you would a tray of appetizers—a nibble here, a nibble there, let it settle in, then return for more later. Or here's an offbeat idea: Put this book in the refrigerator, right next to the beer and leftover fajitas. Every time you open the door, you'll be reminded to open the book. Assimilate one or two tips per visit. We guarantee that in time you'll come to look less like an Amana side-by-side

One of the biggest weight-loss myths is that you need a comprehensive eating plan to be successful. The truth is all that's necessary is some rudimentary knowledge of nutrition and an affinity for small change. Forgoing the Snapple you normally have with lunch, swapping mustard for mayonnaise on your next sandwich, ordering take-out pizza with light cheese . . . little modifications like these, which you eventually won't even notice, can have a major impact on your stomach and hips. Any of the tips you're about to read has that trouser-altering power.

Pick one.

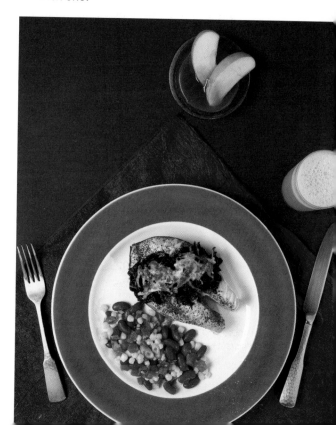

Make Small Changes to Lose Big

To take weight off and keep it off, make small, gradual changes you can live with. We're talking changes so innocuous, it won't seem like you've started a diet at all. When ordering fast food, for instance, get the same burger but tell them to leave off the cheese and you'll save 100 calories per meal, more than half of them from fat. Get your breakfast sandwich on a bagel instead of a fattier croissant and save 200 calories. Use low-fat mayonnaise and "lite" margarines in a tub; most taste as good but have half the fat of regular products. Avoid fatty salad toppings like eggs, olives, and regular dressing. And drink skim or 1 percent milk instead of 2 percent or whole.

Try the Never-Be-Hungry One-Day Meal Plan

Try this simple meal plan to kick-start your healthy eating lifestyle.

Breakfast

½   cup oatmeal, topped with 4 ounces skim milk and 1 tablespoon brown sugar

1   grapefruit

2   tablespoons peanut butter on 1 slice whole wheat toast

620 calories, 22 grams fat (3.5 g saturated fat), 23 protein, 91 g carbohydrates, 18 g fiber

Lunch

Low-fat cheese quesadillas, made with two 6-inch corn tortillas

8   ounces beef minestrone soup

550 calories, 18 g fat (7 g saturated fat), 34 g protein, 74 g carbohydrates, 16 g fiber

Snack

12-ounce strawberry-banana smoothie

160 calories, 0.5 g fat (0 g saturated fat), 6 g protein, 36 g carbohydrates, 4 g fiber

Dinner

Chicken-vegetable shish kebabs (6 oz boneless, skinless chicken breast)

8-inch baked potato with ¼ cup light sour cream

830 calories, 37 g fat (11 g saturated fat), 47 g protein, 76 g carbohydrates, 10 g fiber

Daily Total

2,160 calories, 77.5 g fat (21.5 g saturated fat), 110 g protein, 277 g carbohydrates, 48 g fiber

Make Weight Control a Habit

Here's another simple menu for one day of healthful eating. Repeat as necessary:

6:30 A.M. The moment you wake up, drink a glass of skim milk. The protein will energize you, dampen your appetite and prime you for a low-glucose carbohydrate breakfast that'll supply long-lasting energy.

7 A.M. You need to eat early in the day or you're doomed to high-calorie, fatty binges later. Stuff down some high-fiber oatmeal. Add brown sugar for flavor or cantaloupe chunks for bulk.

10:30 A.M. Have a piece of fruit—an apple or a pear. The goal is to never get hungry.

12:30 P.M. Midday meals need to be protein-heavy to keep you mentally alert and to ward off the afternoon slump. Think fish, chicken, or beans.

4 P.M. Mid-afternoon is when your natural cravings for food hit their zenith. Any fat you eat will quickly fire up your appetite for a high-fat dinner. So eat a high-fiber mini-meal that delivers some protein. Two hundred to 400 calories well invested here can keep you from eating a thousand in the evening. Our favorite is a whole wheat quesadilla with black beans, but you could try mixing raw oats and a sliced banana into a cup of plain, low-fat yogurt, or have a cup of bean soup. Dehydrated soups are great snacks you can take almost anywhere (just watch the sodium). They're especially good for plane rides.

7 P.M. When you dine out, send back the bread basket and start with a high-protein appetizer, such as a shrimp cocktail. Or simply skip to the main course and order some broiled fish. This will help curb your urge to pig out by taking advantage of the naturally satiating effect of protein. Once you have a taste of it, your appetite will start to wane. To finish out your main course, eat like an Asian. Use meat only for flavor and fill your plate with vegetables and other high-fiber foods.

8:30 P.M. You may crave sweets after dinner. Perfectly natural, and if you ignore it, the craving will disappear. But if it's just killing you, suck on a small piece of milk chocolate.

Estimate Serving Sizes

Doling out food portions for a recipe or a diet plan is always a crapshoot; we can barely tell 3 ounces from 10. Worse, we simply shovel down restaurant chow until we're asked to leave. Nutritionists helped us compile a dozen easy conversions for standard servings. (The nutritional information may vary by brand and type of food.) Remember, you eat the stuff on the left.

Food Portion	Calories	Fat (grams)	Same Size As
1 ounce sausage link	54	5	shotgun shell
1 ounce cubed Swiss cheese	107	8	4 dice
½ cup ice cream	143	7	tennis ball
1 tablespoon blue cheese dressing	77	8	½ golf ball
1 teaspoon butter	34	4	tip of thumb
½ cup cooked spaghetti	99	1	fist
8 ounces lasagna	270	8	2 hockey pucks
½ cup mashed potatoes	112	5	½ apple
3 ounces beef	219	13	deck of cards
1 cup chicken noodle soup	175	6	baseball
1 ounce mozzarella	80	6	Ping-Pong ball

This will satisfy your craving more than eating three pieces of cake with frosting. That's why the chocolate-covered dinner mint is a brilliant, time-proven idea.

11 P.M. After a great day of fat-burning (you did make it to the gym, didn't you?), don't blow it by wolfing down a midnight snack. Honor your mom's disciplinary tactic and go to bed hungry. This will set you up perfectly for burning fat overnight.

Eat Like Brando, Look Like Rambo

It takes 3,500 calories to make a pound of fat. So shave off 230 calories a day, and you'll lose nearly 2 pounds per month. For the record, that's roughly equal to a handful of potato chips, 2 tablespoons of olive oil, or a 16-ounce bottle of iced tea.

Request a Table for One

Want to eat less? Dine solo. The more people seated at the table, the more food each person consumes. Psychologists found that eating with one other person increased the size of each diner's meal by 28 percent. Two extra diners increased everyone's intake by 41 percent, and six or more dinner partners led folks to eat 76 percent more food. Eating with a group may cause people to linger over their food, consuming more than they would when alone.

Keep Serving Plates off the Table

Placing 9 pounds of meat loaf in your line of sight guarantees that you won't be satisfied with two pathetic slices.

OBSERVE THE ¾ PLATE RULE

Three-quarters of your dish should contain fresh produce and grains with the last quarter saved for fish, meat, or chicken. This combo will supply longer-lasting energy and fuel you for a good 5 hours.

Bag the Bagel

Bagels are low in fat, but most are so refined that they're almost devoid of nutritional value. They can also trigger a bad metabolic response in the body, reducing beneficial HDL cholesterol and raising triglycerides and insulin levels. This can increase your chances of developing diabetes and heart disease. Eat more whole grains instead.

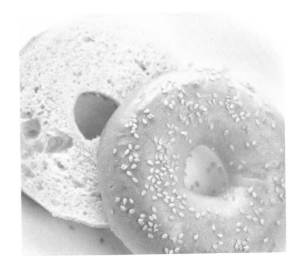

Eat Twice As Much

Cutting calories doesn't have to make you feel like you're starving yourself. Here's proof:

For breakfast, you can eat this . . .

½ dry bagel (200 calories)

9-ounce fat-free, sugar-free muffin (720 calories)

6 ounce corn muffin (530 calories)
1 large skim caffe latte (no sugar) (180 calories)

Or this . . .

2 light waffles, 2 tablespoons light syrup, berries (200 calories)

1 pineapple, ½ cantaloupe, ½ kiwi, ½ papaya, handful grapes, 2 pears, 2 whole-wheat rolls (720 calories)

4 English muffins (530 calories)

6 large hazelnut coffees, each with low-calorie sweetener and 2 tablespoons milk (180 calories)

For lunch, you can eat this . . .

1 chicken nugget (80 calories)
Turkey sandwich with 2 tablespoons mayo on rye (8 ounces turkey) 740 calories

2 slices cheese pizza (900 calories)

About ⅕ bacon cheeseburger (210 calories)

Dish of crispy Chinese noodles (400 calories)

Or this . . .

1¼ cups vegetable lentil soup (80 calories)

2 turkey, lettuce, and tomato sandwiches with mustard on rye (3 ounces turkey each) 620 calories

1 slice cheese pizza, 1½ cup minestrone, salad w/artichoke hearts and tomatoes (600 calories)

1 whole Boca burger on bun with tomato, onion, pickle, ketchup, and relish (210 calories)

Bowl of Chinese vegetable soup, 4 ounces shrimp, 1½ cup broccoli, 1 tablespoon hoisin sauce, ⅔ cup brown rice, fortune cookie (400 calories)

For a snack, you can eat this . . .

1 fat-free cookie (60 calories)
2⅔ ounces potato chips (400 calories)

Or this . . .

1 small cantaloupe (60 calories)
10 cups popcorn (400 calories)

For dinner, you can eat this . . .

1 meatball (100 calories)

2½ oz vodka and ½ cup mixed nuts (740 calories)

2-ounce hot dog, 2-ounce sausage, ⅓ cup macaroni salad (530 calories)

3 to 4 ounces assorted cookies (460 calories)

7-ounce square of cornbread and 1 tablespoon butter (820 calories)

Or this . . .

1¼ cups black-bean soup (100 calories)

1 cup consommé, 5 ounces scallops, asparagus, red cabbage, tossed salad, semolina roll, berries, 3 ounces wine (490 calories)

5 ounces shrimp, red peppers, onions, 2 portobello mushrooms, potato, zucchini, corn on the cob, 2 pounds watermelon (530 calories)

Mixed salad with dressing, marinated hearts of palm and artichoke, 3 ounces salmon, asparagus, oven-browned potatoes, poached pear in red wine (460 calories)

2 ears corn, roll with jam, baked potato with salsa, sweet potato, 2 slices raisin bread (820 calories)

For dessert, you can eat this . . .

1 black-and-white cookie (640 calories)

1 sundae with 3 scoops ice cream, 6 tablespoons chocolate syrup, 2 tablespoons chopped nuts, 2 tablespoons whipped cream and a maraschino cherry (1,360 calories)

1 raspberry tart (440 calories)

1 pint light ice cream (800 calories)

Or this . . .

2 frozen-yogurt cones, large plate of fruit, 6 hard candies, 8 chocolate mint sticks (640 calories)

4 sundaes, each with 3 scoops fat-free frozen yogurt, mixed fruit, 1 tablespoon chocolate syrup, 2 tablespoons whipped cream, and a maraschino cherry (1,360 calories)

8 cups raspberries with whipped topping (440 calories)

32 low-calorie Creamsicles (800 calories)

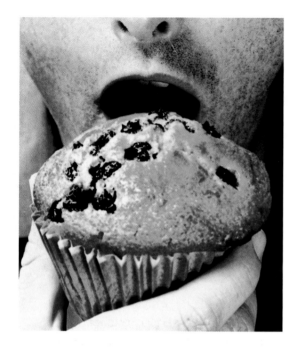

Cake Donut (310 calories, 19 grams of fat). You could slug down six small chocolate shakes at McDonald's for that much fat. Instead, go for a Bavarian Kreme Donut. It has a more tolerable 210 calories and 9 grams of fat. Tastes better, too.

Stop for the Egg McMuffin

Believe it or not, you can eat two Egg Mc-Muffin sandwiches from McDonald's and get less calories and fat than having a bagel with two tablespoons of cream cheese. The McMuffins have 580 calories, 24 grams fat, and 34 grams protein. The bagel delivers 643 calories, 28 grams fat, and 20 grams protein.

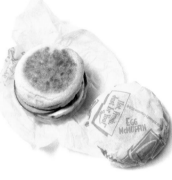

Forgo Muffins for Breakfast

The word "muffin" was coined so people wouldn't feel guilty about eating cake for breakfast. The regular ones, which can seem like they're the size of cauliflowers, can contain 500 calories and a lot of fat—up to 60 percent of calories. It's basically the same recipe as cake.

Be Careful of Coleslaw

This "vegetable" has as much fat as a large milk shake and fries. The creamy variety averages 36 grams of fat per serving—more than half what you should eat in a day. Pepper slaw is a much better choice. It's made of finely chopped cabbage and green peppers, but it has a vinegar-based dressing instead of mayo. A serving has only 1 gram of fat, and it's low in calories and sodium, too.

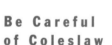

Don't Die at Dunkin' Donuts

The worst possible snack combination you can grab at Dunkin' Donuts is a large iced Coffee Coolatta with Cream (615 calories, 33 grams of fat) and a Whole Wheat Glazed

Cancel the Croutons

Most commercially prepared croutons are loaded with oil. Instead, add melba toast to your salad to provide crunch without lots of calories. Two slices of toast crumbled into a salad add only about 35 calories.

Dip Your Fork First

Whenever you have a salad, order the dressing on the side. Dip your fork in the dressing first, then spear a piece of lettuce, then eat it. Sound dumb? In fact, it's one of the smartest habits you can have. Four tablespoons of, say, honey-mustard dressing can have 60 grams of fat—nearly an entire day's worth for an average guy.

Don't Hail Caesar

Because its dressing contains so much oil, Caesar salad can be 70 to 80 percent fat. (One tablespoon of oil is 120 calories of pure fat.) And since it's usually tossed before it's served, you can't control the amount of dressing that's applied. Order the house salad with dressing on the side instead.

Behold the World's Most Dangerous Salad

A chef's salad is a meal—and a big one. Topped with turkey, roast beef, ham, cheese, a hard-boiled egg, and a few olives, what most dieters order as an exercise in restraint is really an act of indulgence. The average chef's salad has about a thousand calories—and that's in the nude. Dress it up in a 5-tablespoon suit of Russian, blue cheese, or Italian, and you're looking at 1,400 total calories—a figure that dwarfs a lot of full-course meals.

ORDER A PROTEIN APPETIZER

A cup of black bean soup or a few pieces of prosciutto-wrapped melon will sharply cut your appetite. That'll stop you from gorging on a high-calorie lunch, which is why your butt usually drags in the afternoon.

Think of Them as Fried Triangles of Death

When you're at a Mexican restaurant, it's common to go through a couple baskets of tortilla chips before your meal arrives. But just one basket of these fried triangles typically contains 1,067 calories, of which 46 percent are from fat (55 grams). Order steamed tortillas and dip those in the salsa instead.

Don't Order This, Hombre

The worst thing you can order at a Mexican restaurant are chiles rellenos. That's Spanish for "fat bomb." These mild to spicy chile peppers are stuffed with cheese and fried in egg batter. A typical two-pepper serving can have up to 800 calories and 46 grams of fat.

Make a Dinner of Appetizers

When dining out, pair a shrimp cocktail and clams casino with a side salad or soup to create your own healthful meal.

Oil Your Appetite

Fifteen to 20 minutes before dinner, soak up 2 teaspoons of olive oil with half a slice of bread (80 calories) and eat it to control your appetite. Olive oil stimulates the release of cholecystokinin, a gut hormone that signals the brain to stop eating. It'll help you eat less during dinner or skip dessert.

Eat Wet Food

Foods filled with water will satisfy your hunger with fewer calories. Go for strawberries instead of peanuts. Or order a cup of soup instead of a sandwich.

Slice Fat from Pizza

Always order your pizza with double tomato sauce and light cheese. Studies show that men who eat a lot of tomato products tend to have less prostate cancer—probably because tomatoes are a rich source of lycopene. Reducing the mozzarella by just one-third (you won't miss it) will save you 20 grams of fat. That's as much as in a McDonald's Quarter Pounder.

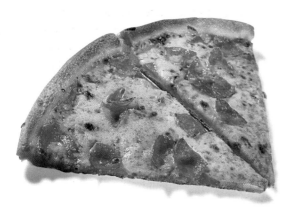

Correct Your Slice

Having lunch at Pizza Hut? Two slices of thin-crust pizza have 30 grams of fat and 722 calories, but you'll actually save about 6 grams of fat if you add ham. When the pizza makers use ham, they cut back on cheese, says a Pizza Hut spokesman.

Blot Your Pizza

By blotting the grease on top of a pizza with a napkin, you'll eliminate at least a teaspoon (4.5 grams) of fat per slice.

Vote Sicilian

Sicilian pizza is better than thin because you get more carb-rich dough and less fat-laden cheese. Watch out for deep-dish, though: The crust can soak up extra fat from a heavily oiled pan.

Grill the Waitress

Don't assume that grilling is a more healthful method of cooking. In many restaurants, the meat is "grilled" in a pan with butter or oil, which can make chicken just as fatty as beef. Ask.

Eat More Loins

Meats with "loin" in their name tend to be lower in fat. Three ounces of pork tenderloin, for example, have a measly 5 grams of fat.

Pass on the Prime Rib

The reason prime rib seems to melt in your mouth is because it's full of tenderizing fat that, unfortunately, can't be trimmed away. Although it's unmarbled and looks very lean, prime rib is the fattiest type of steak—typically 982 calories and 78 grams of fat for a broiled 1-pound, king-cut portion. That's the equivalent of almost two Big Macs.

Wash Your Meat

Here's an easy way to cut the fat content of your secret chili recipe: As soon as you finish browning the ground beef, pour it into a dish covered with a double thickness of paper towels. Then put another paper towel on top and blot the grease. If you want to remove even more fat, dump the beef into a colander and rinse it with hot (but not boiling) water. The water will wash away fat and cholesterol. Using these methods together can cut 50 percent of the meat's fat content. And in chili, you won't taste the difference.

SNEAK IN SOME TURKEY

Hamburgers made entirely of ground turkey tend to be dry, but a little mixed with ground beef is hardly noticeable. Ground turkey makes an excellent substitute for beef in chili, though. You'll never notice the difference. When buying ground turkey, make sure it's ground turkey *breast*. Regular ground turkey can include fattier dark meat and even some skin, which gives it almost as much fat as lean ground beef.

Give Bacon the Boot

Bacon prices have been extremely low, so fast-food joints have been adding it to everything. "Would you like a bacon shake, sir?" Pass on it; four strips add 12 grams of fat and 144 calories to a burger.

Make a Better Fish Stick

Fish sticks are the seafood version of hot dogs. Here's a healthier do-it-yourself version: Pick up a salmon or tuna steak and cut it into finger-size portions. Dip the sticks into an egg-white batter and roll them in a bowl of bread crumbs. Freeze and then bake when hungry.

Fork Out the Chinese

When you order out for Chinese, instead of using a spoon to scoop the food out of the carton, use a fork or chopsticks. That way you'll be more likely to leave behind the fatty, artery-clogging sauce.

Be a Portobello Fellow

For a meaty dinner entrée, substitute portobello mushrooms for a T-bone. One portobello (roughly the size of a saucer) has less than 1 gram of fat, and when it's grilled it tastes like a tender steak. Slice a few portobellos to ½-inch thickness and brush with a mixture of fat-free Italian dressing, thyme, and Worcestershire sauce. Grill for 3 or 4 minutes on each side over a medium-hot flame. Garnish with grilled onions and peppers.

Eat This Junk

For the occasional splurge, go with Wendy's Classic Single with Everything (410 calories, 19 grams of fat). It beats Burger King's Whopper with Cheese (760 calories, 48 grams of fat) and McDonald's Quarter Pounder with Cheese (530 calories, 30 grams of fat).

Order This at Wendy's

A Wendy's plain baked potato and a small chili contains 92 grams of carbohydrates, 22 grams of protein, and only 7 grams of fat. Pour the chili on the potato for a hearty lunch.

Don't Get Hooked on Fast Fish

Fish has a health food reputation, but let it swim by at fast-food franchises. McDonald's Filet-o-Fish has 450 calories and 25 grams of fat, twice the calories and three times the fat of the basic burger.

Curd the Fat

Use small-curd, low-fat cottage cheese instead of high-fat ricotta in lasagna, manicotti, and other Italian dishes.

FEEL THE BURN

Eating spicy foods will make you eat more slowly, fill you up more quickly, and slightly increase your metabolism so you burn more calories—three strong reasons to sprinkle some cayenne on your chicken.

Instead of Seconds, Have Gum

When sanity dictates that you stop shoving food into your face at the buffet or dinner table, pop mint-flavored gum into your mouth. It changes the flavor of everything, and it makes that third helping of linguine almost impossible to swallow.

Don't be a Bottom Feeder

Fruit is good for you, so the best yogurt must be the kind with fruit in it, right? Not necessarily. For the most nutritious yogurt, skip the "fruit on the bottom" varieties. The "fruit" may be mostly jam, which packs the equivalent of 8 or 9 teaspoons of sugar per cup—nearly as much as a can of soda. Instead, choose plain fat-free yogurt or flavors such as lemon, which don't contain fruit, and add your own berries. Fresh berries will provide a healthful dose of fiber as well.

Can Your Sweet Tooth

Canned pineapple, mandarin oranges, and peaches are all great sources of prime nutrients, and they can satisfy a sweet tooth. Buy 'em packed in light syrup or water.

Oil Your Potato

To save calories and fat, put a splash of olive oil on your baked potato instead of butter or sour cream.

Cool Your Cans

Refrigerate canned meats, soups, gravies, and other canned foods containing fat. The fat will collect and rise to the top so you can scrape it off.

Order the Steak Fries

If you love french fries, always order the steak fries. Large cut fries don't absorb as much oil as shoestring or curly fries, which lowers the fat count.

Freeze, Mister

One of the easiest ways to improve your diet is to stock your freezer with bags of frozen vegetables. Not only do they provide a variety of nutrients, but they're also convenient. Throw a handful in soups, stews, stir-frys, and instant rice dishes. Frozen vegetables are usually frozen within a few hours of harvest, so their nutritional quality can actually be better than fresh.

Know Your Nuts

As any man with a long dating history knows, it's impossible to avoid nuts completely. Although most nuts are high in fat, some are better than others. The most healthful nut is the almond. A handful (that's 2 ounces) contains as much fiber as an apple (7 grams), almost as much potassium as a banana (436 grams), and 10 milligrams of heart-protecting vitamin E. But don't get carried away; that handful has 15 grams of fat. The death nut is the macadamia. It contains very few nutrients (almost no vitamin E) and is loaded with fat (21 grams per 2 ounces).

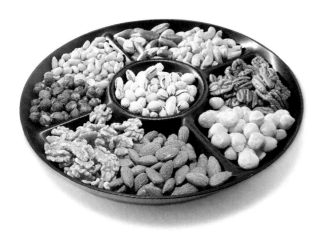

Don't Have Any of This

Coconut. It's about 76 percent *saturated* fat.

Choose Marinara over Pesto

Pesto makes you plump with 320 calories and 31 grams of fat in a quarter-cup. Marinara has only 50 calories and 2 fat grams for the same amount.

Get Rice, Not Pasta

You can't put a lot of rice on your fork. So you eat more slowly. With pasta, you can devour a plate in 10 minutes. And that's including the pasta.

Use Whipped Butter

When nothing but butter will do, buy whipped butter. The whipping process mixes in air and increases volume, so you'll use less. Just remember that if you melt it, you're back to the same high calorie and fat count as the stick stuff.

Hold the Mayo

The ultimate eating blunder is using full-fat mayo. One tablespoon contains 100 calories and 11 grams of fat. Instead, substitute mustard or our favorite healthy brand: Hellmann's Light Mayonnaise (50 calories, 5 grams fat).

Buy This Peanut Butter

Besides being great rat bait, peanut butter is nutritious. It's a potent source of protein, potassium, fiber, and carbohydrates, and it contains very little cholesterol. Unfortunately, with 16 grams of fat and 190 calories in every 2-tablespoon serving, peanut butter sticks to more than the roof of your mouth.

We taste-tested some of the new lower-fat brands to see how they compare. Reduced-fat. Natural. Creamy. Chunky. We tried 'em all.

Our favorite is Peter Pan Whipped Creamy peanut butter. It has a light, airy texture and is smooth, not oily with a honeylike sweetness and ballpark-peanut saltiness. Plus, this peanut butter has fewer calories and less fat per tablespoon than most "natural" and re-duced-fat varieties (just 140 calories with 110 from fat, compared with 200 total calories and 150 calories from fat for Smucker's Natural, and 190 calories, 110 of them from fat, for Reduced Fat Jif.)

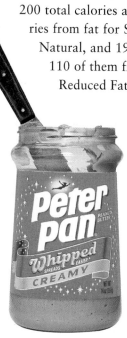

Share a Kiss after Dinner

A tiny taste of chocolate will satisfy your sweet buds just as thoroughly as several large handfuls.

It's Not Just for Breakfast Any More

Whenever you get a craving for sweets, have a bowl of kids' cereal instead. Sugary cereals have relatively low calorie and fat counts, so an occasional bowl won't hurt. Our three favorites—Lucky Charms, Count Chocula, and Frosted Flakes—supply 25 percent of your Daily Value of thiamin, riboflavin, niacin, vitamins B_6 and B_{12}, folate, and zinc in a single serving. Frosted Flakes also offers 15 percent of your Daily Value of vitamin A and 25 percent of vitamin C. With skim milk, it has fewer than 300 calories, compared to a large chocolate candy bar which packs more than 500. That change alone can save you close to 1,500 calories a week. To get more vitamins, drink the leftover milk in the bowl.

Crunch One of These

Quaker Chocolate Crunch Rice Cakes are the best way to calm a sudden chocolate craving. That's partly because they're so filling. Researchers found that foods that have been puffed with air are better at satisfying hunger than lower-volume foods that pack the same number of calories. Just 60 total calories and 1 gram of fat in one.

Get Your Chocolate Fix

Chocolate biscotti sounds foo-foo, but it's low in fat and great for dunking in coffee. Keebler Chocolate Grahams are also tasty and low in calories.

Prioritize Your Vices

If your weakness is cheesecake, then don't settle for the second-rate stuff revolving in some diner's pie case. Indulge in nothing but the best. If this means you have to overnight a Baby Watson for $50, so be it. You'll savor it more and eat less. The same holds true for any fatty food you love: Find the one place where it's been elevated to an art form, and eat it only there.

Order Cake over Ice Cream

Both are similar in fat and calories, but ice cream is more habit forming. If you have cake on Monday, you won't usually be craving more on Tuesday. But open a carton of Ben & Jerry's, and it's only the beginning of a month-long orgy.

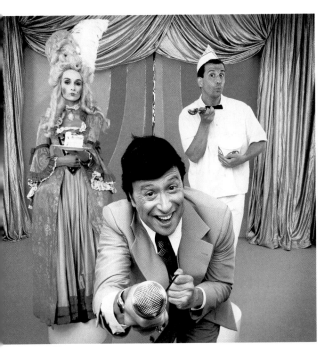

SAY YES TO FUDGE

One homemade brownie with nuts will run you more than 300 calories and 21 grams of fat. Better you should pass it up for . . . fudge. Remarkable, yes, but at 1 ounce, fudge carries only 112 calories with 3 grams of fat.

Watch the Cookie Crumble

A cookie's crumble indicates its fat content. In general, store-bought cookies have a higher fat content to give them a softer texture. Harder cookies like gingersnaps and vanilla wafers have about half the fat of their softer cousins. To be doubly sure, rest your favorite cookie on a napkin. If it leaves a grease stain, don't eat it.

Pass the Bar Exam

These six frozen treats passed our test for great taste and low fat:

Nestlé Crunch Reduced Fat Vanilla Ice Cream Bar. 240 calories, 2g protein, 15g carbohydrates, 8g fat. Love those crunchy bits.

Klondike with Oreo Ice Cream Bars. 160 calories, 2g protein, 17g carbohydrates, 10g fat. Clever cookie concept, smooth ice cream.

Tropicana Orange Cream Bar. 70 calories, 1g protein, 14g carbohydrates, 1g fat. Great combo, rich, sweet, citrusy, low-cal.

Starbucks Frappuccino Mocha Bar. 120 calories, 4g protein, 22g carbohydrates, 2g fat. It'll perk you up, not weigh you down.

Hershey's Vanilla Ice Cream Sandwich. 210 calories, 4g protein, 30g carbohydrates, 9g fat. Low-fat bliss.

Fudgsicle. 90 calories, 3g protein, 18g carbohydrates, 1g fat. A guilt-free, satisfying classic.

Have a Milky Way Lite

Despite having a reasonable 170 calories and 5 grams of fat, Milky Way Lite is just as creamy, airy, and delicious as the original Milky Way, which weighs in at 11 grams of fat and 280 calories for a 2.15-ounce bar. The light bar gives a great caramel chew, but it's also a half-ounce smaller than the real bar, or about three bites less.

Reward Yourself at Dairy Queen

While it's no lean treat, the Banana Split at Dairy Queen isn't that bad. With 510 calories and 12 grams of fat, it has only half the fat of an ice-cream cone with a chocolate shell. The bananas give you 467 milligrams of potassium, 10 mg of vitamin C, and a few grams of fiber, too.

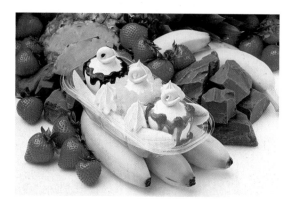

Pop Up Some of This

The best microwave popcorn is Pop-Secret, the "94% Fat Free" version. It's the tastiest brand we've tried, and if you split a bag with someone, you get only 110 calories and 2 grams of fat, plus 4 grams of fiber. Inhaling the whole bag? Even then, you're getting 60 less calories and 7 grams less fat than one Milky Way bar.

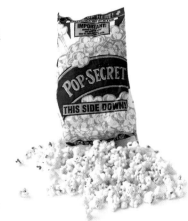

Don't Be Fooled by Energy Foods

Sports drinks and sports bars are all over health clubs. But unless you skip a meal somewhere, these items will add hundreds of calories to your daily intake. If you're doing extreme endurance sports in hot weather, you may need sports drinks. Otherwise, water quenches thirst just as well, and there's nothing an energy bar can give you that real food can't. Have a banana instead.

Always Eat a Little Dessert

Here's why: Sweets such as cookies and low-fat ice-cream bars signal your brain that the meal is over. Without them, you might not feel satiated, which might leave you prowling the kitchen all night for something to satisfy your sugar jones.

Cure Midnight Cravings

If you're the type who wakes up hungry in the middle of the night, keeping a glass of water and some grapes on a bedside table will save you a trip to the kitchen, where the last piece of chocolate cake awaits.

Have a Mineral Water Chaser

At a party, follow each drink with a glass of mineral water or soda. You'll always have something in your hands to sip, but you'll be getting half the liquor and calories you otherwise would. No-calorie, carbonated mineral water and lime looks just like a 170-calorie gin and tonic.

Pour Yourself Some Chocolate Milk

Nestlé Nesquick delivers only ½ gram of fat per 2 tablespoons. The key is to use skim or 1 percent milk instead of whole milk. Chocolate syrup is just as low in fat.

Skip This Juice

Apples are a terrific source of vitamin C and fiber. But apple juice is little more than sugar water.

Chill Cans in Minutes

The quickest way to chill soda or beer is to submerge the six-pack in chopped ice or a soup of water and ice. This method works even faster than putting it in a freezer.

Know Where a Beer Belly Comes From

Alcohol suppresses your body's ability to burn fat. When you drink alcohol, your body combusts fat much more slowly than usual. In one study, for example, researchers found that 3 ounces of alcohol reduced the body's ability to burn fat by about one-third. The unburned fat may go to your waist, creating a beer belly. So it is not just the calories and the fact that alcohol is converted into simple sugars that make it fattening, but also the way that alcohol throws off your body's normal disposal of fat in your diet.

Eat This, Then Go Out

Eat an apple before you head to your local tavern. This will prevent you from inhaling three bowls of beer nuts and a plateful of nachos when you sidle up to the bar.

WHEN ALL ELSE FAILS

KEEP A BOTTLE FROM STICKING TO A COASTER

Here's a great use for salt. Sprinkle a little salt on a coaster to keep it from coming up when you pick up your bottle of Bud.

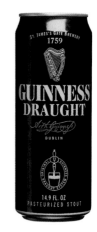

When You Booze, You Can Lose

Some drinks can make you fall right off the weight-loss wagon, while others aren't so bad. Here's a quick primer:

Beverage	Calories
The Good	
One ounce of any 80-proof alcohol and club soda	65
A glass of red or white wine (4 ounces)	85
One light beer	95
Any coffee drink with an ounce of alcohol (no whipped cream)	100
The Bad	
White Russian	245
Piña colada	329
Daiquiri	422
The Ugly	
Any ice-cream concoction	

Lighten Your Brew

For a light beer without a watery taste try Molson Canadian Light. Just 690 calories in a six-pack.

Have a Guinness

Although Guinness looks heavy, it's actually lower in calories than many watery light beers. There are only 149 calories in 14.9 ounces.

Drink Your Coffee Black

A cup of black coffee has 10 calories and no fat. The caffe latte you buy at the coffeehouse has 210 calories and 11 grams of fat. Multiply the difference over a year, and you save 73,000 calories—21 pounds.

Lighten Your Own Coffee

Half-and-half contains 2 grams of saturated fat per 2 tablespoons, but when coffeehouse servers lighten your coffee, they typically use anywhere from 4 to 8 tablespoons. That's as much as 9 grams of saturated fat—more than you'd get from eating a beef hot dog. It's better to add the stuff yourself or switch to skim milk.

WHEN ALL ELSE FAILS

WATCH SLUGS DIE

If a legion of slugs is assaulting your garden, here's a vicious option: Buy a case of cheap beer. Pour a can into a pie plate. Now sit back with the other 23 cans and watch the fun. By the time you come to, every slug in North America will be in the tin plate, dead. Like you, they can't resist the stuff.

Belly Up to the Bar

When you're having a few brews at the local tavern, here's which snacks to enjoy and which to avoid:

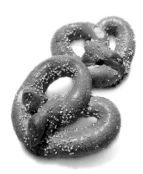

	Calories	Fat
Eat This		
3 big, hard pretzels	300	0g
Not Bad, but Go Slowly		
Cheddar Goldfish (2 ounces or 2 big handfuls)	260	10g
One slice of cheese pizza	140	3g
One crab cake	160	10g
Two Slim Jim Giant beef jerky snacks	140	8g
Two mozzarella sticks	110	6g
A bowl of chili	229	7g
Loosen the Belt		
Four onion rings	220	11g
Two pickled eggs	210	11g
15 popcorn shrimp	210	12g
Four buffalo wings	280	18g
Two potato skins	260	12g
Buy Yourself a Caftan		
A handful of peanuts	336	29g
Seven pigs in a blanket	320	26g
Plate of nachos with the works	569	31g
Six to eight fried shrimp	454	25g
Fried breaded clams (¾ cup)	451	26g
Four breaded and fried jalapeño poppers or other vegetables	360	24g

Open Bottled Beer (Without an Opener)

If you find yourself with a beer but no opener, you have our condolences. But if you have a key, all is not lost.

1. Choose the longest key in your bunch.

2. Grab the bottle around the neck with your left hand, allowing the neck of the bottle to extend above your index finger and thumb.

3. Align the shaft of the key so that the left edge is just under the cap of the bottle. The tip of the key should lie across the bottom half of your left index finger. (Tip: The key should extend far enough onto your left finger that you don't pierce your skin.)

4. While levering off your left index finger, use your right hand to pop the top off of the bottle.

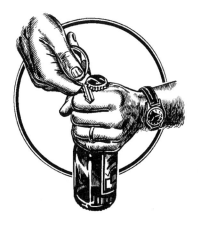

Make a Skinny Irish Coffee

Irish coffee with heavy cream has 176 calories and 11 grams of fat. Make it with fat-free whipped topping—not cream—and it drops to 76 calories and no fat.

Don't Diet with Diet Soda

Be careful with diet sodas. They're low in calories, but one study found that people who drink beverages loaded with artificial sweeteners may actually eat more food. Limit yourself to two per day.

Hit the Snacks Instead of the Shower

The quickest and most effective way to maximize the results of lifting weights is to have a snack immediately after you finish your workout. Research shows that men who eat after exercising gain more muscle than men who don't. Munch immediately—ideally within 30 minutes of working out—and swallow the right food. The perfect post-weight-training snack has about 400 calories, with 20 to 30 grams of protein (to build new muscle) and 50 to 65 grams of carbohydrates (to repair old muscle). Peanut butter and jelly sandwiches or energy bars fit the formula. Or pick up one of these on your drive home:

• Taco Bell Steak Burrito Supreme (without sour cream) and a diet soda (420 calories, 16g fat, 19g protein, 50g carbohydrate)

• Arby's Light Roast Turkey Deluxe sandwich and an Arby's orange juice (400 calories, 5g fat, 24g protein, 67g carbohydrate)

• KFC Honey BBQ chicken sandwich and a small soft drink (410 calories, 6g fat, 28g protein, 64g carbohydrate)

Melt the Ice Cream

Here's a list of favorite foods and how much time you need to spend on a stair-climbing machine to burn off the calories they pack:

Food	Time (minutes)*
1 chocolate-chip cookie	5
6½ ounces orange juice	9
12 ounces light beer	10
10 potato chips	10
1 cup plain yogurt (whole milk or low-fat)	14
12 ounces Coca-Cola	14
3-ounce T-bone steak	18
Snickers bar	28
Hamburger	40
1 pint Ben & Jerry's ice cream	104

Based on 10-calorie-per-minute average burn off by a 150-pound man on a typical stair-climbing machine.

Don't Get Fat Eating Fat-Free

If your new crash diet entails eating nothing but fat-free foods, rethink your strategy. Study subjects who replaced 20 percent of their fat intakes with fat substitutes were not only ravenous by day's end, they stuffed down almost twice their normal quota of fat-laden foods the next day. Real fat slows digestion, but fat substitutes don't. The result: You're hungry sooner after eating.

WHEN ALL ELSE FAILS

PUT THE BEER IN THE WASHER

The average washing machine can hold 24 cans of beer and a couple of bags of ice. So put your machine to good use at your next party! This strategy keeps your refrigerator clear during parties and saves you from having to drain a cooler the next morning.

Vend Off Hunger

Don't make a habit of it, but if you ever find yourself stuck in a Des Moines motel with $2.80 in change (long story), here are a couple of healthful dinner alternatives:

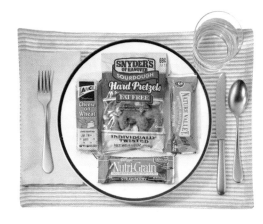

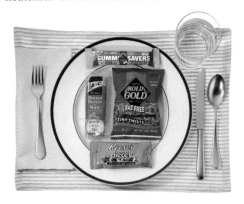

Meal 1

Lance Peanut Butter on Malt Crackers (1.3 oz): 190 calories, 10 g fat, 6 g protein, 18 g carbohydrates

Reese's Pieces (1.6 oz): 230 calories, 10 g fat, 6 g protein, 28 g carbohydrates

Fat-Free Rold Gold Tiny Twists (1 oz): 100 calories, 0 g fat, 3 g protein, 23 g carbohydrates

Gummi Savers (1.5 oz): 130 calories, 0 g fat, 2 g protein, 32 g carbohydrates

Total: 650 calories, 20 g fat, 17 g protein, 101 g carbohydrates

Meal 2

Lance Cheese on Wheat Crackers (1.3 oz): 190 calories, 10 g fat, 4 g protein, 21 g carbohydrates

Strawberry NutriGrain Bar (1.3 oz): 140 calories, 3 g fat, 2 g protein, 27 g carbohydrates

Snyder's Fat-Free Pretzels (2 pretzels): 220 calories, 0 g fat, 6 g protein, 44 g carbohydrates

Nature Valley Peanut Butter Crunchy Granola Bar (1.5 oz): 190 calories, 6 g fat, 5 g protein, 28 g carbohydrates

Total: 740 calories, 19 g fat, 17 g protein, 120 g carbohydrates

Cultivate Permanent Change

Don't make temporary changes to your diet with the idea that you'll stop them when you've lost some weight. Permanently change your eating habits and the way you think about food. That's the way you'll keep the pounds off for good.

Color Your Diet

Besides weight loss, the food choices that you make affect every process in your body. Good nutrition starts with smart shopping. Buy the brightest colored vegetables that you see. Vibrant colors usually correspond with more vitamins. This means go easy on iceberg lettuce, celery, and cucumbers and load up on carrots, tomatoes, red bell peppers, and sweet potatoes. They're higher in vitamins such as A and C. Or go for darker shades of greens. Romaine lettuce, for example, has nearly seven times the vitamin C and twice the calcium of its paler, iceberg cousin. The same holds true for fruit. Pink grapefruit, for instance, has more than 30 times the vitamin A of white grapefruit.

Pick a Perfect Avocado

When choosing an avocado, apply gentle pressure with your thumb. Feel for a little give, but if you leave a dent, it's overripe.

Make the Most of Your Produce

Cut and wash fruits and vegetables *just before* cooking or eating them. This keeps vitamin levels at their max. And don't cut them into tiny pieces. The more surface area exposed to oxygen, the faster vitamins lose their potency.

Drink Your Breakfast

Every meal you eat is a choice—you can choose good health or not. Choose right, right from the start with breakfast. Our favorite morning drink is Carnation Instant Breakfast. Each shake has just 1 gram of fat and supplies up to 50 percent of your daily requirements of 21 of the most important vitamins and minerals for men. We like the variety pack, which supplies five flavors: milk chocolate, vanilla, chocolate malt, strawberry, and cappuccino.

UNCOMMON KNOWLEDGE

POUR THE PERFECT BEER

By pouring beer into the center of the glass, you get more bubbles, which release the aroma of the beer and enhance its taste. Optimum pouring is a matter of balance. Begin by letting the beer flow down the side of the glass, then move the stream into the center in order to top off the beer with a half-inch head. You know what to do next.

Swap Out Snacks

You don't have to quit snacking entirely to lose weight, just substitute more healthful snacks. Here are a few suggestions:

Instead of snacking on ...	Snack on ...	And save ...
Pringles Cheezums (1 oz or 1 small can)	Combos Cheddar Cheese Pretzel snacks (1 oz or ⅓ cup)	160 calories
2 Twinkies	2 Tastykake Chocolate Cupcakes	100 calories
3 Pecan Sandies	3 Chips Ahoy cookies	80 calories
1 5th Avenue candy bar	1 Whatchamacallit candy bar	60 calories
1 Pop-Tart (Frosted Blueberry)	1 Nutri-Grain Bar (blueberry)	60 calories
Twix (2 cookie bars)	Kit Kat (4 sticks)	60 calories
3 Musketeers (candy bar)	100 Grand Bar (2 pieces)	60 calories
Cheez-It Snack Crackers (30)	Cheese Nips Air Crisps (3)	56 calories
Wise Premium Original Butter Popcorn (3 cups)	Orville Redenbacher's Microwave Movie Theater Popcorn (3 cups)	40 calories
Goldfish Snack Mix Honey Roasted (½ cup)	Wheatables Snack Mix Toasted Honey (½ cup)	40 calories
Fritos Corn Chips (1 oz or 32 chips)	Nacho Cheesier Doritos (1 oz or 11 chips)	20 calories
Sprite (12 ounces)	Ginger ale (12 ounces)	20 calories

Drink the RDA

To get your recommended six servings of fruits and vegetables daily without munching on any fruits and vegetables, do this:

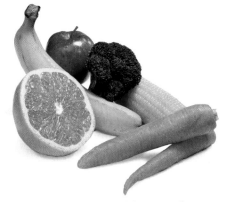

At breakfast: Drink one tall (12-ounce) glass of a 100 percent red-grapefruit/orange juice blend. (Tropicana makes one.)

At lunch and dinner: Drink one tall glass of low-sodium V8.

That's it. You just drank the

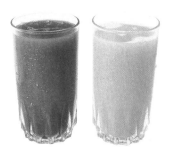

equivalent of six servings of fruits and vegetables and also swallowed some extra protection from prostate cancer, thanks to the lycopene in the tomatoes and red grapefruit.

Squeeze More Calcium Into Your Diet

The best orange juice you can drink is Tropicana Pure Premium with Calcium. Many men don't get enough calcium, which is why our nutritionist panel unanimously recommends calcium-spiked OJ. (According to one recent study, the calcium in just one glass daily will cut your risk of certain colon cancers by close to 50 percent.) Our tasters said the Trop was tops when it comes to flavor.

Steam the Dream

Broccoli is the king of vegetables. It's high in fiber and more densely packed with vitamins and minerals than almost any other food. In fact, a cup of steamed broccoli delivers more than 150 percent of the recommended dietary allowance of vitamin C, almost half of vitamin A, 22 percent of calcium, 18 percent of iron, 9 percent of thiamine, and 7 percent of niacin—a real bargain at only 46 calories. Ounce for ounce, steamed fresh broccoli contains nearly 90 percent as much vitamin C as fresh orange juice and half as much calcium as milk.

Steer Clear of Trans-Fats

According to a Harvard University study, you could cut your heart-attack risk in half by eating just 4 grams less of trans-fat each day. You'll find it in stick margarine, crackers, cookies, cakes, and many deep-fried foods, especially french fries. Look for the phrase "partially hydrogenated vegetable oil" on nutrition labels. The closer to the top of the ingredient list you find this, the more trans-fat the food contains.

Order Soup as an Appetizer

Eating vegetable and noodle soups before a normal meal can help you lose weight. The fiber causes food to go through your digestive system faster, and the water helps dissolve the fat. Add a potato to the soup, and studies suggest that you're likely to consume about 20 percent fewer calories over the course of the meal. Tomato soup has the same effect. You'll eat less during the meal, and you'll feel full longer.

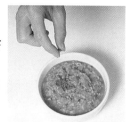

Doctor Yourself with Pepper

Sweet red peppers often cost two times more than green ones, but they might be worth it. Red bell peppers contain nine times as much vitamin A as green peppers do. Vitamin A is a disease-fighter known to speed the healing of wounds. Also, red peppers have more than double the vitamin C of their green cousins.

SNACK ON A STALK

Celery is pretty much the answer for any man whose doctor has told him "You have high blood pressure; cut down on salt." Celery's natural salty flavor can help quash your sodium jones, whether noshed raw or added to a wide variety of dishes. And as a bonus, it contains potassium, a mineral that's been shown to help fight hypertension.

GROW MONSTER TOMATOES

Turn a leaf blower on your tomato plants for 2 seconds every other day. One study showed that tomatoes from plants pollinated this way were about 17 percent heavier than those exposed only to natural wind. The higher-powered machinery helps get the pollen into the female organ.

Spend Your Bread Wisely

Shopping in the bread aisle, you naturally grab a loaf of something brown—it surely must be higher in fiber than Wonder Bread, right? Well, actually no. That dark complexion may be courtesy of molasses or food dyes. Likewise, a loaf with seeds or oatmeal flakes gracing its top isn't necessarily high in fiber, either. The seeds or flakes could be just decorations. To be sure you're a bread-winner, look for the phrase "100 percent whole wheat" or "whole-grain" on the package.

Brownnose General Tso

The next time that you're lunching at Chew Sum Fat, ask the waiter to substitute brown rice for white. Your fortune cookie's note should read: "You will increase fiber by more than 200 percent."

Pour Milk on the Fire

If you're a lover of chile peppers, you've probably already discovered that even a tall glass of ice water won't douse the flaming pain. That because capsaicin, the stuff that makes hot peppers hot, isn't soluble in water. Instead try milk, sour cream, or yogurt. Alcohol dissolves capsaicin, too, which is why beer and Mexican food go together so well. Rice and bread are also effective.

Have Another Pint

Blueberries are one of the most healthful foods you can eat. They beat out 39 other fruits and vegetables in the antioxidant power ratings, making them a great hedge against cellular damage that contributes to heart disease and cancer. One study also found that rats who gobbled blueberries were more coordinated and smarter than rats who didn't. Make it your goal to eat a pint of blueberries every week.

Avoid Fancy Chocolate

As a general rule, the darkest European chocolate is highest in fat, because it has the highest concentration of cocoa butter. Milk chocolate, on the other hand, is higher in sugar but often lower in fat.

Skip the Crust

You can eat your pie and have it too by forking out the filling and leaving the crust—especially the thick stuff around the edges. A standard pastry crust contains 18 grams of fat per slice—almost twice the amount in a regular Milky Way bar.

Change Your Oil

Before you cook foods in oil, learn which oils won't gunk up your insides. The worst are those high in saturated fat, such as coconut oil and lard. The best are olive, safflower, and canola oils, which are high in monounsaturated and polyunsaturated fats. These are heart-healthier fats that can help you lower your total cholesterol and raise your HDL (good cholesterol).

	Calories	Total Fat (grams)	Saturated	Monounsaturated	Polyunsaturated
Butter	68	7.7	4.8	2.2	0.3
Canola	124	14.0	1.0	8.3	4.1
Coconut	120	13.6	11.8	0.8	0.2
Corn	120	13.6	1.7	3.3	7.9
Lard	115	12.8	5.0	5.8	1.4
Margarine	67	7.6	1.3	2.7	3.3
Olive	119	13.5	1.8	10.0	1.2
Peanut	119	13.5	2.3	6.2	4.3
Safflower	120	13.6	1.2	1.7	10.1

Serving size: 1 tablespoon for oil and lard; 2 teaspoons for margarine and butter

---

Drink Milk after Eating Steak

Here's a way to feel better about eating that occasional juicy steak: Wash it down with a tall glass of skim milk. According to research, calcium may help reduce the amount of saturated fat your body absorbs. Like fiber, calcium binds with fat molecules and helps flush them out through the intestines.

Wash It Down with Grape Juice

The best health drink for guys with heart trouble is a glass of purple grape juice after a daily aspirin. Aspirin protects your heart by preventing blood clots, but this effect can be blocked by adrenaline produced by exercise and stress. Flavonoids in grape juice may stymie that response.

Sip Water after Soda

Diet soda is highly acidic, and it can erode your tooth enamel over time. The problem is compounded if you drink soda without eating food, because the acid stays on your teeth longer. Prevention is simple: Just rinse your mouth with water after you've slugged your soda. That'll wash away the damaging acid.

Don't Touch the Jugs

Choose a paper carton of milk over a plastic jug and you'll get more nutrients for your money. Studies show that in 24 hours under the fluorescent lights of supermarket display cases, skim milk in semiclear plastic jugs can lose up to 90 percent of its vitamin A, which is sensitive to light. Because cardboard blocks light, vitamin A losses are minimal. Fortunately, no matter which container your milk comes in, you'll still get a full complement of calcium and vitamin D.

Try These Ideal Meals

There's no question about it, what you eat affects your health. Try these meals to build muscle, ward off heart attacks, and lessen stress.

The Perfect Meal
for Building Muscle

Steak: Meat builds twice as much muscle fiber as other protein sources such as tofu and tuna. Make your meat beef, and you'll also get testosterone-boosting amino acids. Testosterone helps you lift more weight and build more muscle.

Almonds: You need your nuts; they're high in magnesium. Researchers found that people taking magnesium were able to lift 20 percent more weight than those taking a placebo.

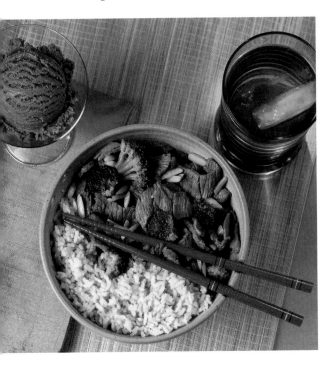

Broccoli: Athletes in one study suffered less post-workout muscle damage when they took a vitamin-C supplement than when they took a placebo. Broccoli is your vitamin-C supplement; half a cup has 60 milligrams, more than any other vegetable.

Brown rice: It has more of the amino acids arginine and lysine than the white stuff you pelt the bride and groom with. Men who took arginine and lysine supplements in one study had 1½ times more muscle-building growth hormone than the saps who got the placebo.

Iced tea sweetened with honey: Researchers found that people who ate honey had higher and longer-lasting levels of glucose, which may help store the muscle fuel glycogen after exercise.

Low-fat ice cream: Scoop out some chocolate for more magnesium. Plus, just a half cup contains 63 milligrams of calcium, the mineral your biceps, triceps, and all your other 'ceps need to contract properly.

The Perfect Meal
for Preventing a Heart Attack

Grape juice: The Concord kind is loaded with flavonoids, compounds that could reduce your risk of heart disease by up to 25 percent.

Salmon: The bear bait is high in omega-3s—good fats that can reduce your risk of heart disease—and the amino acid arginine. Research shows that extra arginine may improve circulation by 30 percent.

Spinach: Nothing you can pull out of the ground and put on your plate has more calcium and potassium, minerals that can lower your blood pressure. Spinach is also high in folate, which may cut homocysteine (that's a compound linked to heart disease) by as much as 25 percent.

Kidney beans: Ignore the name; this is heart food. Researchers found that eating beans four times a week can lower the risk of heart disease by 19 percent

Onions: They come with two compounds—quercetin and kaempferol—that inhibit LDL cholesterol oxidation, the process that leads to heart disease.

Apples: All apples are high in pectin, a gelatin-like substance that helps keep cholesterol out of your blood.

The Perfect Meal
for Beating Stress

Papaya: Stress sucks potassium, vitamin C, and manganese out of your body, resulting in fatigue, sore muscles, difficulty concentrating, and a rise in blood pressure. Get those nutrients back with one papaya, the best fruit source of all three.

Ricotta cheese: Researchers found that people who ate a daily 2.8 grams of whey (the liquid in the cheese) produced fewer stress hormones. They also had 48 percent more tryptophan, the substance that tells your body to release more of the feel-good chemical serotonin.

Whole wheat pasta: It'll give you extra tryptophan and the steady supply of energy you need to fight off stress-induced fatigue.

Turkey: Turkey is a good source of tryptophan and pantothenic acid—a B vitamin vital to the production of stress-fighting hormones. Plus, the zinc in turkey may help keep you from being worried and weak. One study found that zinc supplements increased muscle strength and endurance.

Make the Perfect Match

Picking the right drink is more than "red with beef, white with fish."

If You're Eating . . .	Have a Drink That's . . .
Barbecue	*Cold and crisp.* Like a Bud. Anything lighter will taste watered down against fiery sauces. Anything darker will cover the flavor.
Chinese	*Slightly bitter.* A Heineken or a whisky drink will go best with the garlic and ginger.
Indian	*Strong or fizzy.* A gimlet (gin and lime juice), a heavily hopped beer, or a pale ale neutralizes the hot curries.
Italian	*Red.* A rich, full-bodied red wine is the best thing to accompany a traditional Italian meal—besides a rich, full-bodied Italian girl. Try a Shiraz.
Mexican	*Citrus-flavored.* Why else do you think so many people order margaritas or lime-plugged Coronas? The fruits cut through the oils and grease.
Seafood	*Mild, citrus-flavored.* It'll mimic a squirt of lemon on fresh fish. Try a sauvignon blanc. For beer, go for a Michelob or a wheat microbrew.

Whole wheat bread sticks: Whole grains are rich in folate and other B vitamins, which help supply your brain with the fuel it needs to keep you sharp when you're stressed.

Dark chocolate: Want a runner's high without the annoying running part? Eat a little dark chocolate; it will give you a shot of endorphins, a natural morphine.

Milk: Even the low-fat kind has protein that will elevate your levels of the stress-fighting hormones dopamine and norepinephrine.

Feed Your Brain

The brain responds to what you eat. Just 3 or 4 ounces of protein at lunch or dinner can send enough of the nutrient tyrosine to the brain to promote the production of chemicals that keep you alert. On the other hand, eating just an ounce to an ounce-and-a-half of carbohydrate-rich, low-fat food such as potatoes, bread, pasta, and dessert can encourage the brain to emit another chemical, tryptophan, which is used to make serotonin. Serotonin quiets communication between brain cells, which is why you tend to feel like napping, not networking, after a lunch high in carbohydrates.

Cure Constipation

If you're constantly clogged up, you need more fiber in your diet—specifically 25 grams per day. Most men only get half that. To make up the difference, eat a bowl of bran flakes every morning, for an extra 5 grams of fiber. Mix in a handful of raisins, and you'll add another 4 grams. Munch on a couple of apples or a handful of carrot sticks every afternoon, and that should keep you regular. Two warnings: Increase fiber intake gradually (5 extra grams per week) and drink plenty of fluid.

CURE FLATULENCE

If you're having an embarassing gas problem, head to the grocery store or pharmacy and buy a bottle of Beano. Sprinkling some of this tasteless substance on fibrous foods before eating them will help break down the sugars that cause gas.

Walk Away Indigestion

Ate too much? Take a walk. A post-meal stroll can help you digest your food 40 to 50 percent faster.

Test for Lactose Intolerance

If you have persistent bouts of diarrhea, gas, and bloating, you may be lactose intolerant. It stems from your body not producing enough lactase, the enzyme necessary for digesting dairy products. Try not eating any dairy foods for a day or two, then slowly add them back to your diet to gauge your body's reaction. If the problem returns with gut-wrenching certainty, reduce or eliminate dairy products, switch to lactose-free milk products, or try one of the over-the-counter lactase preparations that make up for the missing enzyme.

Beat Kidney Stones with Beer

Researchers found drinking one beer per day was associated with a 40 percent lower risk of developing kidney stones. One explanation: The hops in beer help to keep calcium from leaching out of bones and taking up residence in your kidneys. Or maybe it's all those bathroom visits.

Shake on Some of This

The best substitute for salt is Mrs. Dash, a concoction of spices and dried vegetables. It doesn't taste salty, but it tastes good enough to make bland foods taste better.

Sharpen Your Skills with Oatmeal

The best food to eat before a big presentation is oatmeal with cinnamon and brown sugar. Researchers found that eating certain carbohydrate-rich foods like oatmeal is the same as having a shot of glucose, a.k.a. blood sugar, injected into your brain (without having to ex-

MR. CLEAN

DO DISHES IN THE TUB

When you need to wash all your dirty dishes fast, pile them in the bathtub and fill it with hot, soapy water. (If you're really in a hurry, bathe with them.) Return later, turn on the shower to rinse, and move everything into a laundry basket. Let the basket sit until the stuff is dry.

Spot the Hidden Sodium

Sometimes it's easy to spot the extra salt in your diet, like the crystals on the rim of your margarita glass. Other stealth foods like these can quickly push you past your daily allotment of 2,400 milligrams of sodium.

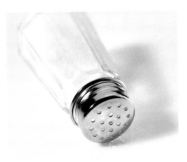

Food	Milligrams of Sodium
1 can Campbell's chicken noodle soup	2,225
8 oz Campbell's tomato juice	750
2 cups Kellogg's Raisin Bran	700
2 slices Velveeta cheese	660
3 or 4 pancakes (6-inch diameter)	590
2 slices whole wheat bread	300
1 medium chocolate shake	300

plain why there's a syringe sticking out of your head). Your body quickly takes glucose out of the carbohydrates and feeds it to your brain to help it function. In other words, the higher the concentration of glucose in your blood, the better your memory and concentration. No oatmeal, or just can't stand the stuff even with cinnamon and brown sugar? Grab a banana or a bagel instead; they turn into glucose fast, too.

Improve Memory with Choline

If you're up late studying for an important test, have an egg-salad sandwich and a glass of milk for a snack. Eggs and milk are the richest sources of choline, a nutrient that will improve your memory. Studies have shown that college students given 3 to 4 grams of choline 1 hour before taking memory tests scored higher than those who didn't receive the choline supplements. It's believed choline increases the release of a neurotransmitter that helps your brain store and recall information.

Be the Duke of Nuking

Heed these tips to microwave your meals with confidence:

• Keep paper towels and brown bags out of the microwave. They sometimes contain metal fibers, which can start fires.

• Move thick foods to the edge of the dish. The heat is more intense there.

• Debone meat. Microwaves can't penetrate bone, so the meat nearby will remain cold. Heat thick meat slowly, at half-power.

• Salt after cooking. Salt granules attract microwaves, burning the food and causing freckles.

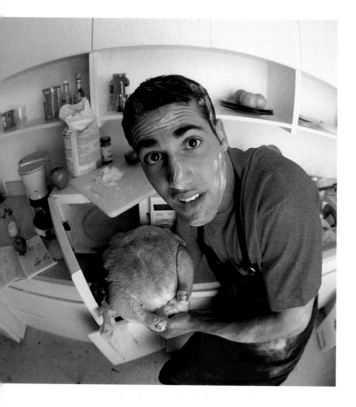

• To microwave a potato, stab two holes in it, one on each side. Too many holes will leak steam and make your baked potato hard. Nuke a medium-size spud at full power for 3 minutes, then remove it and wrap it in a cloth for 5 minutes.

• Microwave vegetables briefly. Heat them for 15 seconds at a time, checking to make sure they don't get too soft. Overcooking destroys nutrients.

Double the Recipe

If you don't have time to cook every night, double your casserole recipes, then eat one and freeze the other.

Wake Up with the Shakes

Here are three easy-to-make blender breakfasts. Match them to what you need to do during the morning.

Change Your Mood with Food

Certain foods can intensify or change your mood. So when you're not feeling your best, try some foods that can give you a lift:

If you feel . . .	Avoid these . . .	Eat these . . .
Tense, anxious, and stressed	Chocolate, alcohol, cake, ice cream, and coffee	Fresh or dried fruit, pasta, whole grain bread, baked potatoes, rice, and veggies
Sleepy and lethargic	Sweets, wine, beer, pizza, and high-fat food	Low-fat, high-protein foods such as broiled or baked fish, veal, and poultry; low-fat cheese; egg-white omelet; or fruit
Depressed	Cake, ice cream, bread, and pastries	Whole grain entrees, such as pasta primavera, and rice and beans

Endurance shake: When the finish line is 10 kilometers away, you need to draw on more carbohydrates than your morning bowl of Froot Loops can provide. You also need protein and fat. In one study, cyclists who drank a prerace beverage consisting of four parts carbohydrates and one part protein cycled 66 percent farther than when they quaffed an all-carbohydrate sports drink. And when researchers added a little extra fat to runners' diets, they lasted 23 percent longer on endurance runs than they did on a low-fat diet.

Ingredients: 1 sliced banana, ½ cup orange juice, 8 ounces low-fat vanilla yogurt, 4 ounces crushed pineapple, 2 tablespoons peanut butter. *640 calories, 20 g fat (5 g saturated fat), 22 g protein, 101 g carbohydrates, 6 g fiber*

Brain builder: You could down a cup of coffee to jump-start your brain. But caffeine depletes your stores of B vitamins, the very nutrients you need to keep your mind sharp. Instead, feed your head with this recipe. Not only does it provide those badly needed Bs, it also delivers a shot of protein to help produce the wake-up chemicals dopamine and norepinephrine. The milk in the mix contains choline to help fire up your memory. Along with the vitamin C in the fruit and orange juice, choline can also help prevent the mental deterioration associated with Alzheimer's disease and Parkinson's disease.

Ingredients: 1 cup skim milk, 2 tablespoons frozen orange juice concentrate, 1 cup strawberries, 1 kiwifruit. *210 calories, 1.5 g fat (0 g saturated fat), 11 g protein, 41 g carbohydrates, 6 g fiber*

Hangover helper: Use this liquid meal to fight alcohol-induced dehydration. It's loaded with

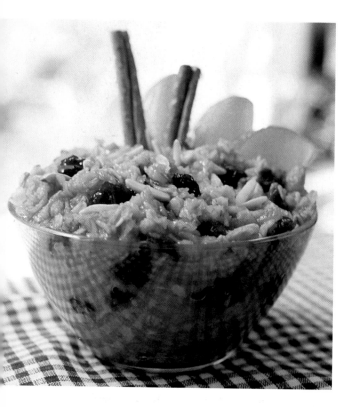

Make Oatmeal Edible

If you avoid oatmeal because it tastes like wallpaper paste, try this recipe.

Edible Oatmeal

1½	cups apple juice
¾	cup dry, quick oats
1	pear, grated (optional)
	Cinnamon and maple syrup to taste
¼	cup raisins
⅓	cup toasted slivered almonds
1	peach, sliced (optional)

Heat the apple juice in a microwave for 1 minute or until it boils, then pour it into a bowl with the oats and pear shavings. Stir until thick. Add the cinnamon, maple syrup, and raisins. Top with toasted almonds and peach slices.

Serves 1

Per serving: 760 calories, 21 g fat (2 g saturated fat), 17 g protein, 131 g carbohydrates, 12 g fiber

vitamin C to help combat binge-related cell damage, and the fructose in the fruit juice helps speed the metabolism of liquor. Upset stomach? The ginger in ginger ale will help quell the motion sickness caused by your spinning bedroom, as will the peppermint. And some experts say that acidophilus bacteria in the yogurt may get your gut back in chemical balance.

Ingredients: 1 cup tangerine/orange blended juice, 1 tablespoon lime juice, ½ cup low-fat vanilla yogurt, ½ cup Canada Dry ginger ale (or any other ginger ale that contains real ginger), sprig of peppermint. *260 calories, 1.5 g fat (1 g saturated fat), 8 g protein, 54 g carbohydrates, 0 g fiber*

Sandwich Aunt Jemima

Aunt Jemima Mini Pancakes have a rich, biscuit-like flavor, plus they're low in calories. One pancake has just 18 calories and less than a gram of fat. Make a sandwich out of them by sliding a slice of Canadian bacon between two frozen pancakes, spearing the whole thing with a toothpick, and microwaving it on high for close to a minute. Since these sandwiches are small, you can eat up to five. Each contains 81 calories, 7 grams protein, 8 grams carbohydrates, and 3 grams fat.

FLIP FLAPJACKS

To turn a pancake over in the air with a flourish, sweep the frying pan forward, up, and around in a smooth looping-the-loop motion.

Crack an Egg One-Handed

Anyone can crack an egg with both hands. Practice this, then make sure your girl is watching. It'll impress her the morning after.

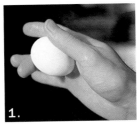

1. Hold the egg with your thumb and middle finger, then rest the back of the egg against the palm of your hand.

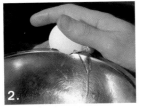

2. Crack the egg against something solid, like a metal mixing bowl, and immediately lift your wrist.

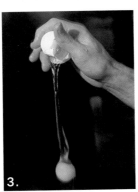

3. Now here's the part that requires practice: In one quick motion, lift both halves of the cracked shell up with your thumb and fingers like a bird's wings. Gravity will take care of the rest.

Flip an Egg

To properly flip an egg, begin by spraying a fair amount of nonstick cooking spray into a skillet. Turn up the range to medium high, and when the skillet's hot, break in your eggs. When bubbles start to appear in the egg white, you're ready to flip. Make sure the egg isn't stuck to the bottom of the pan. Use a spatula to gently pry it loose before you flip it. Move the pan away from the burner and, in an even motion, draw the pan back toward you so that the egg slides back toward the far end of the pan. Just as it gets there, shoot your arm forward with an even motion ending with a slight flick of the wrist upward. The egg will slide just off the end of the pan, roll over, and come down easy.

Make a Leftover Chinese Breakfast

Take about two-thirds of a cup of leftover white rice and combine it in a bowl with one-third of a cup of skim milk. Add some raisins. Add a little maple syrup and some ground cinnamon if you've got it. Pop it in the oven and you're 2½ minutes from hot porridge heaven. Enriched white rice delivers carbohydrates and good amounts of the vitamins thiamin and niacin. The raisins pack a good fiber punch, plus potassium and vitamin B_6.

Turn Over a New Leaf

The masculinity of salads has always been suspect. Sure, they're cool, crunchy, and packed with nutrients, but salads have never quite overcome their association with quiche, finger bowls, and ladies who lunch. Except for this one:

Thai Beef Salad

Salad

1	10-ounce bag mixed salad greens
½	pound London broil
1	small red onion, finely chopped
½	small red bell pepper, thinly sliced
1	small cucumber, sliced
½	pound cherry tomatoes
¼	cup chopped cilantro
2	tablespoons chopped mint leaves
1	clove garlic, finely chopped
1	small red chile pepper (2 if you like it hot), seeded and finely chopped

Dressing

3	tablespoons lime juice
3	tablespoons light soy sauce
1	teaspoon finely chopped lemon peel

1. Rinse and drain the greens.

2. Grill the meat 5 to 6 minutes each side, turning once. (It should be about medium-rare.) Allow to cool slightly, then slice thinly. In the meantime, combine dressing ingredients in a small bowl and stir well.

3. Combine the sliced beef, onion, bell pepper, cucumber, tomatoes, cilantro, mint, garlic, chile pepper, and dressing in a large bowl. Divide the salad greens onto two plates and top with the beef mixture.

Serves 2

Per serving: 320 calories, 13 g fat, (5 g saturated fat), 29 g protein, 24 g carbohydrates, 7 g dietary fiber

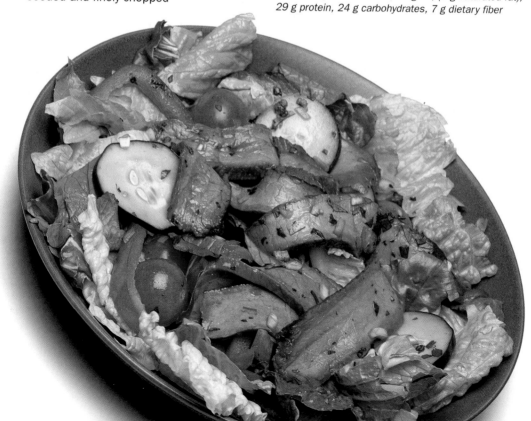

Dress a Salad for Success

Your salads don't need fattening dressings to taste great. Try making these toppings:

Thick and creamy: Whisk ½ teaspoon of freshly squeezed lemon juice into ½ cup fat-free yogurt. Stir in dill and chopped cucumber to taste.

Thousand Island: Fold 2 tablespoons of tomato paste into the previous dressing. Add minced garlic, pickles, shallots, and celery to taste.

Green goddess: Fold minced garlic, chives, scallion, parsley, and tarragon into the Thick and Creamy dressing.

Ranch style: Combine ¼ cup of buttermilk with 1 teaspoon of Dijon mustard and minced garlic, parsley, and chives.

Make Some Weight-Loss Soup

Here's a real recipe for weight loss: One serving packs a mere 154 calories, only 17 percent of them from fat. At that rate you could eat the whole pot. But you won't need to. Soup suppresses hunger, so you'll consume fewer calories during the meal. You'll also feel full longer, thanks to the fiber in the brown rice.

Weight-Loss Soup

½	cup diced onions
½	cup diced celery
½	cup diced carrots
1	clove garlic, chopped
1	tablespoon olive oil
2	28-ounce cans plum tomatoes
1	cup quick-cooking brown rice
1	cup reduced-fat chicken broth
1	teaspoon dried parsley
½	teaspoon dried thyme

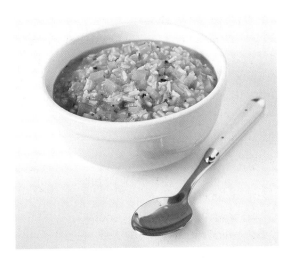

1. In a 4-quart pot, combine the onions, celery, carrots, garlic, and oil. Cover and cook for 10 minutes over medium heat, stirring often.

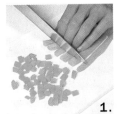

2. Put the tomatoes (juice included) in a blender and blend until smooth. Add the tomatoes to the pot and bring to a boil.

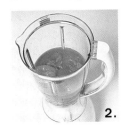

3. Reduce the heat to medium and simmer for 20 minutes. Then add rice and broth, cover, and simmer for another 20 minutes. Sprinkle dried herbs over the top before serving.

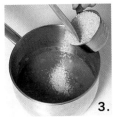

Serves 6

Per serving (1½ cups): 154 calories, 3 g fat (17% of calories), 5 g protein, 27 g carbohydrates, 3 g fiber

TRIM YOUR WINGS

How about some spicy low-fat buffalo wings? But instead of using chicken wings, make them with skinless chicken-breast tenders. Marinate them overnight in a mixture of Louisiana hot sauce, olive oil, lots of garlic powder, and red wine vinegar. (Experiment with the amounts to suit your taste.) Then roast the chicken "wings" at 400°F for 15 minutes.

Heat Your Oil

If you heat your skillet before adding oil, less fat will be absorbed by the food. Warm oil cooks more efficiently; cold oil tends to soak into meats and vegetables.

Put a Lid on It

You can dramatically reduce the amount of oil needed to pan-fry foods simply by keeping the lid on the pot. The lid catches and returns moisture that would normally escape, thus preventing the need for more oil.

Stop Pasta from Boiling Over

If you've blown it, blow on it—literally, right on the surface of the water. This will buy you about 15 seconds to dump a tablespoon of oil into the pot, which will calm the raging waters.

Say Goodbye to Rubbery Cheese

To prevent low-fat cheese from turning to rubber in the microwave, spritz your nachos with a quick blast of cooking spray, such as Pam, before nuking them. Or spray the inside of a grilled cheese sandwich before you toss it in the pan. This adds just enough fat to make the cheese stay creamy when it melts.

Grate Your Cheese

When it comes to cheese, get handy with a cheese grater. Grate some Parmesan or other hard cheese on your sandwich, and you'll save boffo fat calories over standard sliced fare. You'll naturally use less.

Throw in the Towel

To reheat pizza in the microwave, put a paper towel underneath the pizza to absorb moisture. This keeps the crust from turning into a doggie chew toy.

WHEN ALL ELSE FAILS

ELIMINATE VIDALIA DIGITS

Get the smell of raw onion off your fingers by rubbing your hands and fingers on a stainless-steel faucet. Just rub and the smell disappears. Honest.

> **MR. CLEAN**
>
> ## BOIL YOUR ROCKS
>
> Twice a year, boil your lava rocks in a large container of water with a tablespoon of low-sudsing dishwashing detergent. This will remove the grease that can cause flames to leap too high, ruining your T-bone, your grill, and your eyebrows. Let the rocks bubble for 25 minutes, rinse, then dry completely before using.

Top Off Your Spud

A potato can be a low-fat belly-filler—just keep off the sour cream and butter. Here are some healthful alternatives toppings:

The Italiano: Blend a tablespoon of grated Parmesan cheese and a clove of minced garlic into ¼ cup of reduced-fat pasta sauce. Rent *The Godfather*.

275 calories, 2 grams fat, 5.9 grams fiber

The theme restaurant lookalike: Crumble a slice of cooked turkey bacon into 2 tablespoons of fat-free sour cream. Add a tablespoon each of chopped chives and minced, roasted red peppers (a.k.a. pimientos).

259 calories, 3.2 grams fat, 4.9 grams fiber

South of the border (pictured): Combine ¼ cup each of diced avocado, thawed frozen corn kernels, and diced tomato, then add a tablespoon of fat-free yogurt, a chopped scallion and a squeeze o lime juice. Don sombrero if desired.

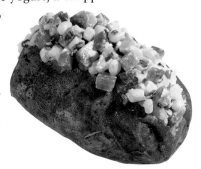

368 calories, 9.2 grams fat, 6.3 grams fiber

The bare fridge: Combine 2 ounces of grated mozzarella cheese, a teaspoon of minced basil, and ¼ cup of chopped tomato. Brown one to two minutes under the broiler, if desired.

371 calories, 9.3 grams fat, 5.3 grams fiber

The really bare fridge: Mix 2 tablespoons of minced red onions and 2 ounces of shredded low-fat Cheddar cheese. Brown one to two minutes under broiler, if desired.

421 calories, 14.2 grams fat, 5.2 grams fiber

Build a Better Reuben

Simulate a cheese Reuben by replacing fatty corned beef with turkey ham and topping it with low-fat mozzarella, mustard, spicy shredded cabbage, and pickles. Slap all that on traditional rye bread and broil until the cheese melts. Fat savings: 10 grams.

Poke the Chicken

Broiled or grilled chicken is tasty, but leave the skin on, and the bird will be as fatty as beef. Peel the skin off, and it'll be drier than melba toast. A quick solution: Poke a few dozen holes in the skin with a fork before roasting. This will let the fat drip out but still keep the meat moist.

Make Chicken under a Brick

Every grill jockey needs a showstopper. This recipe makes you look as if you really know what you're doing, but it's incredibly easy.

Chicken under a Brick

2	large boneless, skinless whole chicken breasts
1	teaspoon coarse salt
1	teaspoon cracked black pepper
½	teaspoon hot red pepper flakes
1	tablespoon chopped garlic
1	tablespoon chopped rosemary
	Juice of 1 large lemon
¼	cup extra virgin olive oil
2	clean bricks

1. Rinse and dry the chicken breasts, then sprinkle them with the salt, black pepper, red pepper, garlic, and rosemary. Place them in a baking dish, pour on lemon juice and olive oil, and refrigerate for 30 minutes to an hour.

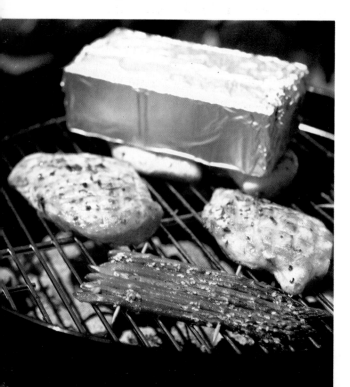

2. Wrap each of the bricks in aluminum foil. Brush the grill with a stiff wire brush. Dip a paper towel (folded into a small square) in oil and holding it with tongs, rub it over the rods of the grill to oil them. Then place the chicken at a 45-degree angle to the rods and put the bricks on top. Cook over high heat for 4 to 6 minutes per side, reorienting each breast every 2 minutes for a crosshatching effect.

Serves 4

Per serving: 260 calories, 16 g fat (2.5 g saturated fat), 26 g protein, 2 g carbohydrates, 0 g fiber

Make Some Unfried Chicken

If you have a craving for fried chicken, steer clear of the Colonel and make this low-fat version at home: Pour a big bowl of corn flakes, then mash the cereal with a spoon. Sprinkle in some black pepper and dried, crushed rosemary (or paprika, oregano, or fried-chicken seasoning). Pour some skim milk into another bowl. Trim the skin and fat off about 3 pounds of chicken. To coat the chicken, dip it in the skim milk, then roll it in the crumb mixture. Place the chicken on a baking sheet that's been lightly coated with nonstick cooking spray. Bake for 45 minutes in an oven at 400°F.

Marinate Steak in Yogurt

Great steaks are made with yogurt. The live bacteria in yogurt produce acids and enzymes that, when used as a marinade, can break down a fillet's fibers. That spells tender. Just spoon ½ cup of plain, fat-free yogurt into a bowl and mix with 2 tablespoons of horseradish, 1 teaspoon of spicy mustard, and 1 minced clove garlic. Spread it over the steak and refrigerate for 1 hour.

CARVE A TURKEY

Come dinnertime on Thanksgiving Day, the duty of carving the turkey is invariably relegated to the gent of the house. Unfortunately, no one ever taught us how to do this task properly. Here's a quick course:

1. Always use a sharp carving knife.

2. Wait 20 minutes after the bird has come out of the oven before carving.

3. Remove the legs and wings first. To do so, plant the carving fork in the breast. Cut at the thigh joint by pressing the leg away from the body and severing the ligaments. Do likewise with the wings. Next slice loose meat off the bones. Place this dark meat on the platter first because it won't dry out as quickly as white meat.

4. Carve the white meat at the table to order. For best results, begin with your knife blade at the tip of the breastbone. Work at an angle, cutting toward the joint where the wing was removed.

Squeeze the Fat out of a Dog

Make a deep slit down the length of the hot dog and pierce it a few times with a fork before slowly grilling it over medium heat. This lets more meat come into contact with the heat for a longer period of time, which burns off more fat.

Juice Up Your Burgers

For burgers that sizzle, add 4 tablespoons of ice water to each pound of lean chopped sirloin. The grill's heat will seal in the extra moisture, making your homemade quarter pounders juicier than the hockey-puck patties you usually churn out.

Build a Better Burger

Make a better burger by cutting the beef one-to-one with mashed firm tofu in a mixing bowl. (You won't even taste the tofu, and you'll be adding B vitamins and calcium.)

Next add chopped onion and whole wheat bread crumbs for fiber. Mix in some egg white, a little ketchup, and dried oregano. Form into patties and cook. Serve it on a whole wheat roll and top it with romaine lettuce and tomato.

Create a Better Kebab

Shish kebabs are great, healthful, manly meals. To make them perfectly, use twin steel skewers. Two prongs keep the chunks more secure when you turn them on the grill. Afterward, put the kebabs in a serving dish, douse them with warm cognac or brandy, and touch a lit match to them. They'll burn for a few minutes, leaving juicy meat under a crusty coating. Delicious!

CLEAN THE GRILL WITHOUT SCRUBBING

Soak your charcoal grill in a plastic wastebasket with hot water, dishwasher detergent, and a little white vinegar. After an hour's soak, the grease should come off easily.

Always Use Tongs

Piercing meat with a fork lets out the juices. That leads to dry meat. This is especially important if you started with particularly lean cuts.

Cook While You're Driving

The only thing better than eating while you're driving is cooking while you're driving, then driving while you're eating what you've cooked. Here's how to get revved up:

Hot dogs: Take a stout piece of tin foil and lay in however many low-fat hot dogs you want. Add 2 cups of ketchup, about ½ cup of water, a handful of onions, and ¾ cup of brown sugar, just to cut the taste of any exhaust fumes. Seal tightly. Secure on the engine block away from moving parts. If possible, tie down with duct tape. Drive. Hot dogs will require about 20 minutes at 60 mph.

Corn on the cob: The perfect accompaniment for engine block dogs is, of course, engine block corn on the cob. Season each ear with a few dashes of hot pepper sauce. Wrap the corn in foil and secure it to the engine block.

Long-haul gourmets know that you can also poach a fish this way. But forget pot roasts, chicken tandoori, venison stew, and all that. Too many miles, not enough heat. The valve covers make an excellent warming tray, incidentally.

Start the Grill in a Flash

When you need to heat up the hibachi in a hurry, use a "chimney." This device, which is available for $10 at home supply stores, resembles a tall metal coffee cup with a wooden handle on the side and small holes in the bottom. You simply stuff in some newspaper, fill it with charcoal, and light. As its name suggests, this mini chimney creates an updraft that ignites the briquettes 30 to 40 percent faster with no lighter fluid.

Switch to This Gyro

For a low-fat gyro, mix some fat-free yogurt with chopped or sliced cucumbers, add a squeeze of lemon juice, and pour over a pita stuffed with grilled chicken or beef strips.

Make Salmon in Your Dishwasher

Hate to cook? Here's a foolproof recipe that's also a blast to make:

Drizzle a teaspoon of olive oil on a 14-inch-square piece of heavy-duty foil. Add two 6-ounce salmon fillets, the juice of one lemon, salt, pepper, and some fresh dill. Wrap the foil around the fish and create an airtight seal by folding the edges over several times and pinching tightly (see illustration). Place the package on the top rack of your dishwasher and run it through the entire wash-and-dry cycle on high heat. Don't try to do a load of dishes at the same time.

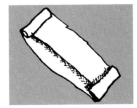

Sear a Shark

Shark is health food. A 6-ounce serving gives you about 75 percent of the Daily Value for protein at a cost of only 298 calories and 11 grams of fat. You also take in a week's worth of omega-3 oils, which protect your blood vessels and heart. Here's how to make it.

Shark Steaks

½	cup teriyaki sauce
¼	cup orange juice
2	tablespoons soy sauce
1	teaspoon garlic powder
4	1- to 1½-inch-thick, 6- to 8-ounce shark steaks

Mix the teriyaki sauce, orange juice, soy sauce, and garlic powder. Marinate the steaks for 5 minutes on each side. Spray the grill rack with non-stick cooking spray (remove it from the heat first) and grill the fish over medium coals for 5 to 6 minutes on each side. Baste the fillets frequently with the sauce. Wear a Hawaiian shirt throughout.

Serves 4

Per serving: 270 calories, 8 g fat (1.5 g saturated fat), 39 g protein, 8 g carbohydrates, 0 g fiber

Cook Tastier Seafood

Thyme is the magical spice for cooking seafood. It eliminates that fishy taste and brings out the creature's unique flavor.

Roast in Peace

Great grillers grill *indirectly*, meaning they move the coals to the sides of the grate and cook over the center. With a gas grill, shut off the center burner just under the meat. This little trick roasts the food without burning it.

Use Healthful Condiments

One important key to weight loss is making bland foods taste good. Slather the right grainy mustard on a fat-free turkey sandwich and it becomes downright delicious. Use Worcestershire sauce to spruce up steamed broccoli and other healthful foods. Brush barbecue sauce on grilled vegetables and you'll actually crave that eggplant.

REAL-LIFE SURVIVAL

PREVENT A GAS GRILL EXPLOSION

When a gas barbecue grill blows up in someone's face, it's usually because the guy kept trying and trying—and trying—to light it. Everyone forgets that natural gas is heavier than air, so it accumulates at the bottom of the grill. If it doesn't light in 5 seconds, shut off the gas and leave the lid open for 5 minutes.

Eat More Vegetables (Without Realizing It)

If you just don't like the taste of vegetables, try sneaking them into foods. Chop or shred veggies and add them to dishes that will hide their flavor. Put spinach in chili, mushrooms in macaroni and cheese, artichokes on pizza, and peppers and scallions in omelets.

Flash-Boil Veggies

Flash-boiling is one of the fastest and healthiest ways to cook vegetables. Just bring a pot of water to a rolling boil, add the veggies, count to 10, and then drain them. This softens them a bit but preserves much of their vitamins and minerals.

Keep Rice Nice

If the rice is cooked, but your guests aren't ready to eat, throw it in a bowl, put a slice of dry bread on top, and cover it. The rice will stay fluffy until dinnertime.

Put Coke in Your Beans

You'll find the secret to kick-butt baked beans in a can of Coke. The syrup in the soda lends a sweet caramel flavor that brown sugar can't match. They're simple to make. Just dump three 16-ounce cans of pinto beans (drained) into a bowl and stir in ½ cup of chopped onion, ½ cup of ketchup, 2 tablespoons of spicy brown mustard, 1 tablespoon each of white vinegar and Worcestershire sauce, and a can of Coke. Pour into an 8 × 8-inch greased pan and bake at 375°F for an hour.

Lord over the Fries

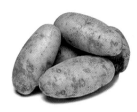

Twenty chicken wings have 140 grams of fat. Eat them during the game, and you'll end up shaped like a football. Instead, try these low-fat, spicy steak fries.

Steak Fries

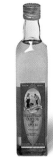

5	medium potatoes (2 pounds)
1	tablespoon olive oil
¼	teaspoon salt
½	teaspoon pepper
⅛	teaspoon onion powder
1	garlic clove, crushed, or 1 tablespoon garlic powder

Preheat the oven to 450°F. Peel the potatoes and cut each one lengthwise into six wedges. Place the wedges flat in a baking dish coated with non-stick cooking spray. Sprinkle them with the seasonings and oil, then stir them around. Bake for 30 minutes or until they're brown.

Serves 6

Per serving: 140 calories, 2.5 grams fat (0 g saturated fat), 3 g protein, 28 g carbohydrates, 2 g fiber

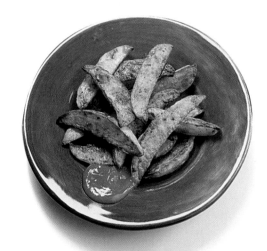

Make Some Zucchini Fries

Want some fries to go with your burger? Try zucchini fries. Slice two zucchini into fry-sized pieces. Sauté the fries in ½ teaspoon of oil in a large pan over medium-high heat until lightly browned. Sprinkle with basil. Or if you like things hot, sprinkle with Cajun spices.

Chip Away Fat

Run the option on Super Bowl Sunday. Instead of serving fatty potato or tortilla chips, bake up your own tasty, low-fat chips using pita bread:

1. Use pocket or pocketless low-fat pitas in your favorite flavor. (Substituting whole wheat pitas will give you 5 extra grams of fiber per eight chips.)

2. Cut each pita into eight wedges.

3. Bake in a 350°F oven on an ungreased cookie sheet for 7 to 10 minutes (or until the tips turn golden brown).

4. Serve warm with guacamole and salsa, or seal in a plastic bag for later.

Set Your Food on Fire

It's called flambéing, and it's not only easy to master, but it'll also make you look like one sophisticated hombre. Here's how to make the classic dessert, banana flambé:

Banana Flambé

1 tablespoon butter

1 tablespoon brown sugar

1 banana, sliced

Dark rum or Grand Marnier

1 cup low-fat frozen vanilla yogurt

1. In a sauté pan over medium heat, melt the butter and brown sugar. Stir until the sugar melts, then add the banana. Toss around pan for 3 minutes. Add a generous splash of dark rum or Grand Marnier, count to five, then touch a flame to the liquid.

2. When the smoke clears, serve over frozen yogurt.

Serves 2

Per serving: 250 calories, 7 grams fat (4.5 g saturated fat), 5 g protein, 39 grams carbohydrate, 1 g fiber

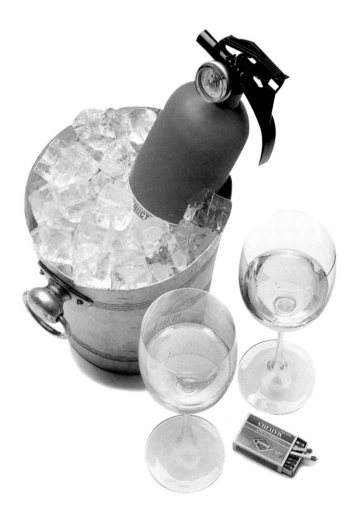

Make Fruit Sorbet

Our delicious sorbet is low in calories, nutritious, and has zero fat. Here's how to make it:

Buy a can of fruit. Peaches or pineapple in light syrup work well. Freeze it overnight. Place the can in hot water for 1 minute. Remove the lid and pour any liquid into a blender. Remove the bottom of the can, slide out the fruit and chop it into 1-inch pieces. Throw it in the blender and puree. Eat immediately.

Improve Your Noggin

Traditional eggnog gets 55 percent of its calories from fat. Our concoction is just as festive, but it gets only 1 percent of its calories from fat.

Old Recipe		New Recipe	
6	beaten eggs		Egg substitute, 6-egg equivalent
2	cups milk	2	cups skim milk
⅓	cup sugar	⅓	cup sugar
4	tablespoons light rum		Light rum to taste
4	tablespoons bourbon		Bourbon to taste
1	teaspoon vanilla	1	teaspoon vanilla
1	cup whipping cream	1	cup fat-free vanilla frozen yogurt
½	teaspoon ground nutmeg	½	teaspoon ground nutmeg

Simply add the ingredients to a blender and mix well. Then chill for at least 4 hours. Serve in small cups, with some nutmeg sprinkled on top.

About 10 ½-cup servings

Old Recipe, per serving: 218 calories, 14 g fat, 167 mg cholesterol, 71 mg sodium.
New Recipe, per serving: 104 calories, 0.1 g fat, 0.8 mg cholesterol, 84 mg sodium.

Save Dying Food

With some quick action, it might not be too late to save dinner if you've had a cooking catastrophe.

Overcooked meat: If the meat's dry, cut it into thin slices and drizzle on a sauce of brown mustard and olive oil.

Wilted carrots and lettuce: Soak them briefly in ice water or wrap them in a damp towel and refrigerate.

Crusty bread: Wrap the bread in a damp kitchen towel and heat it in a 250°F oven for 10 minutes to soften it.

Burned bread: Scrape off the worst of the charcoal and brush the slices with olive oil. Sprinkle with Parmesan cheese and, *voilà*, you're serving *crostini*.

Salty sauce or soup: A dash of sugar, lemon juice, or vinegar neutralizes excess salt. Or simmer half a raw potato in the sauce or soup for 5 minutes, then discard it. It'll absorb the salt.

Sticky pasta: You forgot to stir the pasta, and now you have a linguini basketball. Put it in a colander and run cold water over it, then toss with a tablespoon of olive oil; it'll separate.

Have More Family Meals

Make eating dinner together a priority. Research indicates that the fewer meals eaten as a family, the higher the level of stress in the family. Another study found that the most common denominator among National Merit Scholars was that the majority eat supper as a family at least five out of seven meals per week.

CLEAN YOUR PIPES

After putting your kitchen to all this good use, your kitchen sink may need some attention. A clogged drain and no Drano isn't a disaster. Just grab the Alka-Seltzer. Drop three of the ol' plop, plop, fizz, fizzers down the drain, followed by 1 cup of white vinegar. Wait a few minutes. Now turn on the hot water and charge yourself $75 for making a house call.

Serve the Kids Blue-Plate Specials

When your wife is away and you're in charge of feeding the kids, make a blue dinner. Keep it simple: Hamburgers and milk. Just add blue food coloring to milk and a few drops to uncooked meat. Kids generally think funny-looking food is a riot. But there's also a lesson to be learned: The fact that something looks weird doesn't mean that it tastes bad.

When to Chuck Food from Your Wagon

Nothing will get you kicked out of the kitchen faster than poisoning the family. Here's a cheat sheet for telling when different types of food have exceeded their life expectancies:

1. **Frozen vegetables and dinners:** Most will have a "best if used by" date on the box or bag, but they're generally good up to a year after purchase.

2. **Frozen yogurt and ice cream:** In this case, rely on the freshness date. The stuff will taste gummy if it has been in the freezer too long.

3. **An opened jar of spaghetti sauce:** Throw it out after 2 weeks, if not before. Mold tends to collect around the cap and the sides of the jar, and these bacteria-carrying spores often wind up in the sauce without being seen.

4. **Milk and butter:** Dates on dairy products do not signify expiration. Rather, they are recommended "sell-by" dates. Milk is usually good for one week afterward; butter lasts a month.

5. **Orange juice:** OJ will last a month, but its vitamin C may not. Juice will lose its nutritional value if it isn't tightly capped or in a glass container.

6. **Cheese:** If you buy the individually wrapped prefab cheese food, it will last beyond the apocalypse. A packaged block of Cheddar or mozzarella will have a freshness date on it, and generally, if there's no mold or odor, you're safe for a few weeks from purchase if it's well-wrapped. If you see some mold, just cut off a generous hunk and salvage the rest.

7. **Eggs:** Despite what the carton might say, unless they smell funny you can use eggs for a month after purchase.

8. Yogurt: It's safe for 2 weeks after the sell-by date.

9. Restaurant leftovers: In general, your doggie bag will last 2 to 3 days if the container is sealed tightly.

10. Cold cuts and lunch meats: They're usually good for a week, though low-salt versions might not last as long.

11. An open bottle of wine: Red wine will oxidize faster, so cork it immediately after opening to guarantee the best taste. (Oxygen makes wine bitter.) Make an occasion to drink the rest of your wine (either red or white) within 2 or 3 days, or it's salad dressing.

12. Condiments: Mayo, ketchup, mustard, relish, salad dressing, jams, and jellies are generally good for a year.

13. A loaf of bread: If you buy bread bakery-fresh, keep it in the fridge, because it doesn't contain the preservatives of commercially prepared breads. If you freeze bread, you won't lose vitamins or nutrients, and it will keep for a month.

14. Leftover pizza: If pizza is wrapped securely, it's good for a week in the fridge or a month in the freezer.

15. Tomatoes, onions, potatoes, and fruit: Don't refrigerate any of them. Chilling destroys their flavor.

Avoid Getting Queasy from Over Easy

You probably already know that eating raw eggs puts you at risk for salmonella poisoning. But you probably don't realize that *undercooked* eggs are just as dicey. A lot of men like their eggs over easy. Usually there's a runny white, and that's the most dangerous part. Bacteria can be having a big pool party in there. It's best if the whole egg is cooked through. Or, at the very least, make sure the white is firm.

The Fridge: What's Out, What's In

She stores a hunk of your wedding cake in the freezer. You chill the fish bait. Each of you thinks the other is nuts. Here are the rules, once and for all. (By the way, keep the temperature between 39° and 41°F, or everyone gets in trouble.)

What Stays Out

Item	Tips
Alkaline batteries	Hot or cold, they'll last 5 to 7 years.
Chocolate	A harmless white film will form if you keep it in the fridge.
Fruit	Chilling stops the ripening process and dulls flavor.
Garlic cloves	They'll last 2 weeks unchilled. Refrigeration weakens flavor.
Medication	Chilling may destroy potency. Unless the label says otherwise, store in a cool, dry drawer or closet.
Olive and canola oil	Keep them in the pantry for 6 months.
Peanut butter	The sugar prevents bacterial growth. But chuck it after 3 months.
Potatoes	Chilling converts the starch to sugar, making potatoes too sweet.
Tomatoes	Cooling destroys the flavor. Refrigerate other veggies, though.

What Stays In

Item	Tips
Jelly	Chilled jams and jellies should be edible for 1 year.
Mustard/ketchup	Left out, both can get moldy. Toss after 1 year.
Film	Chilling prolongs its life. Freeze if not used for longer than 3 months.
Cayenne/chili powder	They lose their punch when stored at room temperature.
Milk	Of course, it stays in. Leaving it out for just 30 minutes robs freshness.
Mixed garlic/oil	This combo invites botulism. Always refrigerate; trash after 2 days.
Hot sauce	The spices don't act as preservatives. Dump after 1 year.
Cream baked goods	Any cream filling needs chilling. Eat within the week.
Coffee beans	Chilling retains flavor.
Bait	We're with you all the way, keep it cool.

D E - S T I N K   Y O U R   F R I D G E
Place fresh ground coffee in a bowl on a refrigerator shelf. After a couple of days, the coffee will absorb all the foul odors.

Get 'em into the Fridge Fast
Freshly purchased vegetables, such as cauliflower and radishes, can carry more than 1 million bacteria per gram. Fortunately, by storing your vegetables between 39° and 41°F—ideal refrigerator temperature—you can stop the bacteria from reproducing and even reduce their number. Put them in there as soon as you get home.

Don't Trust Prewashed Greens
Even if that package of fancy mixed greens in your supermarket is labeled "prewashed," don't trust it. *E. coli* and other harmful bacteria can thrive in lettuce just as they do in meat, fish, and eggs. Always wash the mixes under cool, running water.

Keep Lunch from Killing You
Food left at room temperature may look and smell okay, but it could contain high concentrations of the bacteria that cause food poisoning. If you don't have an office fridge, minimize the risk by packing your lunch with a reusable frozen gel pack. Or use a frozen juice box. It'll give you two benefits: The juice will be thawed by lunch, and your food will last a few extra hours out in the open. The following chart shows how long typical lunch foods will survive a morning on your desk at room temperature.

Food	Hours Safe at Room Temperature
Tuna salad sandwich	1
Beef, bologna, leftovers with meat	2
Macaroni salad	2
Pudding	2
Soup	3
Yogurt	4
Hard cheeses like Cheddar	5
Salad with oil-based dressing	6
Fruit pies	7
Peanut butter and jelly sandwiches	8
Cake	8
Bread, raw vegetables, cookies, dried fruits or meats	All day

Hate Liver Even More
Many of the residues from chemicals and hormones fed to livestock end up in their livers, which filter their blood. Like most organ meats, liver is also high in fat and cholesterol. One type: polar bear liver, is lethal. It contains toxic levels of vitamin A.

Press Your Luck

The fact that your beef is brown doesn't necessarily mean it's safe to eat. Meat that's old or has been exposed to too much air can brown prematurely, making it appear properly cooked. Press down on the burger and note what color liquid emerges. If the juice is nearly yellow, with no trace of red, it's safe. If not, send it back.

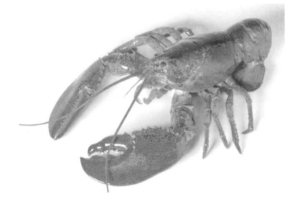

Check Lobster for Freshness

To make sure the lobster on your plate is the same one you fingered in the tank, look at the tail. Is it curled? If not, then the lobster you're looking at was dead before it was boiled.

Buy the Best Berries

Before you buy strawberries or raspberries, flip the carton over. You're looking for nature's expiration date: juice stains. Dripping fruit is one step away from rotten fruit. If you've already bought berries that are going soft, place a single layer of them on a baking sheet and freeze them for 20 minutes.

Let Her Smell the Milk

Not sure if the milk's gone bad? Women have a better sense of smell than men.

Make Fish the Dish

Fish, especially cold-water fish, contain tremendous amounts of a class of polyunsaturated fatty acids called the omega-3 group. The omega-3s seem to be genuine superstars when it comes to protecting your heart and blood vessels. They "thin" the blood, slowing down the potentially dangerous clotting process, and lower cholesterol levels. They also reduce triglycerides, another blood fat considered almost as important as cholesterol in determining heart-disease risk.

Pick Up Beer

Check your fridge. See any beer lying on its side? If so, you're sabotaging your good time by increasing the surface area of the beer exposed to the air trapped in the bottle or can. The longer your brew is exposed to air, the weaker it'll taste.

Avoid the Fly Seasoning

Never eat food that's displayed beneath one of those electric bug zappers. When the little guys hit the electrified grid, they explode, scattering bug guts for several feet. The potato salad has plenty of seasoning already.

TEST YOUR VITAMINS

Even with all this food know-how, you still may decide to take vitamins for some nutritional insurance. If a vitamin doesn't break down within 20 to 30 minutes, it will bypass the first part of the small intestine, where most nutrients are absorbed. To see how well your vitamin is being absorbed, drop it in a glass of vinegar. If it doesn't break down in 30 minutes, try another brand.

Don't Pump Iron

If you're taking a multivitamin, make sure it has low or no iron. Iron buildup has been linked to heart disease in men. You don't need more than 10 milligrams a day.

Eat More C for Longevity

Men with high vitamin C intakes live longer than men with low intakes. A 35-year-old man who takes in 300 milligrams or more of C a day has a life expectancy 5.5 years longer than a man whose daily intake is less than 50 milligrams.

Be on the Lookout for Multivitamins in Disguise

You may already be taking a multivitamin without knowing it. If you're eating a fortified cereal every morning, such as Total or Life, you don't need a supplement. Many energy bars also contain 100 percent of the RDA—the recommended dietary allowance—for lots of vitamins and minerals.

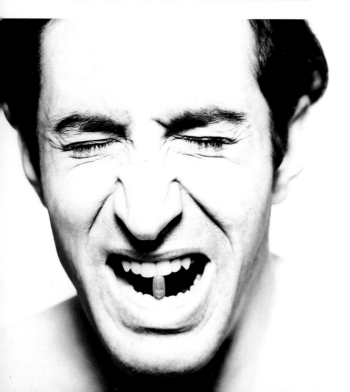

Calculate How Much Food You Need

So much food, so little time. Here's an easy way to calculate your daily calorie needs, which usually has little to do with your daily calorie wishes:

1. Your weight in pounds: _____

2. Basic calorie needs. Multiply line 1 by 11:

_____ × ___11___ = _____

3. Physical activity. Multiply line 2 by .2 if you get no exercise, .3 for light exercise (2 hours a day on your feet), .4 for moderate exercise every day, or .5 for intense exercise 3 or 4 days a week:

_____ × _____ = _____

4. Your daily calorie needs. Add line 2 and 3:

_____ + _____ = _____

5. If you'd like to lose weight, subtract 500 (so you can lose 1 pound a week). The result is your ideal daily calorie intake:

_____ − ___500___ = _____

Figure Out Your Fat Budget

You may think that dietary fat is your sworn enemy when you're trying to lose weight, but it's not. You must have a little fat in your diet if you want to lose weight. Nobody is going to stay on a diet that leaves him hungry all the time, and nobody is going to stay on one that just doesn't taste good. It's better to figure how much fat you can get away with, and then ration it out over the course of a day. Here's how to do that:

1. Your ideal daily calorie intake (from line 5 in the previous formula):

_____

2. Multiply line 1 by your desired percentage of fat calories (0.2 for 20%, 0.3 for 30%):

_____ $\times$ _____ = _____

3. Divide by 9 (the number of calories in a fat gram). This is your daily fat budget, in grams:

_____ $\div$ ___9___ = _____

See If You're Fat

Here are some easy tests.

1. Measure the circumference of your relaxed waist (around your belly button). If it's more than 40 inches, you're carrying too much belly fat. This rule holds true for men of all heights and frames.

2. Stick a finger in the collar of your dress shirt and lightly whisk it around your neck. If you can't do this without grazing skin, you're getting fat.

3. Look at your penis. If it seems shorter, you've probably gained weight. As you gain fat in your lower abdomen, it obscures the base of your penis, making it look shorter. In the worst-case scenario—what doctors called "buried penis"—your entire willy disappears.

4. Calculate your Body Mass Index (BMI). To do so, divide your weight (in pounds, naked) by your height (in inches) squared, then multiply by 705. For a man who's 180 pounds and 5-foot, 9-inches tall (that's 69 inches, which, squared, equals 4,761), the formula would look like this:

$$69 \times 69 = 4,761$$
$$180 \div 4,761 = .0378$$
$$.0378 \times 705 = 26.7$$

If your BMI is 25 or over, you're overweight. A BMI of 30 or more means you're obese.

Weigh Yourself Daily

The biggest health risk for adults is weight gain, so monitor your weight daily. You cannot sense a 3- to 5-pound weight gain without a scale. When you step on the scale each morning, compare what you're seeing today to yesterday, this week to last week, this month to last month, this year to last year. If you see an increase, immediately begin portion control and increase physical activity.

Drop and Gimme 2!

For safe, lasting weight loss, don't lose more than 2 pounds per week. The biggest drawback to rapid weight loss is that you're far more likely to regain the weight. People who drop pounds quickly typically rely on extreme exercise programs or very low-calorie diets, which are tough to maintain for more than a few weeks. Rapid weight loss also involves losing a lot of fluid, which can be dangerous, especially if you're engaged in serious exercise. Often, those who lose a lot of weight quickly eventually rebound to a weight even greater than they started with.

Be Strong for 3 Months

Three months. Just 90 days. If you can hold out that long, you may win the age-old battle of the bulge. It seems 3 months' time is what it takes for a guy to lose his cravings for fatty food.

Eat with Your Left Hand

Holding your fork in your nondominant hand will slow down your eating and help you ingest less.

Scour Out Fat with Fiber

Research shows that if you double your daily fiber intake from 18 to 36 grams, you reduce the absorption of fat and protein from other foods by 130 calories per day. In one year that comes to 13 pounds of weight loss—without eating less.

Put the Tub Down, Tubby

Never eat foods out of their original containers. How many times have you dipped into a pint

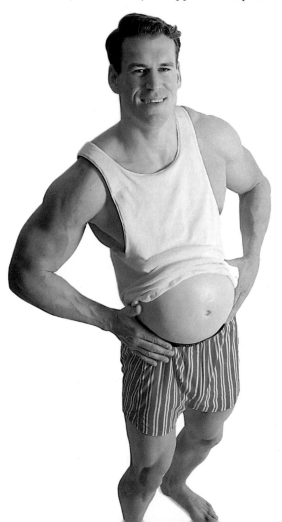

of ice cream with the intention of having "just a tad," only to find yourself staring at the bottom of the container 15 minutes later? You're much less likely to do that if you dish out the food in a measured portion. Or purchase single-servings of packaged snack foods. It's hard to stop when you're buried elbow-deep in a family-size bag of corn chips.

Wet Your Appetite

Drink two glasses of water before every meal. This will do two things: keep you hydrated and make you eat less.

Never Let Yourself Get Hungry

Rather than three big meals per day, eat five or six smaller ones. The trick, however, is to not eat any more calories than usual but to spread them more evenly throughout the day. This strategy prevents overeating, since you're never ravenously hungry. It also keeps your body from lowering its metabolic rate and conserving fat. Plus, it eliminates those dips in mood and performance you typically feel around 10 A.M. and 3 P.M.

Splurge One, Diet Two

It's okay to splurge once in a while for dinner. But if you do, remember this formula: Figure two days of eating light for every time you eat a high-calorie meal.

Keep Your Abs from Turning to Flab

When and *how* you eat are just as important as *what*. Eating large meals, for example, can stretch your abdominal muscles. Stuff yourself on a regular basis, and your abs will become so stretched they'll lose the ability to restrain your gut. Eating a large meal before bed is even worse. When you sleep, the muscles that hold in your gut relax. Your stuffed stomach presses on them, and they stretch in response to the pressure. (Turns out your mom had the right idea when she sent you to bed hungry.) Eating more frequent, smaller meals is an easy answer.

Try Dim Lights and Small Plates

Dim lights make you want to eat less than bright lights do. You can also reduce the amount you eat by using smaller, patternless dishes. You're programmed to eat more when you use large or patterned plates.

Learn to Crunch

Hard foods make hard bodies. Foods that digest slowly will kill your hunger, cut your glucose load, and turn off the hormones that make you hungry. Think raw vegetables and hard beans.

Eat in Slow Motion

Most overweight men don't eat their food; they inhale it. One way to slow down is to never have a spoon or fork in your hand while there's food in your mouth. Take a forkful of food, put it in your mouth, and then put the fork down by the side of the plate, chew, swallow, then pick up the fork again.

Listen to Music While You Munch

Studies have shown that people who listen to relaxing music during meals chew at a more leisurely pace and eat less.

TURN YOUR APPETITE OFF

Many people eat while watching TV, whether they're hungry or not. To break this habit, you have to learn to separate food from entertainment. Try either not watching some of the shows where you gobble the most, or videotape them and stop whenever the snacking urge arises. Keep doing this until you get over the desire to eat with the TV on.

Brush Your Teeth When You're Hungry

Sometimes the toothpaste flavor can take the edge off a sugar craving. Worst case: You'll have a dazzling smile.

Pinch Your Ears to Stifle a Craving

In Oriental medicine, the little bud of cartilage directly above your ear canals (called the tragus) is the acupuncture spot that controls hunger. Lightly pinching that area for 1 minute should cause food cravings to subside.

Teach Your Dog to Guard the Fridge

If you have a problem with midnight snacking, try teaching your dog this new trick:

1. Teach the dog to bark on command by holding a treat and saying, "Speak!"

2. Go to the refrigerator after dark, tell the dog to "Speak!" then open it and give him a treat. Eventually, he'll run to the fridge and bark when he sees you heading there, which will serve as a reminder not to snack.

Think Little, Not Big

Instead of a big, revolutionary goal, like eating more healthfully, give yourself a specific goal—like eating one additional piece of fruit each day, or avoiding beer on weeknights. By keeping things simple and focusing on specific tasks, you'll increase your chances of losing weight and keeping it off.

Stop Hunger Pangs

Tighten your stomach muscles as firm as possible, and slowly count to 10. You'll help curb the flow of stomach acid that causes the sensation.

Beat Sweets with Vanilla

Sniffing vanilla can fight a dessert craving. Among 160 volunteers, those given vanilla-scented skin patches lost an average of 4½ pounds. Vanilla may trigger the release of serotonin, making you less likely to crave sweets.

Take a Good, Long Whiff

Part of the reason men gain weight as they age is because their sense of smell fades. Your sense of smell controls about 90 percent of your sense of taste. So as you get older, food naturally tastes blander, and you crave more sugar and salt. To get around this, chew your food twice as long. The more you chew, the more aroma reaches your nose. This can help heighten your sense of taste and trick you into feeling fuller faster.

PUT ON YOUR "FAT" CLOTHES

Keep your old fat clothes around. Every month or so, put them on and let them drop to your ankles.

Clothes Out This Excuse

Ever weigh yourself while clothed, then subtracted, oh, 10 pounds or so to compensate for what you had on? We weighed some outfits on a postal scale to find out just how heavy clothes really are. A suit, dress shoes, socks, shirt, tie, belt, and underwear came in at 5 pounds, 8 ounces. Street clothes, jeans, T-shirt, belt, socks, sneakers, and underwear weighed just 3 pounds, 15 ounces. Stop kidding yourself.

Laugh Your Way Thin

It's estimated that 100 belly laughs gives an aerobic workout similar to 10 minutes on a rowing machine.

Don't Scare Yourself Fat

Avoid scary films if you're trying to lose weight. In a study of how stress and mood affect eating, suspenseful chase scenes made dieters eat twice as much popcorn as dull travelogues.

Find Out What's Eating You

If you're depressed and depression is making you gain weight, get it treated. What makes you fat isn't necessarily what you eat—it's what's eating you.

Cycle Away Your Inner Tube

If you want to burn fat by riding a stationary bike at the gym, avoid the automated program that says "fat-burning." It's just a long, slow workout. You'll burn more calories if you do the "interval" workout instead, which forces you to pedal at varying intensities. In the long run, you'll chew up more fat.

Follow the Sound-Sleep Diet

Sleep deprivation decreases the odds of shedding blubber and keeping it off. Researchers found that healthy men who snoozed only 4 or 7 hours a night for 6 nights in a row had higher glucose and insulin levels in their blood. This is a terrible state of metabolism for a man who's trying to lose weight, because surplus insulin boosts body-fat storage. Hit the sack for 8 hours each and every night.

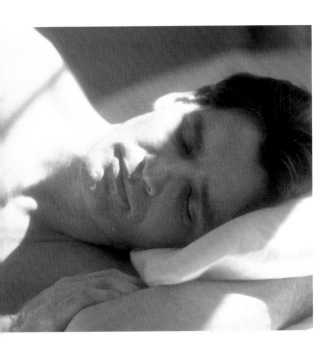

Lift Weights to Lose Waist

Weight training builds muscle, and muscle takes more energy to sustain itself than fat does. The more muscle you have, the higher your metabolism idles, not just after exercising, but *all* the time. Every pound of muscle you add raises your calorie needs by 30 to 50 per day. Over the course of an 8-week weight-training program, if you gain 3 to 5 pounds of muscle, which is typical, you could be burning 250 extra calories per day just by sitting still. This metabolic afterburn from weight training is one third greater than what you deliver from aerobic exercise.

Stretch Away Your Gut

If your hamstrings are tight, you may develop a habit of leaning backward to relieve the pressure. This posture tends to thrust your gut forward, making it look even bigger than it is. Stretching your hamstrings a few times a week should help.

Burn Fat in Bed

If you're lucky enough to have sex three times per week—nothing fancy, just a modest merger—you'll burn about 7,500 calories every year. That's the equivalent of jogging 75 miles.

Schuss Do It

If you want to lose weight, winter is the best time to get outside and exercise. In the cold, your body needs to burn more calories to maintain its normal temperature. Cross-country skiing is one of the best calorie-burners. A 150- to 160-pound man will typically combust 700 calories per hour.

Fidget Yourself Thin

Do you bounce your leg while you read, pace while you wait, or tap your fingers while you think? Good. It's possible to burn up to 800 calories a day through these purposeless movements.

Shop after Dinner

Always shop on a full stomach. Then your good sense won't have to fight bad advice from hungry taste buds.

Be More Physically Active

If you just can't stick with an exercise program, stop trying so hard to exercise. Instead, attempt to be more physically active in your daily life by taking the stairs, riding your bike for around-town errands, or using a push mower. This subtle shift in mindset is key. It's the way to achieve permanent weight loss.

Know the Best Exercises for Fat-Burning

Cross-country skiing is the fastest fat burner and is more strenuous than running, yet it has a low risk of injury because its movements are gliding rather than bouncing. Rowing, either indoors or outdoors, is the second best. Like cross-country skiing, it exercises most of the large muscle

Burn Fat Quicker

At home, you flick between 103 TV stations. At a barbecue, you sample six kinds of meat. So why, at the gym, do you sweat all over the same piece of cardiovascular equipment for your whole workout? Instead, try switching machines during one session. You can prevent your body from adapting to the workout, and force it to work harder and burn more fat. Short on time? Try this 20-minute high-intensity workout. A 185-pound man will burn 250 to 300 calories—that's 35 to 50 percent more than if he spent the entire time on a stationary bike.

Warmup:

Bike 5 minutes

Workout:

Jump rope 3 minutes

Treadmill 5 minutes

Bike 3 minutes

Rowing machine 5 minutes

Jump rope 3 minutes

Cooldown:

Bike 5 minutes

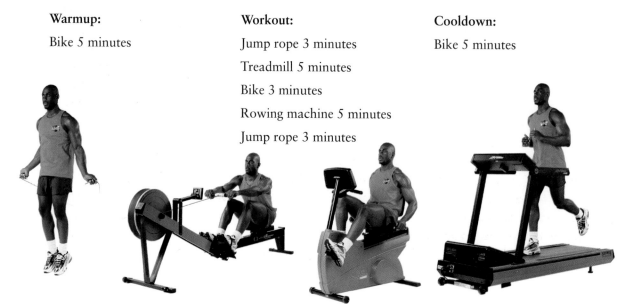

MEASURE WHAT MATTERS

Here's a simple way to measure your weight-loss progress:

1. Measure your waist.

2. Measure your neck.

3. Subtract your neck size from your waist size.

Repeat this calculation every 4 weeks. If the number is going down—if your waist is getting smaller relative to your neck—you're losing fat. If it's going in the opposite direction, you need to beef up your workouts and slow down your fork.

groups without stressing joints. Swimming is the most deceptive. Although it provides an excellent cardiovascular workout, tones muscles, and has a very low risk of injury, it is not a great fat-burning activity. Swimmers consistently carry more fat than runners or cyclists.

Exercise Less to Lose More

Three 30-minute exercise sessions burn twice as much fat as two 45-minute workouts. Why? Every exercise session speeds up your body's metabolism and decreases hunger. Men who exercise three times per week enjoy these advantages an extra day.

Get Yourself Moving

One guy we know dupes himself by eating one bad thing a day—a Twinkie, a doughnut, a bag of Chee-tos. The guilt drives him straight to the gym. The extreme version: a man who stops at the all-you-can-eat buffet to see all the huge people. In fear and revulsion, he hustles off to his workout.

Stop Crunching to Lose Weight

Don't try to lose your gut by working your abs. Researcher found that it takes 250,000 crunches to burn 1 pound of fat—that's 100 crunches a day for 7 years.

Scare Yourself Thin

For this trick, you'll need a camera and a mirror—or a friend. Put on your swim trunks. Shirt off. Let out the gut. Now take your picture in the mirror, or have your buddy take it. This, my flabby friend, is how you'll look in summer beach snapshots unless you get your act together. Make a copy and tape it to the rice pudding.

First On, Last Off

The first commandment of weight loss is this: The first place thou hast gained weight is the last place thou shalt lose it. For most men, this is around the waist. Be patient. Be persistent.

2

LOOKS

and

STYLE

No man is perfect—not even a *Men's Health* cover model. Before his image is sent to the printing plant to be duplicated nearly a million times, our art department "cleans him up," as it's called in magazine parlance. This might involve electronically excising a mole, whitening his teeth, taming an errant hair, or even adding a bit of shadow between his abs so they look even more *there*. (By the way, these are trade secrets. If you tell anyone about this, we'll find a way to put even more blow-in cards in your next issue.) Honestly, though, none of this should surprise you. We all have our flaws and phobias, our blemishes and inadequacies, little wiggles of lint on our dark-blue suits, smudges on our character. It would be great if some guy with Photoshop software would be there to clean us up every time we left the house, but in case you haven't noticed you're no *Men's Health* cover model—at least not yet. So here's the next best step. This chapter contains 165 of the most useful tips the editors could collect on the subject of looks and style: how to dress, how to talk, how to charm . . . basically, how to be a gentleman. It's the finishing school you never attended. It's the veneer of sophistication that's applied to a body resurrected.

One of the most impressive men we ever met was not a professional athlete, a billionaire executive, or even a Hollywood celeb, although he regularly partied with all of them. Rather, he was a 70-year-old Romanian butler, who instead of sipping the Tattingers, served it. He had a confidence about him that you instantly recognized and desired. He was all about manners and grace and looking good and, perhaps most important, revering the details. He'd spend hours polishing silverware and crystal, then burnish himself the same way in front of the mirror. Few of us can be perfect in the grand scheme, he'd lecture, but everyone can be peerless when it comes to the particulars.

That's good advice. And you know what? While at first it doesn't seem worth the time or effort to iron a perfect crease into a pair of pants or polish your shoes to a gleam, you eventually find delight and even a small patch of peace in doing so. Maybe it stems from gaining a fingertips's worth of control in this crazy world. Or perhaps it comes from finally finding a simple way to set yourself apart that doesn't involve money, success, or even having a lot of smarts. Whatever the reason, what initially feels like a dis-

guise eventually becomes your cherished prize. Before long, you realize that to earn respect, you must first respect yourself. That's another lesson the butler taught us.

We'll leave you with one more thought. A buddy of ours, an ordinary-looking guy who doesn't make much money and, in fact, is losing his hair, has a knack for dating beautiful, younger women. One is always on his arm. When we asked him to share his secret, he just smiled and said we wouldn't believe it. "All you have to do," he said, pausing for dramatic effect, "is make sure you wear really nice shoes. That's one of the first things women look at when they meet you."

Polish, friend, polish.

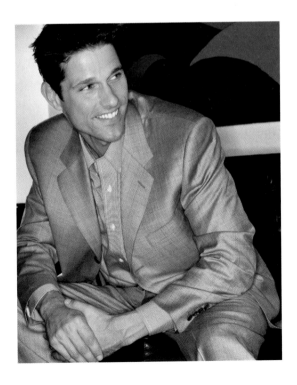

Think Yourself Handsome

To be handsome, dress handsome, talk handsome, act handsome. If you believe it, if you radiate it, women will see you that way.

Take the Balding Test

There are 100,000 hairs on the typical male head and on any given day you lose 50 to 100 of them, whether you're balding or not. If you're unsure whether the amount of hair coming out in your comb is worth worrying about, try this simple test. Grab a clump of hair and tug gently but firmly. It's normal for six or fewer hairs to come out. More than six could be an early warning that you may someday be bald.

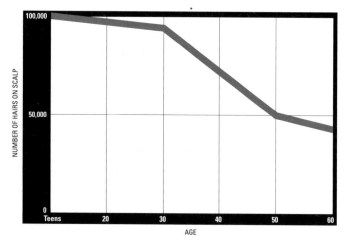

Don't Blame Mom

A single, dominant gene does not cause baldness. (The belief that hair loss is inherited from the mother's side of the family is a myth.)

Rather, it's a combination of genes, and their influence is cumulative. The more domes that are shining in your family, the more likely it is that you'll thin. First-degree relatives have the most impact—namely your father, brothers, and uncles.

Strive for Good Health

Drinking, smoking, and not exercising can all contribute to hair loss. If you have a genetic risk of balding, bad lifestyle factors can make hair loss happen faster and more severely.

Thicken Your Hair

So called "hair-thickening shampoos" actually work. They coat your hair with protein and seal in moisture, increasing the diameter of each strand by as much as 50 percent and creating the illusion of thicker hair. For a do-it-yourself alternative, mix 1 tablespoon of white vinegar with 1 pint of water and massage it into your hair after shampooing. Wait a minute or two, then rinse. It changes the chemical balance of your hair to be slightly more acidic; for some reason that makes hair appear thicker.

Keep the Sun off Your Head

A bad sunburn on your head can do more than make combing painful; it can make an already wispy pate become even more sparse. Sunburn irritates skin, which responds by creating a natural inflammatory compound called *superoxide*. This is also the messenger that tells hair follicles to move from a growth phase to a shedding phase. Sun exposure also

SAVE MONEY ON MINOXIDIL

Buy cheap minoxidil. It doesn't matter if it's CVS brand or Walgreens, generic minoxidil is FDA approved to help grow hair. Pick up the 5 percent extra-strength variety, but trash the enclosed spray applicator. You'll end up spraying most of your dosage on your hair instead of your scalp, and it won't have its full effect. The medicine dropper allows you to get the product directly onto your scalp. And if you fertilize post-shower, towel your head off first. If there's too much water, the solution will be diluted, and it won't work as well.

makes hair shafts more fragile. The hairs may grow back after a sunburn, but they won't be as hardy.

Don't Trigger a Shed

Younger men with a genetic susceptibility to male-pattern baldness can trigger it prematurely by crash dieting or subjecting themselves to too much stress. The condition is called "shedding." If you're trying to lose weight, make sure your diet contains ample protein, which is essential for hair growth.

Eat Less Fat, Grow More Hair

Eating a traditional American steak-and-potatoes diet can not only plug up your arteries; it might lead to hair plugs, as well. After reviewing 30 years of hair loss and heart disease data collected from more than 2,000 American men, researchers found that those with the least hair also had the highest risk of dying from heart disease. The connection is likely due to nitric oxide, a naturally occurring chemical that prevents blood clots and dilates blood vessels

(two keys to avoiding heart attacks). Nitric oxide also seems to foster hair growth and erections. When atherosclerosis damages the walls of your blood vessels, it causes them to produce less nitric oxide.

Spot Bogus Baldness Treatments

Beware, buyer. Steer clear of these baldness treatments:

• Any that are not minoxidil or finasteride. These are the only two drugs that science currently recognizes as influential in reversing hair loss. If someone promotes another substance, ask him why all the world's dermatologists have missed it.

• You found it on the Internet. Cyber-ads can be pure fiction. While reputable publishers and broadcasters screen their advertisers, anything goes on the Web.

• The infomercial is staged as a talk show. The acting's better than most of what you see on TV, but then the guys are better paid.

WHEN ALL ELSE FAILS

GET RID OF DANDRUFF

Dip a cotton ball in castor oil and rub it on your scalp—the flakes will dissolve. Wait 5 minutes, then wash your hair thoroughly. Or, shake 1 tablespoon of salt into dry hair, massage, and shampoo.

• It has roots back to Mesopotamia and was perfected in Istanbul. Few scam artists align themselves with places like Boston University. It's too easy to pick up the phone and check. Desperate men are suckers for the ancient and exotic.

• They claim it will give you hair in minutes. Magic is pretty scarce nowadays. The "too-good-to-be-true" law applies.

• The promoter or label promises "amazing results." The shampoo costs $80 and didn't grow a single hair. Isn't that amazing?

• It's a "secret formula." If it really worked, the secret would be out—evidence attached—overnight.

• It's guaranteed to grow hair. No legitimate product will make this claim. Not even God grows hair on every head.

Disguise a Thinning Head

Fortunately, hair doesn't thin uniformly. It usually thins most from the top of the head. To disguise this, let the hair on top grow out a bit while reducing bulk at the back and sides. It'll make your hair look balanced and more consistently full.

Brush before a Shower

To really clean your hair, brush your hair *before* you wash it. A few brushes will loosen dirt, grooming products, natural oil, and environmental pollutants that build up over the course of a day.

Don't Give Yourself Dandruff

Dandruff shampoos can cause dandruff. Steady use can dry your scalp and cause more flakes. To be safe, dilute it with baby shampoo and use it just a few times per week.

Heal Your Scalp

If you have dandruff, try preshampooing with honey, a natural antifungal. In one study, dandruff sufferers who washed their scalps with honey (diluted with warm water) daily had no more flakes or itching after 5 weeks.

Look Younger Longer

At about age 50, the oil glands that in your youth worked overtime to bless you with acne start retiring, and your skin gets dry. To keep your face from looking parched as a Dead Sea scroll, use a moisturizer containing lanolin or the oils of wheat germ, safflower, or coconut. Apply it right after a shower or wet shave. Upping your water intake can also help combat dry skin. Drink at least a quart of water a day.

Look Younger Instantly

The simplest way to hide lines in your face is to get a short haircut. The lines around the face are downward, and long hair accentuates those creases. Clip your hair to a length of 1 inch. Keep your sideburns and the hair on the back of your neck (not to mention your ear and nose hair) meticulously shaved and trimmed.

Never Get Wrinkles!

Tone your facial muscles by doing these exercises repeatedly each morning.

1.
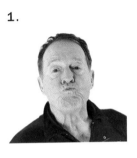

2.
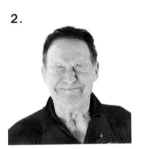

3.
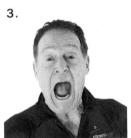

4.
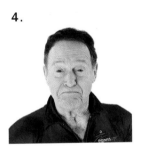

Shave after a Shower

Instead of shaving first thing in the morning, have breakfast, shower, then shave. Your face won't be as puffy, and the warm water will open pores and soften hairs. You'll get a closer shave.

Spot a Sinister Mole

A precancerous mole tends to have an irregular border and usually exhibits a variety of colors. A harmless mole has a clearly defined border and is uniformly brown or tan. If you spot a mole that looks suspicious, see a dermatologist. Caught early, it can be easily removed. But if left to grow, it can be life-threatening.

Fade Sun Spots

Use a cotton swab to dab fresh lemon juice on your sun spots twice a day. The citric acid safely and painlessly peels away the skin's uppermost layer. Be patient. You should see results within a month or so. If you use sunblock, you'll help keep new spots from forming.

Erase Age Spots

Once a day at bedtime, apply a skin cream that contains the spot-erasing ingredient kojic acid. It's just as effective as popular over-the-counter skin-bleaching agents containing hydroquinone, but it causes much less irritation. Check your drugstore for Pro-Cyte Kojic Complex Gel. And to prevent new age spots from forming, start basting your face with sunscreen now.

Zap Zits

Use a drop of calamine lotion or rubbing alcohol to absorb excess oil. Then hold an ice cube wrapped in a washcloth against the skin for 60 seconds.

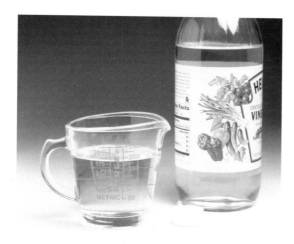

Get Rid of Oily Skin with Vinegar

A few drops of vinegar dabbed on a tissue and rinsed away with water will kill the shine.

Bring a Boil to a Boil

Get rid of a Godzilla-size pimple with a warm compress. Soak a washcloth in warm water, wring it out, and put it on a dish in the microwave. Now nuke the cloth for 15 to 30 seconds, then (after making sure it's not too hot) take it out and apply it to the boil for a few minutes. Repeat until the boil ruptures. Apply an antibiotic ointment and slap on a bandage; you should be completely healed in 3 to 5 days.

Prevent an Eruption

Hold an ice cube to your lip next time you feel a cold sore coming on, and you may keep it from blossoming.

Be Ruddy or Not

If you return from the gym or happy hour with red, puffy cheeks, it could be the beginning of rosacea, a common skin disease that causes the blood vessels in your face to dilate. If left untreated, rosacea can give you a bulbous nose and even permanently mar your face with spider veins and scratchy, pus-filled patches. See a dermatologist immediately. While there's no cure, quick treatment can help. A few months of tetracycline followed with a topical gel or cream will usually control it.

Unpack the Bags under Your Eyes

You shouldn't have had that V8. Vegetable drinks and tomato juice are loaded with sodium, which can cause your body to retain water. The bloating that results will often announce itself around your eyes.

Protect Yourself at the Beach

Use a shot glass worth of sunscreen for full-body protection. Most people use less than half that amount. Apply waterproof sunscreen 30 minutes before heading into the water, so your skin can absorb it. "Waterproof" means it keeps its SPF after a person stands in a pool for about 40 minutes. If you're rubbing yourself off with a towel, diving in the waves, or rolling around in the sand, you're going to lose the waterproof qualities much faster.

Erase Calluses

Some women find callused hands sexy—until you start sanding their bare breasts with those 60-grit mitts. Before any future foreplay, crush five or six aspirin tablets and mix the powder with a half teaspoon each of water and lemon juice. Coat your calluses, and then cover them with a warm, damp washcloth for 10 minutes. Acids in the aspirin will soften calluses, so that they will come right off after a few strokes with a pumice stone.

Square Off Your Toenails

Never cut your toenails in a rounded shape so that the leading edge curves down into the skin at the sides. This can lead to ingrown nails. Instead, always leave the outside edges of the nail parallel with the skin.

Buy a Wardrobe Maker

Here's one simple rule for clothing your body. Lay out some cash for a classic piece or two—they'll make even the less expensive stuff you own look good. For instance, make sure you own one great sport coat. Then buy more affordable pants, shirts, ties, shoes, etc. that match it.

Calculate "Price per Wear"

To gauge the true cost of clothing, calculate the "price per wear." For example, a $200 pair of shoes, worn twice a week for a year, costs about $2 per wear. A $25 pair, worn for two special occasions, costs $12.50 per wear. An item's versatility and durability can be more important than its purchase price.

Deal with a Well-Dressed Salesman

When shopping for clothes, find a spiffy-looking sales guy. You don't want some poorly dressed sap telling you how to look. Or call ahead for a personal shopper, which most large department stores offer. They'll lend you color sense if you're a bit lacking.

Disguise a Big Adam's Apple

If you're looking to hide a prominent Adam's apple, wear open-collared shirts. This creates a distraction that helps pull eyes away from the center of your throat.

Bolster a Weak Chin

To compensate for a weak chin, wear a collared shirt that contrasts with the clothes that surround it. For example, the classic combo of a dark blue suit, a white shirt, and a burgundy tie hides a weak chin perfectly.

UNCOMMON KNOWLEDGE

AVOID SUDSY SOAPS

The very soaps that tend to give you the most suds are also the worst for your skin. People associate suds with cleanliness, but that's not the case. Actually, sudsy soaps usually contain harsh detergents, which dry you out like beef jerky. Instead, go with a gentle cleanser such as Dove or Cetaphil or a soap containing moisturizer.

Collar Yourself

Your shirt collar can have a huge impact on how you look and how others perceive you. Here's the scoop.

Button-down: The most conservative look. Despite the buttons, the collar tends to bulge outward during the day, so keep an eye on it.

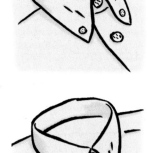

Tab collar: Best for ultra-traditional occasions such as weddings and funerals. Use a tight four-in-hand knot; nothing else fits correctly under the collar.

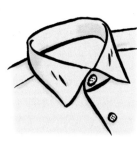

Spread collar: If you have a round face, a spread collar is probably not a wise choice; it will make your face look even rounder. The bulky, half-Windsor knot best complements the spread.

Straight collar: This is the most common shirt collar, with the greatest variations in point length. It complements almost any countenance

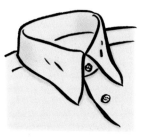

except an exceptionally long, thin face. The four-in-hand is the best knot.

British spread collar: An extra-wide, virtually horizontal spread between points makes this the most formal type of collar. Once again, the tie knot of choice is the half-Windsor. Also,

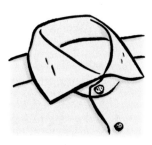

same caveat as above regarding round faces— unless you're a member of Parliament.

Untuck and Cover

Any shirt that can be worn untucked helps hide heft. Two important caveats: First, any shirt that's left untucked must be flat-bottomed. And second, avoid any upper-body gear (sweaters, windbreakers) with elastic bottoms. They cause the material to bunch up at your waist, making even a thin man look like a heavy one.

Say Goodbye to Your Old Crew

If you're overweight, relegate crewneck sweaters to the closet; they round out the face and give you that Charlie Brown look. The point of a V-neck makes you appear taller and leaner and helps reduce any creeping jowl formation.

Keep Collars from Curling

If you lose a stay from your shirt collar, replace it with a paper clip, temporarily at least.

Fold a Shirt

If your shirts aren't professionally folded, here's the best way to do it: Button all the buttons and lay the shirt out, shirtfront down. Fold the sleeves back from the shoulder seam. To prevent the shirt from creasing across your stomach, fold the tail up from the bottom buttons.

MR. CLEAN

DRESS UP YOUR WHITES

Contrary to popular belief, most white cotton dress shirts do not need to be professionally laundered. You can do it yourself, at home. Here are the simple steps:

1. Get all your grungy clothes out of there—even other white stuff. You want to wash your dress shirts separately to prevent any color or grime from tainting them.

2. Rub a stain remover or swish a little detergent around the inside of the collar and the edges of the cuffs. Let it sit for a minute or two.

3. While the stain remover is soaking in, turn on the washing machine to cold or lukewarm. Wait until the machine fills with water, then add the detergent with or without bleach. No more than a capful or two of bleach, please—too much can actually yellow the shirts.

4. Close the machine lid and let the water and detergent mix for a minute. This helps ensure the shirts are cleaned evenly and protects them from bleach stains.

5. Toss the shirts in. Wait.

6. When they're done, don't throw them in the dryer—that could shrink the cotton. Instead, hang them up to dry. Press them before you hang them in your closet.

7. If you like a little starch, you can buy spray starches to use during the ironing process. They're not as stiff as the commercial kind, but they'll help the shirt keep its shape.

Get Rid of Shoulder Nipples

These are the protrusions in your shirt caused by a clothes hanger. To remove them, moisten your fingers and rub them on the protrusions until the shirt is wet. (Just make sure your hands are clean.) When the shirt dries, the nipples will be gone.

Tuck Your Shirt

If your dress shirt is always coming untucked, here's a simple solution. Tuck it into your underwear.

Stop Being Hot Under the Collar

Get your shirts starched. Despite their uptight image, starched shirts are actually more comfortable. They'll hold their shape better, meaning they won't cling to you and soak up your sweat. The result: You won't feel like an overdressed sponge.

Dress to a Tee

Some T-shirts are dressy enough to wear solo with a suit. The white ones that come in three-packs are not. Your rule: If you want to wear a

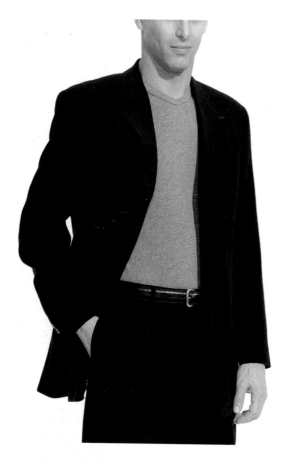

Fold a Sweater Better

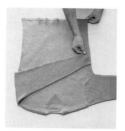

Hold the sweater up by each shoulder, with the front facing you. Or lay the sweater flat, front side down, on a flat surface. Fold each sleeve diagonally across the back.

From the shoulder, fold the sides of the sweater in toward the back so the points of the shoulders meet in the center.

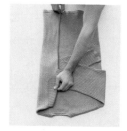

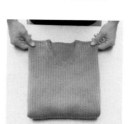

Fold the sweater in half. Now, fill out that application for the Gap.

stand-alone T-shirt under a jacket, buy one with a ribbed knit. Neutral or dark colors work under most jackets. Avoid pastels and bright colors.

Take Care of Your Ties

In the evening, drape your tie over the closet bar for a day to let the creases relax. Then roll it and store it in a drawer. Ditch the tie rack—gravity deforms. When traveling, slip your rolled ties into the inner breast pocket of your suit. And never iron a tie. Doing so sets the dirt and squashes the silk shell into the lining. Get a dry cleaner to steam it.

Buy a Great Tie

To judge the quality of a tie, tie one on. Nice knot equals nice tie every time.

Tie It This Way

The point of your tie should come to just below the belt.

Dot Your Blades

Tired of guessing how to make your necktie blades come out just the right length (front a tad longer, brushing the belt buckle)? Put a tiny dot on the back of the wide blade marking how low the narrow end should hang when you start tying the knot.

Understand Suit Styles

Some suit styles defy understanding—the ones worn on Miami Vice spring to mind. Here's a primer for the others.

American: This straight and full-cut suit says you're conservative. The jacket's lightly padded shoulders and flat front form a square that continues into the hips. Usually single-breasted, with one vent in the back, American-style suit trousers typically have no pleats or cuffs.

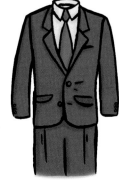

This suit style is comfortable if you're sporting a few extra pounds, or if you're just one big dude.

European: Contoured to the shape of a V, this suit is a snug fit ideal for tallish guys in great shape. Vents are on the sides of the jacket, which may be single- or double-breasted. Pants are typically pleated but not cuffed. If you want to exude the image that you're "fashion forward," this is your number.

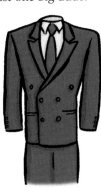

British: A form-fitting suit style that follows the lines of your body, the single-breasted jacket has a nipped-in waist and two deep vents in the back. Pants are typically pleated and cuffed. It's a sophisticated look. If you want to invoke images of an English gentleman, this is your cut.

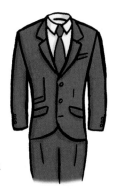

Understand Jacket Styles

Here's the lingo to know if you're wearing a sport coat.

Double-breasted: This type of jacket conveys a formal, elegant image. It should always be buttoned. It should be part of a suit, or a blue blazer—otherwise, stick to single-breasted.

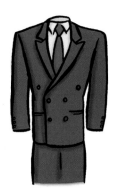

Single-breasted: This traditional design with two or three buttons can be worn buttoned or unbuttoned and is always appropriate. Always leave the bottom button undone.

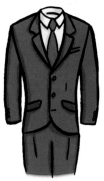

Single vent: This style creates a boxy, conservative image. If you're sporting this type of jacket, don't put your hands in your trouser pockets—the spread will expose your butt to everyone in the room, which is hardly the apex of style.

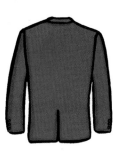

Double vent: This type of coat adds shape to your suit by emphasizing the outside lines of your body, which also makes you look taller. You can move around easily while wearing it, so you'll also appear more graceful.

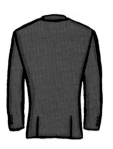

No vent: Having no vents at all streamlines suits and gives them a modern look. The jacket hugs the body and is very form-fitting. The lack of vents makes the jacket a bit uncomfortable when you sit down. This style looks best on a very lean man.

Make Your First Suit Black

If you're just starting out in the Suit World, make your first purchase a black suit. You can wear it to an interview or a funeral or even a party if you slap on a festive shirt.

Pocket It Elsewhere

The reason suit jackets and sport coats come with sewn-up pockets is to discourage you from using them as storage bins for keys, matches, wallets, and other bulky items. This stretches the material and spoils the shape. Instead of making your jacket function as a backpack, carry your essentials in a briefcase, exchange your wallet for a billfold, or just try to travel a bit lighter.

Get Smoke Out of a Sport Coat

Put the coat and a fabric-softener sheet in the dryer and set it to "air fluff"—that means no

Tie Knots

Half-Windsor

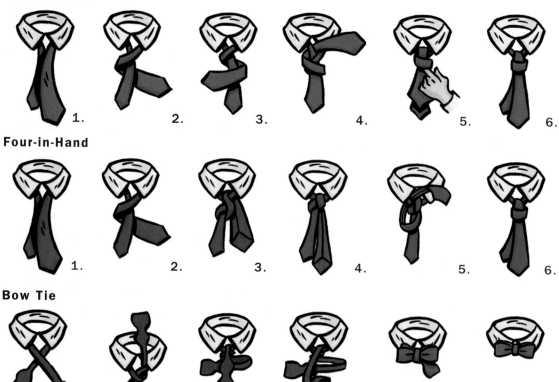

heat—for 5 minutes. The interaction between ozone and static electricity helps eliminate odors. Hang up your jacket immediately, and it should naturally fall back into shape. Don't do this too often; too much tumbling might cause the fibers to knot together. Then you'd have to wear your cape.

Get Rid of Secondhand Smoke Stench

If you're away from home and covered in secondhand smoke, duck into a restroom and plant yourself in front of the hand dryer. Switch it on, and it will raise the temperature around you, vaporizing smoke molecules. Blowing air over the surface of your clothes picks up and carries off any remaining odor-causing molecules. Tousle your hair in the heat stream for a few minutes, then blast your jacket until it's smoke-free.

Size a Sport Jacket

The sleeve of a suit jacket or sport coat should come down to that prominent bone at your wrist. Most men wear their jacket sleeves too long. The sleeve should be short enough that ½ inch of your shirt cuff sticks out below it.

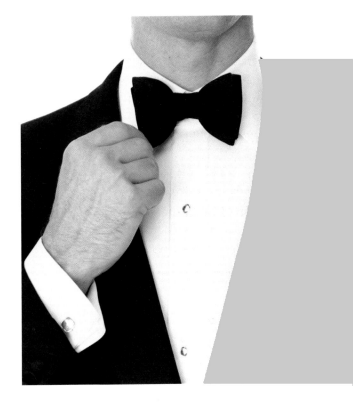

Decide to Rent or Buy

If you attend more than three or four black-tie events a year, buy a tuxedo. Don't worry about it going out of style: The tuxedo has a way of transcending current fashion.

Solve the Cummerbund Conundrum

Unsure which way to wear the cummerbund? The pleat openings should point up. (It was originally designed for use as a ticket pocket, but it also helps catch crumbs and phone numbers.) You don't have to wear a cummerbund with a tuxedo, though. In fact, only do so if you have a small waist. Nothing looks worse than a beer belly doing battle with a cummerbund.

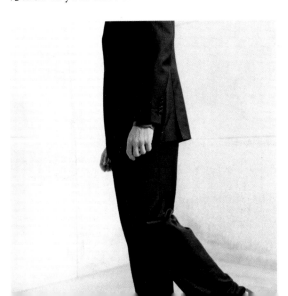

Look Good in an Overcoat

Most men wear overcoats that are too big and look sloppy. Buy a coat that's just one size larger than your suit size. It should follow the contour of your shoulders. The down-to-the-knee fit is a good casual look. For business, go with the traditional mid-calf length. Shrug off padded shoulders.

Choose Gloves Carefully

If gloves are tight, they're won't keep you warm. They'll inhibit blood flow, and the insulation will get the air flattened out of it. Air in the glove is the key to cozy digits. One simple fit trick: Put one on and make a fist. There should be no binding or tightness in the fingers.

Come Hell or High Waters

Your trousers are the proper length when your socks don't show while you're walking in full stride. The front of the trouser leg should rest on the top of your shoe; the touching of fabric to shoe will form a slight fold. That fold is called the *break*. It refers to the break that's created in the neat line of a crease.

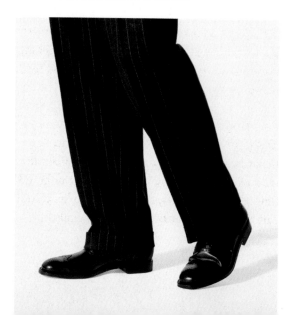

Wear This with Khakis

Save the gray shirt for jeans. Gray doesn't work with the color of khakis because they're both neutral shades that are made of similar colors. Your best bet is to wear shirts that contrast with both the pants and your skin tone. A blue shirt is the safest choice because it never fights with anyone's skin color.

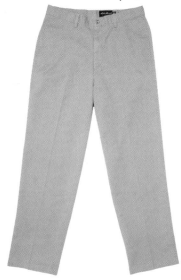

Try 'em On, Then Sit Down

When you try pants on, don't just stand in front of a mirror. To tell if they really fit, sit down. Since your waist and hips get bigger when you sit, if you're uncomfortable in a sitting position, the pants are too small. If you're buying jeans that aren't preshrunk, allow an extra 2 inches in the waist and 3 inches in the inseam.

Give Your Pants Another Chance

Most men dry-clean their trousers too often. To stave off premature aging, dry-clean them once or twice a season and have them professionally steamed when they look rumpled. Frequent fliers might also consider purchasing a small portable steamer.

FLOSS YOUR PANTS

A button pops on your khakis and, wouldn't you know it, it's the important one. No safety pin? Then zip up, pinch the top of your trousers together, and go find someone with decent oral hygiene; dental floss is actually stronger than the toughest thread. Run one end of a 6-inch length of floss through your buttonhole and feed it through the tiny hole in your zipper tab. Loop the floss around itself, pull it tight, and tie it off.

Heed the 7 Rules of Denim

Our jeans ask for so little and give so much. Keep these hints in mind:

1. If we catch you in creased denim, we'll mock you.

2. Jeans are worn at your hips, not an inch above your belly button like dress pants.

3. Jeans don't have a break on top of the shoe. They just brush the middle of the laces.

4. We've never seen a tie work with jeans.

5. Bring a pair of black jeans on every trip you take. They're versatile.

6. If you're deciding between two waist sizes, choose the bigger one.

7. Jeans can be worn with anything from a T-shirt to a cashmere sweater.

Tighten Your Jeans

For form-fitting jeans, pull them on while they're still damp after a washing. Denim has a memory, and it will conform to your body.

Save Your Jeans

To reduce fading, turn jeans inside out before washing them.

Do the Wallet Test

When buying jeans, see if you can easily slide your wallet out of your back pocket. If not, they're too tight; have the saleswoman remove them immediately.

Staple Split Pants

So you're at work and you split your pants. Take them off. Turn them inside out. (Have you closed your office door?) Now staple along the inner seam. There's extra fabric where the stitching is, so your handiwork won't be seen and, more important, won't be felt.

Lose the Socks, Then the Pants

A man in his socks and underpants is a man at his worst. If there's somebody else in the room, always take your socks off before you lose the pants.

Stop Calf Balding

Years of wearing socks that are too tight, particularly support hose, can kill hair follicles in the lower legs by reducing the amount of blood that reaches them. So, if you'd like to keep your calf hair, choose socks that aren't so tight.

Press a Pair of Pants

If all else fails and you have to break out the iron, here's how to press a pair of pants.

1. Warm a heavy iron to high heat and dampen an old cotton sheet that either you or a wild girlfriend has previously ripped into a 3-by-3-foot square rag.

2. Lay your trousers straight out on the board, and fold back one leg as shown.

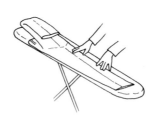

3. After making sure that the crease is straight, drape the rag over the fabric (as protection) and begin ironing.

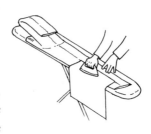

4. Press firmly and use short, horizontal strokes, working from the middle seam outward. When the rag dries, that's your signal to move to the next section.

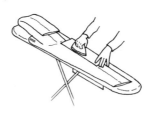

5. After the top half of this leg is done, use the same technique to press from the middle seam inward. Throw back the other leg on top of the pressed one and iron it in the same way.

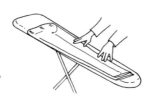

6. When you're finished, shake out the pants and hang them immediately

to cool. Regardless of how good it feels, never wear warm, freshly ironed pants: You'll destroy the crease.

Get Rid of Any Stain

Here's how to minimize the damage when a spill happens, and what to do later to get rid of it for good:

Blood: Rinse with cool salt water, then apply a mixture of soap and cold water. Rinse and repeat. *Later:* If traces remain, mix soap and water with a few drops of ammonia and dab at it. Then wash it in a cold-water cycle.

Butter: Ask a coworker for some nail-polish remover. (Make sure it says "non-acetone" on the bottle.) A greasy stain like this should dissolve with a few drops. Then rinse the spot with cold water. *Later:* If traces remain, wash it in cold water or take it to a dry cleaner.

Chocolate: Scrape away as much as possible, then rinse the area with room-temperature water until the chocolate breaks up. Attack what remains with a paper towel and a solution of a few drops of soap in half a cup of water. *Later:* When the shirt is dry, put some laundry detergent directly on the stain and let it sit for a few minutes, then wash it in a warm-water cycle.

Coffee or tea with milk: Boil water in the microwave. Take off your shirt and pour the hot water through the stain. *Later:* Rub in a few drops of vinegar or peroxide then wash it in hot water.

Crayon: Place the shirt stain-side down on paper towels, and spray the back of the mark with WD-40. Let it sit for several minutes, then turn it over and use the WD-40 again on the front of the stain. Gently work in some liquid dishwashing detergent. *Later:* Machine-wash in warm water, with ¼ cup of color-safe bleach.

Egg: Egg will set deeper into the fabric if you rinse it with hot water. (Protein + hot water = a worse stain.) Scrape away the excess egg, then sponge with room-temperature water and rinse away as much as you can. *Later:* Wash it in cold water.

Gravy: Scrape away the excess, then rinse with hot water until the stain begins to dissolve. When no more will rinse away, rub it a few times with bar soap and continue rinsing with hot water. *Later:* Pat a few drops of ammonia or vinegar and warm water into the shirt and rinse it. Then wash in warm water.

Gum: If you've ever spent an evening scratching and clawing to remove a gum spot, you'll kick yourself for not knowing the simple, elegant solution: Rub it with ice until it hardens. Scrape clean.

Ink: Don't even try to get this out yourself. You'll just make it worse. *Later:* Take it to the cleaner; he has an arsenal of chemicals that may help. Take the pen, too, so he'll know what type of ink he's dealing with.

Iron scorch marks: If the burn is extremely light, immediately wash the shirt with detergent in your regular laundry cycle. If the mark is still

there, sponge it with a solution of peroxide diluted with water and a few drops of ammonia. *Later:* Start sending your shirts out to be laundered—in most places it's only a buck a shirt.

Ketchup: Ask the waiter for some white vinegar, and head to the men's room. Rinse the spot under cool water. Then blend a few drops of the vinegar with water and a small amount of soap, and dab at the spot, continuing to rinse it with cool water. *Later:* Squirt on a spot remover, such as Shout. Blot and rinse with cold water. Then wash it in cold water.

Mud: Let it dry and brush off as much as you can. Then gently it rinse with cold water, rubbing a little to loosen the dirt. *Later:* Make a paste of powdered detergent and water. Rub it on the spot, and let it sit for 10 minutes. Then rinse with cool water and throw it into a warm wash.

Mystery stains: Whatever it is, let it dry, scrape off anything that's dangling, then rub in some soap and room-temperature water. (Hot water sets some stains, cold water sets others; when you don't know what you're dealing with, your best bet is somewhere in between.) *Later:* Soak it in a solution of ¼ cup of bleach and 2 quarts of water. (If the garment isn't white, you'll need color-safe bleach.) Then wash it in a warm-water cycle.

Pasta sauce (water-based): Rinse lightly with cold water, rub in a few drops of liquid soap, then rinse with more cold water. *Later:* Plunge the shirt into cool, soapy water then let it dry. Is there still a ring where the stain was? Sponge it with hydrogen peroxide and rinse with cold water. Still there? It's professional-cleaner time.

Red wine: Blot away the excess wine and rinse the area with cold water. *Later:* Wash it in cold water.

Salad dressing: Put soap and hot water on the spot as fast as you can. Continue to rinse with hot water until the stain is gone. *Later:* Wash it in a hot-water cycle.

Sweat: Blotches at the armpits are a blend of perspiration and deodorant. They form over time and there's no quick fix. Keep your jacket on. *Later:* Ask a professional cleaner to pretreat the area. And start wearing undershirts.

Feel Like a New Man

If you spend a lot of time on your feet, try changing into a new pair of socks midway through the day. This simple technique works wonders. Wipe your feet with a towel and then put on fresh socks. It's very refreshing. It feels just like you've had a shower.

Hang It Right

To keep your clothes looking better longer, treat them like this:

Jackets: Hang your jacket on wooden hangers—not wire, not plastic, and definitely not those frilly padded jobs. The wood—preferably cedar—should be between ½ and 1 inch thick. If the jacket has shoulders that slope gently down toward the sleeves, pick a hanger with a similar curve. Linebacker shoulders? Use a straighter hanger. And don't button when you

---

CLEAN OUT YOUR CLOSET

Throw open the door and follow these six steps:

1. Ask someone to help you—preferably someone younger whom you neither sleep nor golf with.

2. Look for dry-cleaning tags from laundries that have closed. Get rid of any clothes to which they're attached.

3. Admit that if you didn't wear it all last season, you never will.

4. Admit that if you haven't lost the weight in a year, you probably won't fit into those snug pieces again while they're still in style.

5. Try it on and ask "Could I dance in it?" If it's too uncomfortable for that, toss it.

6. Let your kids pick out five items apiece to donate to charity.

hang. The fabric won't be able to relax to its natural shape, and it'll wrinkle.

Pants: Any method of hanging pants is okay, but the best way is to clip them at the cuffs. Make sure you use a hanger with clips that are covered in rubber or felt; plain metal clips could leave marks. If you hang the pants folded, don't button or zipper them, or you'll stress the shape.

Suits: Don't run in after a hard day selling siding and hang your suit in the closet. Your whole closet will smell like your pits. Let the suit air out for an hour or longer. Then, when you hang it, leave a buffer zone of an inch around your suit to keep it from wrinkling. And whatever you do, don't leave it covered in a plastic garment bag. The plastic doesn't allow the fibers to breathe, and eventually they'll deteriorate.

Make Belt-Buying a Cinch

Before you buy a belt, flex it and assess the size of the wrinkles in the leather. If it's the good goods, the wrinkles will be fine creases, like the skin folds at your wrist when you bend your hand back. If they're wider, it's a poor-quality piece. When buckled, the end of your belt should pass through the trousers' first belt loop but not run past the second. It should match your shoes.

Match Socks to Pants

Fred Astaire always wore brightly colored socks when he was dancing because it drew attention to his feet. You don't want to do that, so match your socks to your pants. The pant leg and sock should form a line of color leading to the shoe.

Make Dead Shoes Walk Again

Over time, even the best leather shoes will develop a crease over the bridge of the foot. To buff this out, insert a shoe tree to maintain the shape and apply some Kiwi polish. Then heat the back of a spoon (not the good silver, please) over an oven burner until it's fairly warm. Moving the spoon in a firm, circular motion, work the melting wax into the creases. Allow the wax to dry, then buff.

Buff with Armor All

You're out of time, and your shoes are out of shine. Before you hop in your car and inflict your dullness on others, grab the ol' Armor All from the garage shelf and spray a little on a soft cloth. Now pretend you're wearing all-season radials and quickly buff your fine Italian rubber to a high gloss.

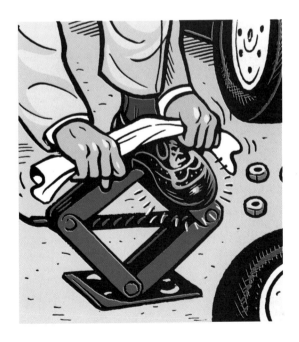

Step Out in Style

Remember what we said before—the first thing a woman notices about you is your shoes. Here's a primer on the different styles.

Wing-tip oxford: Wing tips have a full brogue, which means they have an extra layer of leather protection over the entire surface of the shoe. Black wing tips go with business clothing; brown go with dressy sportswear.

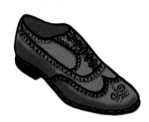

Wing tips are less formal than plain toes, but they're still very traditional. They look best with textured or heavy fabrics such as tweed or flannel.

Plain-toe oxford: The basic business lace-up, plain-toe shoes have no extra lines, leather, frills or decorations. The only visible stitching on the shoe is for re-

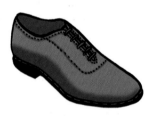

inforcing the eyelets on the upper. The look is appropriate for all business situations, but it works best with serious, dressy suits and fabrics.

Cap-toe oxford: So named because of an extra layer of leather across the toes, the cap can be plain, or it can have perfo-

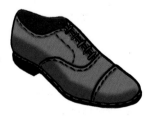

rated or other cut-out decorations. Cap toes are the dressiest business shoes you can wear—and the most popular.

Tasseled loafer: These shoes are appropriate for most business settings but not recommended if you wish to convey a super-serious first impression.

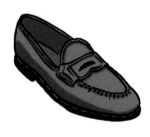

Very dressy tasseled loafers may even be worn with suits— but again, it's not recommended unless you're very certain of the style ground upon which you walk.

Penny loafer: Wear brown or cordovan penny loafers only with casual clothes or sportswear. Black loafers may be worn with dressy casual wear, like trousers with an open-collared shirt, a sport coat, and a tie. Loafers are never appropriate with a suit.

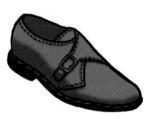

Monk strap: This European shoe has a plain toe with a buckled strap that crosses the instep. It looks best in formal settings, with a dark brown or black business suit. Depending on its styling, it can also work with casual wear.

De-Stink Your Shoes

To keep your tootsies smelling sweet, just slip a dryer sheet into each shoe. It'll last forever and instantly make it smell better.

De-Scuff Your Shoes

To get scuff marks off shoes, apply a little toothpaste to a damp rag and wipe away.

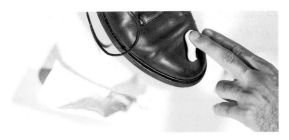

Lace 'em Up for Good

If the laces on your dress shoes are always coming untied, substitute a pair of waxed laces. The wax is impregnated into the weave of the lace, and they come in round styles. They're sticky and hold beautifully.

Dry Out Those Gunboats

To dry shoes and boots, stuff a piece of newspaper into them overnight.

Stuff Magazines in Your Shoes

If you want to wear the same shoes 2 days in a row, roll up two magazines and insert one inside each shoe at the end of the day. When you let go, the magazines will expand to help stretch the leather back into shape. They'll also do a better job of absorbing the day's moisture than plastic shoe trees.

Look Great in Trunks

The only time we think about swim trunks is when we're escorted off the beach for not wearing them. But to accentuate your body type you need to find the right pair. Match your body type to your best suit type as shown.

Tall and thin: Look for board shorts and long bathing suits that reach almost to your knees (about 23 inches along the outer seam). The trunks should tie or snap in front. Wild patterns and loud colors look fine on lean guys.

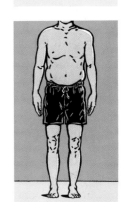

Big in the belly: Skip board shorts. They tend to ride low under a gut. Your best bet is a pair of "volley shorts"—they're similar in style to boxer shorts (about 16 inches along the seam) and have a drawstring waist. The shorter length draws attention away from your midsection; a dark color will also help. Don't buy oversize trunks—they'll make you look fatter.

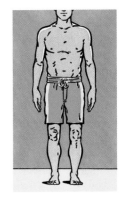

Short: Go with modified board shorts about 20 inches in length. Anything longer will make your legs look short. And look for a solid color, which can add the illusion of height. Skip loud patterns—they emphasize the division of your body at the waist and knee. This midsection distraction somehow makes you look even smaller.

WEAR CLEAN UNDERWEAR ON SATURDAY

If you are determined not to humiliate your mother—or yourself—make sure your undergarments are particularly fresh on Saturday, far and away the most dangerous day of the week on which to drive. You can be considerably more careless about your hygiene on Monday and Tuesday, both nearly twice as safe as Saturday.

Shine Shoes Without Polish

For an emergency shine, rub leather shoes with the inside of a banana peel. Clean the surface and buff with a cloth or a paper napkin.

Pick the Perfect Shades

How do you know how dark your sunglasses should be? Slip on a pair and look in the mirror. You should just be able to make out your eyes. If so, you're wearing the best-density lenses for driving and most outdoor activities.

Build an Eyewear Wardrobe

You wouldn't wear the same pair of shoes to the office that you would to play sports or to go to the movies. Glasses are among the few accessories men have to work with, so vary them.

Pick the Perfect Pair of Glasses

In eyewear, image is everything. If you think you've found a pair you like, have someone else in the store try them on. What is the immediate perception you have of him? That's what people will think of you. Here are a few guidelines:

Color: The iris of your eye contains a few different hues. Look for a frame that matches one of them, and your eyes will stand out. Black frames will do the same for you if you

have a thin black outline around your iris.

Shape: If your eyebrows are arched or rounded, look for frames that have a little lift at the top. If your brow is flat, look for flat-top frames. Also, try to match the shape of your face. If you have a long face, look for glasses that are longer than they are wide. If you have a round or square face, select wider frames.

Polish Your Appearance

Glasses fog up whenever *she* walks by? Smarten up and spray your lenses with Pledge furniture polish. Not only will the stuff clean and polish like an expensive housekeeper, but it'll also fill in all the tiny scratches in the glass and leave behind a water- and dirt-repellent finish.

Spot a Fake Watch

If you take the bracelet and roll it over in your hands, it should adapt nicely to the curvature of your hand or fingers. A cheap watch doesn't do that. Another test: tap the crystal with your fingernail. If you hear the dull sound of Plexiglas rather than the clink of glass, the watch is counterfeit.

Pick the Perfect Watch

When it comes to watches, thinner, shinier, and smaller generally means more formal, while a thicker, duller finish, and more bells and whistles means more casual. The just-right watch shows attentiveness to detail, which marks you as a guy to both hire and desire.

Stop Dribbling

If you tend to dribble on your underwear or pants after peeing, try this trick: Simply run your finger along the underside of your penis to force out remaining liquid.

Give Your Showerhead a Bath

If you notice that your showerhead ain't spitting like it used to, try soaking it in vinegar. This will remove the calcium deposits that have built up inside the thing since the Carter administration.

Stop Showering So Much

The reason your skin turns armadillo-like during winter is that the humidity level in the air is so low, just 15 to 20 percent. As your skin's natural moisture is sucked away by the atmosphere, it also becomes less flexible and more itchy. Use warm water to shower instead of hot, which helps to retain body oils. Avoid scrubbing with a washcloth, and have your geisha pat you dry.

De-Grease Your Hair

Nothing beats a little dishwashing liquid for emergency grease control. But it's too drying to use every day. For daily mop-up duty, use Aqua Glycolic shampoo and body cleanser. The glycolic acid cuts through and dissolves much of the extra oil.

WHEN ALL ELSE FAILS

MAKE A LAST-MINUTE HALLOWEEN COSTUME

Don't go as a transvestite again. Pull together a costume in seconds with items lying around your house.

Laundry basket: Make a hole in your laundry basket (you never use it anyway). Wear the basket around your waist, fill it with laundry, and use an old Tide box as a hat.

Thermometer: Cover your head in aluminum foil. Wear white long johns. Paint a red line that goes from your feet to your neck, and add numbers along the way.

Windblown guy: Put on a dress shirt and loop a straightened wire coat hanger under the collar. Leave 18 inches of the hanger free on the right side. Tie a necktie and insert the hanger through the back of the tie. Now, bend the tie (with the hanger wire inside of it) up and over your right shoulder. Tape some leaves to a trench coat and hat. Turn an umbrella inside out, and put it over your right shoulder. Lean forward slightly as you walk into the party.

Survive with One Contact Lens

If you lose a contact lens and don't have a backup, put the remaining contact in whichever eye is stronger. It will take over more of the work. That should make you less likely to fall down a flight of stairs.

Keep Your Contact Out of Your Mouth

There's a speck on your contact lens and it's driving you nuts. But you don't have any water or lens solution handy, so you clean the lens by putting it in your mouth. Bad move. Your mouth contains lots of bacteria and transferring that to your eye is not a good thing. It can cause conjunctivitis.

Attack Plaque with Silica

Next time you need a new tube of toothpaste, check the label for the ingredient silica. One study found that after 6 months of twice-daily use, patients brushing with silica toothpaste had 44 percent less plaque and tartar than patients using pastes without the ingredient.

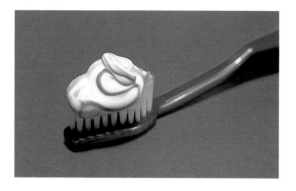

Try Dry-Brushing

People who dry-brush their teeth have significantly less tartar buildup and gum bleeding than those who brush only with paste. It seems that certain toothpaste flavors can be so overwhelming that they reduce brushing time. The best strategy is to dry-brush, rinse, then brush again briefly using a small amount of fluoride paste. It should take you 3 minutes to brush your teeth. Most people spend only 30 to 40 seconds.

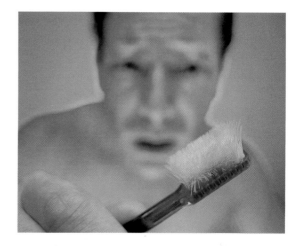

Hang Up Your Toothbrush

Replace your toothbrush every 3 to 4 months, or whenever the bristles become curled or discolored.

Get Rid of Garlic Breath

You eat garlic for lunch then learn there's an unexpected meeting. Before you leave the restaurant, go to the bar and dip a lemon twist in a pinch of salt and chew on it. The lemon oil and salt will help break down the garlic. The tequila's optional.

DON'T LET PASTE GO TO WASTE

Here are 8 alternative uses for toothpaste:

- Removing scratches on glassware.
- Cleaning crayon from walls or piano keys.
- Erasing juice mustaches from kids' faces.
- Relieving itching caused by mosquito bites.
- Removing scuffs on shoes.
- Filling small holes in walls.
- Stopping the bleeding when you nick yourself shaving.
- Polishing chrome in the bathroom.

An Apple a Day Keeps the Dentist Away

Too rushed to brush at the office? Grab an apple after lunch. Apples crunch between the teeth, dislodging food and stimulating saliva flow to counteract plaque. It'll get rid of that piece of spinach stuck there, too.

Banish Bad Breath

You have a date, and your breath is god awful. Quickly concoct your own dental rinse for temporary relief. Mix 2 ounces of 3 percent concentration hydrogen peroxide with 2 ounces of water. Swish a mouthful vigorously for 30 seconds. Spit. You're good to go. For a quick cure in a restaurant, try swishing some water, biting into an orange or lemon wedge, or chewing parsley.

Chase the Alcohol Smell

If you smell like a hangover, drink two glasses of pink grapefruit juice. It activates the liver enzymes that cause alcohol to metabolize faster. Increasing your liver metabolism makes the liquor smell leave your body sooner.

Carry Some Listerine

Listerine PocketPaks Oral Care Strips provide an intense halitosis fix in a quick-dissolving sheet that you place on the back of your tongue. You can immediately start talking without fear. The nifty dispenser is also perfect for bedside.

Shave with Olive Oil

You're out of shaving cream. Go for a few drops of olive oil. The next-best option is petroleum jelly. Hair conditioner and hand lotion work, too.

Stop Up Shaving Cuts

There's a product from France called Alum Block. Alum is a natural antiseptic used by the Egyptians more than 4,000 years ago. All you do is moisten it and apply it to the cut with a little pressure, and it will stop bleeding almost immediately. Another alternative is a styptic pencil. It costs under a buck in drugstores and will last your lifetime. The key ingredient is an aluminum salt, and all brands work equally well.

H O L D   Y O U R   L I Q U O R

For every drink, there's a proper glass. And for every glass, there's a proper way to hold your alcohol:

Champagne flutes; wine, cocktail, and martini glasses: Hold the stem with your thumb and your middle and ring fingers. For balance and support, rest your pinkie on the base of the glass, and place your index finger where the stem meets the bowl. This holding pattern avoids warming the drink with your sweaty hand. Also, you can see the champagne bubbles or the color of the wine—what snobs call "presentation."

Pilsner and highball glasses: Hold 'em as close to the bottom as possible. For a highball, use all five fingers. For a pilsner, use four and let your pinkie rest on the base of the glass. Just use the ends of your fingers; don't grip the glass in your fist. That way you won't warm the drink.

Margarita glass: Support the bottom of the bowl with your index finger and hold the stem with your other fingers. Index-finger position is critical, because the glass is top-heavy and tips easily. (There's a lesson in there somewhere.)

Brandy snifter: Place the stem between your ring and middle fingers and wrap the rest of your hand around the bottom of the bowl, cupping as much as possible in your palm. Brandy snifters are usually used for cognac, which is best served slightly warm. The warmer the cognac, the better it smells.

Beer stein: Place your thumb on top of the handle (many steins have a thumb rest) for balance. Use only the ends of your fingers. Keep your pinkie firmly wrapped around the handle.

At parties, it's best to hold all beverages with your left hand so that you can still shake hands with your right.

Keep Your Razor Sharp

Your whiskers don't dull a razor, rust does. To make your razor last longer, keep it in a cup of rubbing alcohol between shaves. Just make sure to rinse it in water before using it.

Let the Vaseline Slide

Skiers and other outdoors enthusiasts often coat their faces with petroleum jelly to protect their skin in frigid conditions. But petroleum jelly can clog pores and cause pimples. Instead, coat your face with a water-resistant SPF-15 sunscreen, let it dry, then rub in some moisturizer. Think of it as an invisible mask.

Put Your Deodorant to the Test

Test-drive a new antiperspirant by wearing it through a tough workout. If it works then, it'll work anytime. Wondering how much you should apply? Four to six swipes should suffice.

Make a Pit Stop

If your shirt armpits are constantly soaked, use a solid deodorant; it contains the least water. Sprays are cleanest, as they harbor no bacteria. Gels give the best coverage, so they're the strongest odor-killers.

Take Zinc for Your Stink

If your sweat is making you smell so bad you're a lonely guy, try taking zinc supplements. Just 25 to 50 milligrams daily has been found to lessen body odor.

Cover Up Your Stink

Eating peppermint or cinnamon can help mask body odor because some of the scent will come out in your body oils.

Put Some Cologne Here

Avoid splashing cologne on your face. It's simply too strong, and your face is too sensitive. Instead, dab it on your upper chest and lower neck. Note that we said "dab," not "pour," "splash," or "dump."

Keep Cologne in the Fridge

Most colognes last approximately 2 years. If you notice the cologne has darkened significantly, it has probably gone bad. Try keeping you scent in the refrigerator instead. It'll last almost forever in there because heat and light are the factors that cause cologne to deteriorate. Also, cool cologne feels more refreshing when you put it on.

Cover Up a Pimple

To disguise an unsightly blemish, steal some liquid concealer or foundation from your girlfriend's makeup case. Try to find some with a slightly green tint. Why? The green combines with the red skin around the pimple to look more flesh-colored. Dermablend, Chanel, and Shiseido are good brands to look for. Resist the urge to try out her eyelash curler.

Make an Entrance

Style is one of many things that separate the Cary Grants of the world from the well, we can't remember the name of a guy with no style, but you get the idea. Here's one more way to make a grander entrance. Pause briefly after you walk through the door. Quickly survey the room, acknowledging those whom you know at the far end first. As you walk toward the people you know, scan nearby, nodding and acknowledging people close to you, being as engaging as possible while still moving. Continue working the room until you catch up with the people at the far end—by then you'll have made a favorable impression on those with whom you chatted *and* on those who were merely watching you.

Be Cool

Cool guys never think "cool." But guys who aren't cool think about little else.

Make a Memorable Introduction

When introducing two people, try to attach a quickie compliment: For example, "George, I'd like you to meet Miranda, who gave me one of the great nights of my life in Dayton last fall. And Miranda, this is George, who is the best speller I know." Okay, that's a joke, but you get the idea. Give each person a hook into the other. The unadorned intro gives G and M no conversational toehold, and more important, it's devoid of enthusiasm for them. A charming guy is enthused about his acquaintances, even his recent ones.

Kiss a Lady's Hand

When a lady extends her hand, grasp it lightly, just as you would if you were going to shake it. Then turn it clockwise and kiss the back of her hand in the middle, making sure your lips are dry. Hold the kiss for 2 seconds, then release her hand. Ask her anything. She is now yours.

Give Her the Treatment

When walking down the sidewalk with a lady, always position yourself between her and the street. This creates a barrier (you) between her and any dust, water, or catcalls created by passing motorists, plus it allows her to window-shop should the conversation hit a lull.

Brush a Celebrity

What do you say to a famous person when you're understandably nervous? You want to say something that doesn't make you sound like another pathetic schmuck. You want to convey a cool, conversational connection that makes you stand out. How does one do this? Never refer to a celebrity's past work. He hears "I loved you in . . . " a thousand times a day. Instead, ask what he's currently working on. Celebs feed off this.

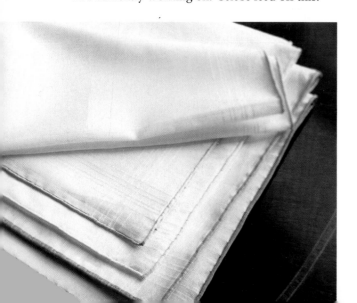

Make the Bentley Gleam

A car's finish should sparkle like fine crystal. The secret to getting that chamois-dried look without the time-consuming buffing is in the rinsing. Working in the shade, hold the hose (without a spray attachment) an inch from the surface. The subsequent sheeting action will prevent the formation of those horrid water spots. Wrap the metal end of the hose with duct tape to prevent scratching.

Walk in the Rain

A man who runs for cover in the rain will end up just as wet as one who walks. Although you spend less time in the rain, researchers found that raindrops, instead of falling directly onto your head and shoulders, hit the front of your body as you run. Because the surface area of your front is much greater than that of your head and shoulders, you end up getting just as wet.

Carry a Linen Handkerchief

Always keeps a folded linen handkerchief stashed in the inside pocket of your sport coat. This is not for blowing your nose or wiping your fingerprints off the gun. In fact, it appears only when a woman needs to dry her tears or when there is a woman around to see you produce a clean linen handkerchief with which to dress the wound of a small child. When does that ever happen, you ask? The rarity of the move is precisely what makes it so sweet. When you're the only man who can offer anything more useful against grief or exsanguination than a crumpled Wal-Mart receipt, you'll emanate Old World manliness.

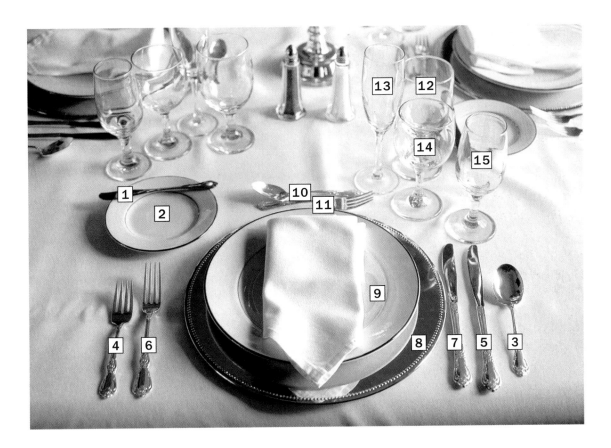

Decode a Place Setting

You've come a long way from sporks. Here's what all those utensils and more are for.

1. Butter knife

2. Bread-and-butter plate

3. Soup spoon (first course)

4. Seafood fork (second course)

5. Seafood knife (second course)

6. Meat and salad fork (main course)

7. Dinner knife (main course)

8. Decoration plate

9. Soup bowl

10. Dessert spoon

11. Dessert fork

12. Water glass

13. Champagne glass

14. Wine glass (for red)

15. Wine glass (for white)

Slurp Soup Right

Always spoon away from yourself. When there's just a bit left in the bowl, you may go after it by tilting the bowl away, too.

C A R R Y $ 5 0

Walking around with $3 in your pocket is beneath your dignity—unless they're your last three. *Men's Health* Rule: A man has at least $50 in cash on him. Why? So he can pick up the tab for a few beers for the boys by tossing some bills on the bar and saying "Thanks, doll." Cash is cool.

Excuse Yourself Properly

Take your napkin from your lap, loosely fold it, and rest it on the seat of your chair. No one wants to look at your soiled linen while you're away.

Leave Him This Much

Tip the waiter 20 percent of the bill minus 2 percent for each instance of poor service minus 5 percent for anything spilled on you.

Get Your Way—Every Time

When you want to have your way, try being mannerly. It's so rare nowadays that it throws people off balance. Don't think of it as merely being nice; think of it as civil war.

Take Command of Your Voice

To find your natural voice, say the word "no" forcefully, as if your dog were about to steal a steak off the kitchen table. It's deep, strong, and

Fold a Fancy Napkin

To add flair to a dinner table, or to entertain your date while waiting for the clams casino, create a bird of paradise out of a cloth napkin.

1. Fold a large, square napkin in half, then in half again to form a smaller square. All four corners should come together.

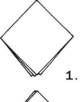
1.

2. Take two of the corners and bring them to the opposite corner.

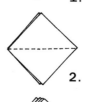
2.

3. Fold the remaining two corners backward to the same corner. You should now have a triangle.

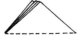
3.

4. Beginning at either end, accordion-fold the triangular napkin.

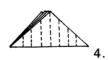
4.

5. Holding the base of the napkin, set it in a wine glass and carefully pull the outer-most material down on each side. Continue with the next layer, then pull the center out slightly.

5.

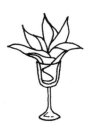

assertive. More important, it lets you speak for long periods without going hoarse. With practice, you can learn to use that commanding voice all the time. One trick is to hum a few bars of "Happy Birthday," then begin speaking with the same tone you used while humming. Your voice will be more resonant than usual.

Deliver a Eulogy

Keep it simple. Don't try to say a half dozen things about the deceased; say one, maybe two. Keep it short. Speak 10 to 12 minutes tops. And remember, a eulogy is not just, or even primarily, a lamentation. It is a celebration of a life. Though it should certainly be reverent, a proper eulogy is never somber. We've all taken a blow, endured an enormous loss. But we're also left with the inspiring example of a life. The eulogist's job is to ever-so-gently fill the survivors' sails.

Stop Swearing in Front of the Kids

Swearing is something most of us do unconsciously, except at tax time. Thus, it's a difficult habit to kick. Enlist your wife as trainer for 2 weeks. Ask her to say "beep" every time she hears your curse in front of the little bastards, er, kids. Hearing her signal will help you become aware of the words you're using, which is a huge step toward controlling the problem.

Be the Perfect Godfather

On every birthday, you should send your ward more money than a kid his age should properly receive. You want him to *think* you're loaded, especially if you're not. A godfather should make the world seem big, loaded with possibilities. His job is to give a child wings.

Give Away Your Daughter

When you're the father of the bride, 2 weeks before the wedding hand-write your daughter a letter declaring your continued devotion. It doesn't matter if you've never written her a letter in your life. In fact, it may be better if you haven't. The letter should be short and simple, with the quality of a vow—a knight swearing fealty to the fair lady. It should make her feel watched over. Message: You are always in my heart; I remain at your service. Then have a man-to-man with the groom. This can take place anywhere. The only requirement is that you issue the invitation. Make it clear that you'd like to talk. He should understand that you and he have one thing in common—you're both crazy about the girl. You want to let him know—without being explicit—that you expect, at the very least, sobriety, probity, fidelity, and an honest manly effort at husbandry. There should be two implications: 1) You'll be watching; and 2) He's got a friend if he needs help. Make it clear you're both judge and ally.

SABOTAGE A SNOOP
You're having friends over for dinner and one of them is particularly nosy. Teach him a lesson. Load up the medicine cabinet beforehand. With marbles.

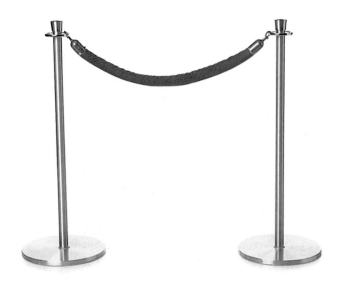

driver lets the passengers out, offer him $20 to give you a ride around the corner to the nightclub. Hesitate for a few minutes before you make your exit, then just walk toward the door as if there's no question that you'll be let in. If there is a question, answer in French.

Get Your Own Place
Cultivate the staff of one ethnic restaurant. Become a regular, chat up the waitresses, ask to see the chef so you can praise him in person. Above all, tip like Trump, which isn't usually too difficult on an $11.38 tab. Then take someone you want to impress to "your" place. As the chef and staff treat you like a king, your guest may well assume you're a hot ticket elsewhere, too.

Get into a Trendy Nightclub
To get past Mr. Biceps and that long line of pathetic schmucks, you need to convince yourself and everyone else that you're "someone," and that no one who's anyone would think of turning you away. Start by skipping the line. Instead, walk a few blocks until you find an expensive hotel. Hang out until a limousine pulls up. (If your wait is more than half an hour, then you didn't pick the right hotel.) After the

Choose Dignity over Dancing
Unless you're appearing in *Cats*, this rule is all-inclusive. We don't care if you have rhythm. We don't care if you're drunk and trying to improve your odds of getting lucky. For men over age 35, dignity is a more valuable commodity than dance-floor abandon. Jitterbugging, shagging, line dancing, yeah, this sort of thing's okay. We're not saying we like it; we're just saying it's okay. At least there's some order to

---

CUT IN LINE AT THE FRONT
Cutting in line at any time probably isn't going to improve your image, but if you must, do it toward the front of the line, not the middle or the back. People are less impatient the closer they are to the ticket booth, so they're less likely to tee off on you. One study found that only 27 percent of people objected when someone broke into the front of the line. But breaking in at the middle or the back brought complaints 73 percent of the time.

UNCOMMON KNOWLEDGE

GET A BARTENDER'S ATTENTION

We hate fighting crowds for drinks, so we asked seasoned bartenders for the best ways to attract their attention. They said a $5 tip on the first round helps, as does knowing the bar's best spots for service:

Under the TV. Nobody stands there, unless they're showing gymnastics. So it's your best shot at getting close to the bar—and drawing the bartender's attention. Hold your bills out so he can see them, but don't wave them.

By the olives. The bartender will always have to retreat for napkins, cherries, and little umbrellas, so stand there and you'll have a chance of getting his attention after every order. Never say, "When you get a chance." That grates on bartenders' nerves. "Hi" works best.

Three feet from where he is the minute you walk in. On busy nights bartenders methodically take orders from one end of the bar to the other, so they can keep track of where they've been. When you enter, see what direction he's heading and burrow your way there.

---

it. But the freestyle stuff is no longer acceptable; more often than not, guys over 30 who do it resemble mimes on steroids pretending to NordicTrack. So knock it off.

Complain the Right Way

The secret to a charming complaint is to suggest that the failure is yours. Everybody knows it isn't, but it keeps a complaint from being an insult. If the Chardonnay tastes like bilge water, say something like, "It may be that I have a cold, but this tastes a little sharper than it should." That small, self-effacing qualifier keeps the complaint from being a personal attack on David, the wine steward.

Stand Taller, Look Younger

A 70-year-old who stands straight, looks alert, and walks with a steady gait looks decades younger. But a 40-year-old who slumps and shuffles looks like he's on his way out. To maintain perfect posture, try this exercise: Stand against a wall, making sure that your shoulders and buttocks touch the wall. Slip your arm into the space between your lower back and the wall, and tilt your hips so that the extra space is eliminated. Hold the position for a count of 20. Do this exercise once a day for 3 weeks to ensure that good posture becomes a habit.

Chill Wine in Minutes

You're motoring to a picnic on a hot afternoon, and your ice expires. Here's a trick: Soak a newspaper in cold water and wrap it around the bottle. Hold it outside the window, angling it toward the sky. Maintain a speed of 60 mph, and the wine will be suitably chilled within 5 minutes.

Display the Cork

Don't stick the cork up your nose the way you did last New Year's Eve. Instead, do this stylish trick:

1. With the bottle upright and its label facing you, use a sharp knife to cut the foil on the top clockwise from point A to point B, leaving about ¼ inch unsliced. Move down about ¼ inch and make the same cut.

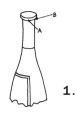

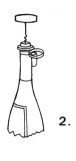

2. Fold the ring and the top circle back at the uncut "hinge." Remove the cork

3. Insert the cork in the ring and fold the excess foil tightly against the cork to hold it in place.

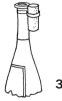

4. Pour with the cork on top of the bottle and the label facing the guest.

Tell If the Wine Is Fine

Sniffing the cork won't tell you anything. Instead, feel the cork to make sure it's moist. A dry cork means air may have sneaked into the bottle and ruined the wine.

What to Drink with What

Let's take it to the next level, past white with fish and red with beef.

Food	Wine
Spicy pasta dishes or red meats	Chianti, Rioja, Bordeaux, Cabernet Sauvignon
Subtly flavored foods such as salmon or soufflés	Beaujolais, Pinot Noir
Naturally rich foods (scallops or lobster) or fish or fowl prepared with butter	Sauvignon Blanc
Grilled veggies or simply prepared fish of chicken	Chardonnay
Chocolate cake	Cabernet Sauvignon

WHEN ALL ELSE FAILS

PULL THE PLUG

Having problems with the wine cork? First, try the obvious. Reinsert the corkscrew at a different angle or place in the cork, and give another pull. If that doesn't work, find a conventional screw—a 3-inch No. 8 ought to work—and screw it into the cork until only about three-quarters of an inch is protruding. Pull it out with a pair of pliers. No screw? No pliers? Shove a couple of flat shish kebab skewers down opposite sides of the cork, then pull them straight out. With luck the cork will come, too. If nothing works, push the rest of the cork into the bottle and strain the wine through a tea strainer or a clean sock. She'll never know the difference, unless you use the wrong sock.

BRING A BASKET TO NEW YEAR'S EVE

There is no more thoughtful gift for the host of a New Year's Eve party then a gourmet basket of bagels, jam, fruit, and pastries. It'll help him, and any stragglers, endure the following morning.

Con Your Way into Any Restaurant

Call to confirm your reservation. Insist that you made one (even though you didn't). The restaurant won't accuse you of lying. It'll view it as an oversight. Or book a room at a fine hotel near the restaurant, and then ask the concierge to call and help free up a table. Once that's done, cancel the hotel reservation.

Make Your Booze Gift Count

A bottled present often says, "I was running late and stopped at the liquor store." Make it say, "I'm so damn thoughtful we should crack open this bad boy right now."

Vintage port: Buy a bottle to match the year of a birthday or anniversary. Popular vintages such as 1963, 1966, and 1970 can be had for $90 to $200 a bottle.

Bordeaux: The French often give new parents a case of Bordeaux wine from the birth year, to be opened when the child reaches age 21.

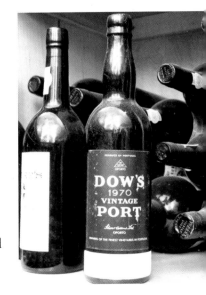

3

SEX

and

RELATIONSHIPS

The two most popular columns in *Men's Health* are "Jimmy the Bartender" and "Ask the Girl Next Door." Each receives thousands of letters and e-mails from men around the world asking advice about sex and relationships. This is particularly interesting because the magazine also has a distinguished advisory board filled with respected experts who have more degrees than a thermometer. Psychologists, marriage counselors, sex therapists . . . you name it. They've studied couples like Kellogg's has studied cereal. They know what makes relationships go snap, crackle, pop, and when they'll start to go soggy in milk. They're listed either prominently on the magazine's masthead or quoted regularly in its pages. And yet, they don't even get junk mail.

Instead, it's the barkeep and the halter-topped neighbor whose counsel is regularly (and passionately) sought. It's as if, when it comes to women, men naturally distrust the advice of "experts." It's as if, from both experience and instinct, we know that love and sex can't be analyzed or dissected in a lab. Rather, love and sex are best figured out over glasses of beer with another guy who's been there, or on an August-evening porch swing with a girl who reminds you of your sister. And even then, all we can hope for is the glint of understanding, a beginning. But that's enough, because their advice is always solid and trustworthy.

Here's an example of what we're talking about: We know this guy—a handsome, hard-charging, thirtysomething attorney with a beautiful wife, a great family, and all the toys you can imagine. Only one day, she cheats on him, and he's devastated by it. Suddenly, their grand life is on trial. She's full of vengeful accusations, while he pleads genuine ignorance. They see all kinds of shrinks, spend a fortune in therapy, but it isn't until one of his colleagues gets talking about her own failed marriage at lunch one day that he sees the error of his ways.

"All I ever wanted from my ex was some attention," is what this colleague said. "Even just a little might have saved our marriage." And from that day forward, our man resolved to give his wife a hug and a kiss before he left the house each morning and another when he came home each night. Although it seemed forced at first, he worked at making it a habit. Five years later, they're still together. That's all it took.

What Jimmy and the Girl Next Door represent is reality. He's a guy, and she's a gal. They're everyday people. And often, as we've seen, that's the wisest kind. What you're about to read are the very best 226 sex and relationship tips ever assembled in one place. Some are from researchers and sex experts, but most are from real people who have either experimented and discovered great truths or screwed up and learned painful lessons. Some are explicit; others are implicit. Through it all, the editors of *Men's Health,* like Jimmy and the Girl Next Door, have been your personal bullshit detectors.

Have fun benefiting from the experience.

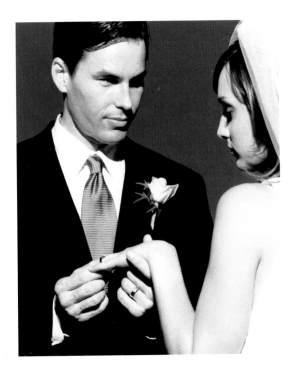

Find Women with Jobs

To locate a high proportion of good-looking (if somewhat bitter and humorless) women, eat and drink in the area surrounding the courthouse. Law offices harbor an astonishing number of female lawyers, paralegals, and legal secretaries. All of 'em eat. Runner-up: hospital cafeterias. Nurses.

Measure Her Eye Contact

Two people conversing naturally look at each other about 60 percent of the time. So if you catch a woman looking at you more than 60 percent, chances are she's more interested in you than in what you're saying.

Scope Out Beach Babes

At the beach, you can assume a woman is looking to meet a guy if her hair is in place and it isn't wet.

Approach the Amazonian

Don't know how to break the ice with that gym babe? Ask her to show you how to do a particular exercise or operate a certain machine. She'll be flattered.

MR. CLEAN

PUT HER IN A LATHER

Forget about fancy cologne. We had women sniff-test a variety of 99-cent soaps (and the freshly washed guys who showered with them) to determine which scent was sexiest. Here's what they said:

Soap	Rating	What Women Said
Lever 2000	5	Strong, clean, subtle. Oh, baby, take it off
Irish Spring Sport	4	An athletic man. Hope he's as good as he smells
Shield	4	Outdoorsy. You definitely know he's showered
Dial	3½	Smells like he likes to chop wood
Coast	3	Strong and cologne-ish. A little fruity
Irish Spring	3	Smells like a frat party
Zest	2	Smells like the hand wash in doctors' offices
Ivory	2	He just did the dishes
Tone	1½	Like pollen. Makes me want to sneeze
Safeguard	1	Like detergent or fruitcake
Dove	½	Guy lives with his parents or grandparents

Get More Sex Appeal

At first glance, women cue in on three things: your teeth, your shoes, and your watch. If any are dirty or missing, or just too cheap to wear in public, she'll drop you faster than a hot coal.

Pat Your Best Spot

When trying to get a woman's attention, identify the body part that you've been told is your best asset—as long as it isn't contained by your underwear. Give that body part a quick pat or scratch when she looks over. The pat reinforces your attractiveness. You're subtly selling yourself to her.

Stop Worrying about Size

Most men think they would get more women if they had 30 pounds more muscle. Not true. When asked to pick the male image they dig most, the majority of women don't choose the big V-shaped hero men think they would. Instead they go for the less ripped guy. Okay, they didn't choose the guy who looked all soft and cuddly. But there's no need to look like Schwarzenegger. It's okay to look okay.

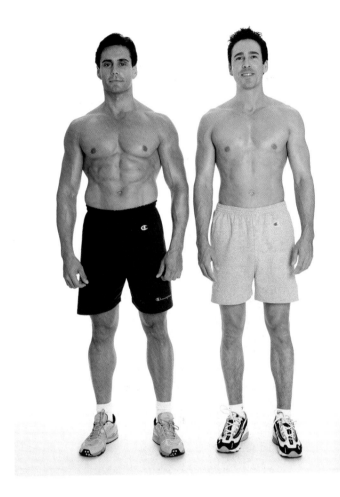

Tell a He from a She in Cyberspace

So how can you tell if the person you're chatting with is a real woman or an Internet imposter—a babe or a bubba? Slip in a few questions that only a woman would know how to answer. For starters: "What's your panty hose size?" (Men shouldn't know that sizes come in A, B, Queen, and Extra-Large Queen, and depend on height and weight.) Or instead

of asking her what she looks like, ask "her" what she looks *for* in a guy. Many men find it tough describing an attractive guy from a woman's perspective.

Flirt Like This

The fleeting glance is the most effective. The idea is to catch her eye, then look away, as if her beauty has nearly blinded you. Then glance back . . . because you cannot help yourself. And, of course, smile.

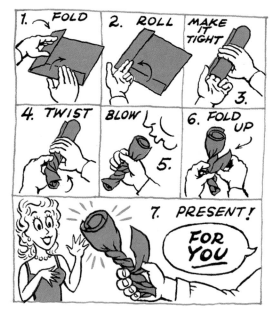

Impress the Hell out of a Woman

Pickup lines rarely work. And when they do, what you've picked up usually requires a 10-day course of antibiotics. Here's a better way:

1. Get a large cocktail napkin. Fold one edge over once, followed by an adjacent side.

2. Lay your fingers over the point where they cross.

3. Roll the napkin tightly over your fingers.

4. Twist the napkin below your fingers to make an upper stem, and then remove your fingers.

5. Blow in the bud to make it bloom.

6. Pull one edge up from the bottom, fold it against the stem to make a leaf, then twist the lower part of the napkin to finish the stem.

7. Present the rose to her and say it's special because it's handmade, it will never die, and it's for her. If she's seen that one before, go younger.

Guess Her Age

Find a pretty girl with a calculator and tell her you can predict her age. Have her punch her age into the calculator. Then have her multiply it by 7, then multiply that product by 1,443. Have her hand the calculator to you. Her age will be repeated three times. Watch: 28 (age) × 7 = 196. 196 × 1,443 = 282,828.

If a woman asks you outright to guess her age, say 25. If she's younger, she'll be flattered that you thought she was more mature. If she's older, she'll sleep with you.

Read Her Dirty Mind

Most people think it's men who initiate flirting, but two-thirds of the time women give off a signal of interest first. If she's doing one or more of the following, she's interested in you:

Flashing her eyebrows. She raises her eyebrows for a second or two, then quickly lowers them. Often combined with a smile and eye contact.

Running her fingers through her hair. Some women make only one hand movement, others stroke their hair.

Smiling coyly. Look for a half-smile, often combined with a downward glance or brief eye contact.

Licking her lips. This could be a simple, subconscious wetting of an upper or a lower lip.

Giving you short, darting glances. The looks usually occur in bouts, with an average of three glances per bout.

Primping. She smoothes out her clothes, even though they're already perfect.

Swaying to the music. While seated, she moves her body to the beat. Get over there and ask her to dance, now!

Caressing an object. She runs her fingers over a glass, an ashtray, a set of keys, or anything else that's handy.

Hiking her skirt to expose her leg. Like we have to explain this?

Move Here

The cities with the highest ratios of young, single women to men are as follows:

1. Baton Rouge

2. Baltimore

3. Memphis

4. Fresno

5. Oklahoma City

Shall we reserve the U-Haul?

Touch Her, Then Stop

Not sure if she's interested? If you've made it to a second round of drinks, initiate contact by touching her arm several times during the next 15 minutes. Then abruptly stop all physical contact. If she's attracted to you, she'll fire a few strokes your way as soon as she realizes you've stopped touching her. Touch is a very important part of courtship. If she touches you back, it's a good sign.

How Low Can You Go?

Sure she looks great, but is she old enough to date?
Take your age (minimum 30)   _____
Divide by 2   _____
Add 3   _____
If her father is older than you, subtract 5 _____
This is the age of the youngest woman you should be dating. To avoid potential embarrassment and certain incarceration, don't go lower than 18 (unless you're going to Utah).

Be the Last One to Leave

As the night wears on, you look better. In a study at a singles bar near closing, women's judgments of men's attractiveness got more generous, as did men's toward women—even after researchers controlled for the effect of alcohol. The reason: As the mating pool thins, what's left looks better and better.

Realize She Could Be Right

In the course of your dating life, there will be women who'll accuse you of being a jerk. Some of them will be right.

See If She's Jazzed Up

While you're waiting for a date in her apartment, scan her CD collection. Research shows that jazz enthusiasts are 30 percent more sexually active than the average person.

Inspect Her Ice Box

You can tell a lot about someone by looking in her refrigerator. Beware if you see obsessively low-fat foods nestled next to tubs of cream cheese. Unbalanced eating means an out-of-balance person.

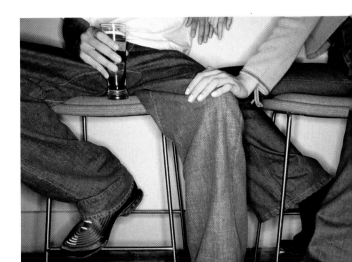

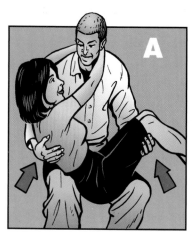
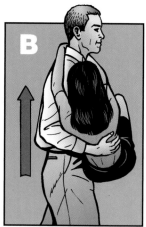
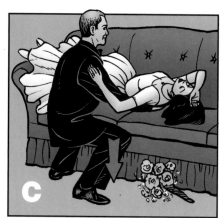

Pick Up Any Woman

She's sick, tired, drunk, or all of the above. Now's your chance to sweep her off her feet:

a. With your feet slightly wider than shoulder-width apart, squat beside your lady in waiting. Have her wrap her arms around your neck. Now slide one arm under the middle of her back and the other under her thighs, close to her knees (not her butt). If she's out cold, cross her arms with her hands at her waist.

b. Slowly stand up by pressing your heels into the ground. Be careful not to arch your back, and try to keep it as close to perpendicular to the ground as possible.

c. Lean back slightly and maintain a wide stance as you walk. When you reach a suitable woman depository—a couch, bed, rug, dorm room—don't bend over for the final delivery. Instead, squat with your legs to set her down. If she's had too much to drink, turn her head to the side to keep her from gagging on your good deed.

Date out of Your League

If you can make a woman laugh, you can probably make her do anything. We recall one instance when an average-looking fellow approached a beautiful woman at a club and offered to buy her a drink. She curtly refused. He then asked her to dance and received the same response. He finally asked, "Well, can I just stand here?" She laughed despite herself, and within minutes he had her name and phone number.

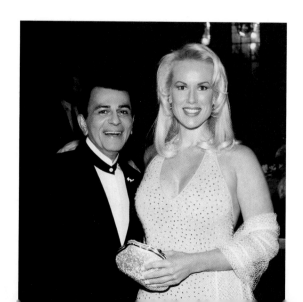

Tell If They're Real

Breast implantation is surgery; surgery leaves scars. Look for twin scars underneath the breasts or around the nipples, or under the arms, close to the torso. It's more fun than an Easter-egg hunt. If she hasn't achieved nudity, check the outline of the top of her breasts. If one or both are perfect semicircles, suspect implants. If all else fails, cop a hug. If they don't compress at all, you're feeling capsules.

Bring a Fake Date

If you have a great-looking female friend, by all means show her off. There are few things more attractive to a woman than the fact that other women are attracted to you. In a study, when people were asked to judge men based on photographs of them with "spouses" of differing attractiveness, unattractive men paired with good-looking women were routinely rated most favorably in terms of status.

Ask Her Out before Lunch

Lusting after a coworker? Ask her out just before lunch—when her mood is likely to be best. People are usually more receptive right before they leave for lunch, because their minds aren't cluttered with what they have to do that day or what they're planning to do when they get home.

Deliver the Perfect Compliment

"You're beautiful" isn't a compliment. "Nice set of helmets" isn't a compliment. Compliment her on what *she's* made not on what God's made. "Lovely dress," "Terrific memo," "Incredible insight," "Great joke!" And don't overdo it. Once is enough. Every compliment after the first one takes away half the value of the compliment that preceded it.

Hang on Her Every Word

You can bestow no greater compliment on a woman than your full attention.

Make a Brilliant Save

When she asks why you haven't called, respond emphatically: "I have! Here's the number right here, 555-6505!" When she says, "No, it's 6506," you're cool.

Imagine You're Proposing

When you're trying to impress a woman, never utter these words at the cusp of an evening: "So, what do you feel like doing?" A true Casanova takes charge. He has a plan. To devise a memorable one, imagine that you're proposing. What would you do to make the night so special she couldn't possibly say no? Then arrange it (minus the ring and bent-knee thing, of course). After all, you *are* proposing—only it's something far more enticing than marriage.

GRILL HER SOME PEACHES

Impress the fetching lass by grilling dessert. Peel some peaches, slice them in half and sprinkle them with brown sugar. Grill them over medium-hot charcoal for 3 to 4 minutes or until warm. Serve with a dollop of fat-free or low-fat frozen yogurt. She's yours.

MAKE THE MOVE

You spot her across a crowded room. She smiles. You smile. Now what?

1. Approach her from the side. This makes you less threatening and increases her interest.

2. Keep your eyes above her neck.

3. Wait for a break in conversation. Forget clever lines. Say "hi." Give her your name. Ask for hers. Talk to her like a relative you actually get along with. She's reluctant? Don't give up. Both men and women are overly ready to think they're being rejected.

4. Leave—briefly. Don't promise to be back; just say "Excuse me a minute, I have to catch up with my friend. It was great meeting you."

5. Return to your pals for 10 minutes. Stay out of her line of sight.

6. Approach her again. If she seems happy to see you, you're in.

Come On Slowly

One guaranteed way to shock and intrigue a woman is to tell her you'd like to take things slowly. Don't sleep with her until the fourth date. Or some nights, suggest the two of you just cuddle in front of the television. That's very refreshing, especially for the young woman who sees all guys as lust machines.

See Her Future

If you want to see how your girlfriend is going to look once the odometer goes around a few times, visit the factory. Family reunions are especially useful in this regard, since older sisters, moms, cousins, and aunts are all produced by much the same design team.

Make It Small but Relevant

You've been dating her for only a month and now it's Valentine's Day. You don't want to appear commitment-mad, but you're not a cad, either. A simple tip: Give her something small but relevant (not warts) that reminds her of how you met. Discovered her at the bikini car wash? Give her a certificate for a free waxing. Met her on a blind date? Give her some Ray-Bans. Think about it—this works for everything!

Give Her Something Unexpected

Women love unexpected gifts. Make hers personal rather than trendy, small rather than large, silly rather than serious—something only she can appreciate, filled with creativity and thoughtfulness. Most important, time your gift's delivery for that critical point in the evening when there remains just one obvious way for her to show her gratitude. And we're not talking about a handshake.

See If You're the Slut

Do you ever wake up wondering whether you're all the man you want to be, or just a Gap-clad pile of cheap, carny trash? Use this scientifically precise slut-o-meter and determine just how right your last girlfriend's analysis of you was. Instructions: Mark each bar on a scale of 1 to 10 (10 is max). Add 'em all up and divide by 10. Mark that number on the last bar, Your Slut Score. Show the results to no one.

10												
9												PURE SLUT
8												
7												AFFABLE
6												TRAMP
5												ROGUE
4												
3												ACCIDENTAL
2												ROMEO
1												CHASTE
0												
	Nameless lovers in previous 12 months	One-night stands per year	Blind date one-night stands per year	Tavern parking lot 1-hour stands per year	Condoms used per month	Barroom make-out sessions	Desperate, unsuccessful passes at cousins, boss's wives, etc.	Number of women's un-dergarments in your per-sonal pos-session	Number of sex toys owned	Her age: How many years older will you go?	Your Slut Score	

TEACH HER CAT TO FETCH

If your girl came with a cat, don't despair. Get some entertainment out of Fluffy at least. Even though their brains are the size of walnuts, you can teach a cat to fetch.

Find a feline-size stick, and rub chicken into the wood. Next, tie on a long length of string and wave your wand under the cat's nose. Now toss the stick. When Kitty picks it up, call her back while you gently pull on the string. As soon as she drops the stick at your feet, feed her face.

Kiss Her Like This Is the First Time

The perfect first kiss is very light. A brush can be better than a full kiss. It leaves her wanting more. Don't give too much away right at first.

Plan a Great Date

Give her a day by herself at an upscale spa. Have her dress there. Pick her up and take her to an elegant hotel so she can show herself off at dinner. Then take her upstairs for champagne and dessert. We guarantee you'll get your money's worth.

Ask for Her Hand

Before you get married, ask permission from you fiancée's parents. This may seem old-fashioned, but research shows that 80 percent of the marriages that fail within the first year didn't have parental approval. Another study showed that 70 percent of couples who divorced in the first year named in-law problems as a big factor.

Deliver a Memorable Proposal

Propose in a way that's memorable, but not overdone. Asking her when she's free-falling out of a Piper Cub is all about you—what a cool guy you are. A proposal is supposed to be about her. Make it romantic. Make it intimate.

Unlock Her Treasure Chest

Every woman has a treasure chest inside her that most men don't know exists. It's that special, secret part of her that she cherishes. Typically, it's a nonbody trait, like her intellectual curiosity, her sense of humor, her outlandishness. But it could be the color of her eyes or even her laugh. It's when a man discovers this, when he comes to appreciate and love that part of her, that he really gets the girl both emotionally and sexually. That's when she feels she's being loved as a complete person. If you don't have a clue what's inside your woman's treasure chest, listen closely the next time she's with her father. Note what he compliments about her and what makes her sparkle.

Find a Wife Who's Full of Life

A successful marriage is one in which it never occurs to you that you've compromised anything.

Pick a Good Wife

It's one of the most important decisions you'll ever make. Here are some key traits of good wives:

• Good wives are interested in being good moms.

• Good wives have that sex trigger you want to keep pulling.

• Good wives drive like guys. Driving is a great measure of competency.

• Good wives understand how to nurture and grow your money.

• Good wives have a sense of humor (or they wouldn't have considered you).

• Good wives are not being treated on an outpatient basis for anything.

Be Wary of This Type

Love is not a business plan. It can't be approached as a goal or as a bottom line, where engagement is slated for the first quarter, marriage for the second, a home for the third, and kids for the close of the fiscal. Many never-married thirtysomething women with ticking biological clocks approach it this way, though. Beware of them. For love to be true, it has to be largely unplanned. It is strongest and most enduring when it is magic.

Work Out to Get Worked Up

An aerobic workout—even a brief one—can help put you in the mood for love and even give your orgasms more punch. Aerobic exercise increases brain activity in the left frontal lobe, triggering positive feelings that can boost interest in sex. Exercise also produces those well-known, feel-good chemicals called endorphins, which can increase arousal and the intensity of orgasms. The effect lasts 60 to 90 minutes after 10 minutes or more of exercise.

Convince Her She's Lustworthy

The biggest single sex blocker among women is insecurity about their physical appearance. Ashamed of being overweight or not good-looking enough, they find it hard to believe their lovers can be attracted to them. So constantly tell your partner how sexy she is. Compliment her. Give her a lustful look. Whisper your desire to lick vanilla pudding out of her navel. Get her to buy the idea that she's lustworthy, and she'll aim to prove it to you.

TALK DIRTY— IN PUBLIC

Quietly whispering, in explicit terms, what you want to do to her in bed that night—especially if you're whispering at the mall—makes it more likely to happen. Why? Sex talk is doubly arousing in public. The mere mention will start her "percolating," a low-grade sexual excitement that can last all day and make her more ready for sex at night.

Analyze a First Date

This self-exam will help you analyze the success or failure of any first date. Simply take a pen and mark a bar on the chart corresponding to how you think you did in each category on a 0-to-10 scale (10 being the best). When you've answered all these critical questions by assigning each a value, add them up and divide by 10. This will give you your final reading on the right-hand side of the chart, Final Date Analysis.

	How much did she . . .	Laugh at your jokes?	Touch your arm?	Fiddle with her hair?	Look at you when you spoke?	Avoid looking at other guys?	Avoid mentioning other boyfriends?	Ask about your job and life?	Feign interest in your favorite sport?	Compliment you on anything?	Swap spit?	Final data analysis	
10													**YOU DOG**
9													
8													
7													
6													
5													**MAYBE NEXT TIME**
4													
3													
2													**SHE LOVES YOU FOR YOUR MIND**
1													
0													

Boost Your Wonderful Rating

Take your calendar and randomly note when it's time to give your lover some unexpected attention. This could be a phone call in the middle of the day, a passionate nibble on the back of the neck, or simply telling her how attractive she is. Such attention will boost you several levels on the wonderful scale.

Be the Horny Husband on Line Two

Call your lover at work and tell her what you'd like to do to her tonight when she gets home. The result: You'll both be thinking about sex for *hours*.

Get Her All Hot in Macy's

Trying on clothing often gets a woman in the mood for sex because she's turned on by enhancing herself—either by being happy with her body or just by buying an article of clothing she feels good about.

Turn Your Good Girl Bad

Here's a sneaky strategy to propose your wildest notion: Portray your fantasy as a dream. For example, if you'd like to take her on the observatory deck of the Empire State Building, but you're nervous about suggesting it, phrase the whole scenario as a dream. "Honey, I had the wildest dream last night. . . ." Dreams are blameless, subconscious thoughts that sneak into our sleep. If she's turned off, simply dismiss the dream. If she wants to hear more, book two tickets to New York, pronto.

Rent One Tonight

Our panel of expert female judges picked five seemingly innocent movies that'll have her undoing your belt before the credits roll.

Bull Durham: (1988) Baseball, sex, and Susan Sarandon. *What the judges said:* "Seeing careless sex on the kitchen table, in the living room, on the bedroom floor, and in the bathtub—all within a 10-minute span—definitely put me in the mood to take my clothes off."

The Mask of Zorro: (1998) Sharp weapons and Catherine Zeta-Jones. *What the judges said:* "The sword fight and the sexual tension didn't let me think about anything else but sex."

Henry & June: (1990) Artsy film, set in 1930s Paris. *What the judges said:* "This movie is just all-out hot. Since it's solely about sexual desire, it really gets you worked up by the end."

The Thomas Crown Affair: (1999) Remake of the classic Steve McQueen heist film. *What the judges said:* "The sex scenes show Pierce Brosnan and Rene Russo laughing and playing together, which make them more romantic and realistic than most movie love scenes. A big turn-on."

The Piano: (1993) Chick flick about, well, a piano. *What the judges said:* "The sequences between Harvey Keitel and Holly Hunter are incredibly slow, naughty, and arousing. Watch for the stocking scene."

Rent a Love Shack

For a bit of sexual intrigue, leave her a note with directions and a key to the hotel room you've reserved for the weekend. The note should tell her to bring nothing—you've taken care of it all.

Administer the Second-Wife Quality Control Test

Before you try to make someone else work in your marital equation, make sure she doesn't add up to the same person all over again. *Directions:* Simple. Rate the prospective missus against your ex, on a scale from 1 to 10.

	Prospective New Wife	Ex-Wife
Her family		
Her friends		
Her sense of humor		
Her mom-ability		
Her interests		
Her basic comprehension of the importance of sports in daily life		
Her scenic value		
Her financial health		
Her affinity for cats		
How well does she travel?		
Is she high maintenance?		
Her moral values (or lack thereof)		
Score:		

Add both columns. If your prospective missus scores better than your ex-missus, you're headed the right way. If not, you're not.

Simmer All Day, Cook All Night

To get yourself really cranked up, try a technique called "simmering." Most men have moments of sexual arousal several times a day: the beauty in the Corvette on the way to work, the cute waitress at lunch, the sexy ad in a magazine, and the phone call from the client with that sultry voice. You can hold onto these lusty moments by simmering.

Whenever you have a sexual feeling toward a woman, go ahead and focus on it for a few moments. Let yourself fantasize about her, guilt-free. Then let go of the thought. An hour later, return to it and relive it. Continue re-playing your fantasies every few hours, but as you get ready to go home, substitute your steady for your fantasy ladies. Simmering keeps feelings of arousal bubbling away until you and your lover are ready to bring them to a boil.

Have Makeup Sex Anytime

Makeup sex is the best. When you fight, anger drives up testosterone in both men and women. If you go to bed with increased testosterone and agitation, the sex drive is going to be stronger. You can reenact fighting—and the emotions that go along with it—without hurting each other. Try something that will create a little physical tension between the two of you. Like:

Miniature golf. You can do anything that's just a little competitive.

Pillow fights. It starts with her hair flying and her breasts moving, and it even gets her gasping a little for breath. There's something very sexual about that.

Naked wrestling. Hint: Let her win.

Play Battle Strip

It's Saturday night. You're snowed in with nothing but old board games and two warm bodies. That's all you need to score:

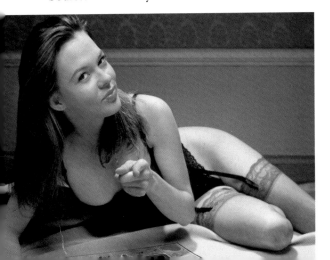

Monopoly: Make up your own Community Chest and Chance cards.

Twister: You've already thrown down the plastic tarp. Now make it slippery.

Battle Strip: Draw your clothes, and hers, on two paper grids. You say E5, she loses her bra. She says F7, you unleash the torpedo.

Get outta Town

For better sex, leave town. A change in setting lets her (and you) adopt a different personality for a while. Case in point, from a longtime (happy) husband: "My wife is inhibited by people and places she knows. A couple of years ago, we went to New Orleans for the weekend. We had sex more often in 2 days than we had in the previous 2 months. She wore this flimsy dress to dinner and returned from the bathroom and handed me her panties."

Leave a Message on the Mirror

While your partner is showering, sneak in and write something romantic on the medicine cabinet mirror. Use a cotton swab and Rain-X antifogger (it's for keeping car windows clear.) Your message will magi-cally appear through the steam, guaranteeing immediate sex. (Unless you write something like, "I've left with Julio, the gardener, for Belize.")

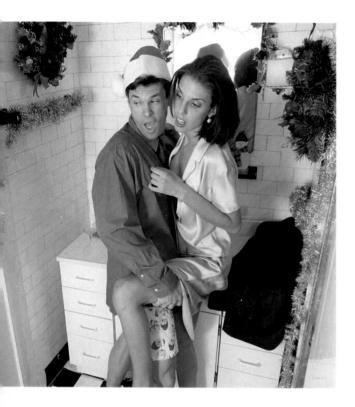

Have a Holiday Quickie

There's only one thing that might—*might*—make the marathon holiday family visits bearable: a little covert sex. Here's the best way to pull it off: Bring the kids' gifts—wrapped, but in a bag. Say you haven't wrapped them yet, and duck into a spare room. Have fun with the bows.

See Who You Brought Home

When walking into a dark room, blink as many times as you can for 5 seconds. It will stimulate your eyes and help them adjust to the darkness faster.

Turn On a Black Light

A black light near the bed really helps get things cooking. It gives bodies a sexy-looking tan without anyone having to destroy their skin by baking in the sun.

Another Use for Old T-Shirts

When a T-shirt gets old, wear it into the bedroom and have your lover rip it off of you.

Shower Her with Flowers

Put flower petals on the top of a ceiling fan. Turn it on when she lies down.

Play Your Song

Play your wedding song in the background while making love. If something has special meaning to you both, bring it to the bedroom because it creates a special connection between the two of you.

Play the Honey Game

You're blindfolded; she hides a dab of honey somewhere on her body. You try to find it—using only your tongue.

Cook Up Some Sex Stew

Share this stew with your honey before an active evening. Oysters are among the most concentrated food sources of zinc, a mineral that's necessary for testosterone production. And celery contains androsterone, a hormone that may act as an aphrodisiac as it's released through perspiration. Garlic will make sure that your blood flows to all the right places—it reduces the platelet clumping that may impede blood flow to your crucial erogenous zones. Plenty of carbohydrates will provide all the staying power you'll need for a wild night.

Sex Stew

1	cup minced onion
1	stalk celery, minced
1	tablespoon olive oil
1	clove garlic, minced
½	teaspoon dried savory
1	baking potato, diced
1½	cups low-fat chicken broth
½	cup bottled clam juice
½	cup frozen corn
1½	cups small oysters, drained
1½	cups low-fat milk
¼	cup minced fresh parsley

In a large saucepan, sauté the onions and celery in the olive oil over medium heat. Add the garlic and savory. Stir for 30 seconds. Add the potato, broth, and clam juice, and bring to a boil. Reduce heat, cover, and simmer for 15 minutes. Stir in the corn and oysters. Simmer briefly (until the edges of the oysters start to curl). Slowly add the milk and parsley, and heat through.

Serves 4

Per serving (1½ cups): 172 calories, 3.4 g fat (18% of calories), 1.4 g fiber, 13 g protein, 23 g carbohydrates.

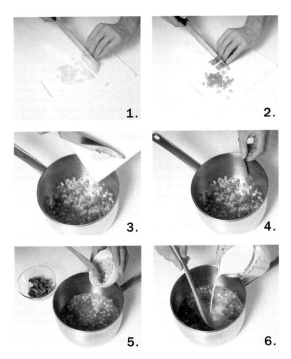

1. 2.

3. 4.

5. 6.

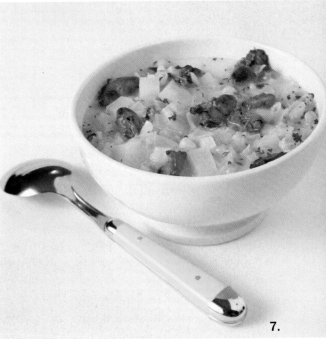

7.

START A ROARING BLAZE

A crackling fire adds romance to any evening. Here's how to spark one with a single match:

1. A fire requires three things: fuel, oxygen, and heat. The trick to building a good fire is giving it enough oxygen, letting it breathe. Most novice fire-builders smother the flames with too much wood.

2. Crumple two pieces of newspaper and stuff them under the grate. Crumple a third and place it in the center, on top of the grate. A fireplace grate helps circulate air under the logs to keep the fire burning.

3. Lean kindling against the ball of crumpled paper, teepee fashion. Use twigs or hardwood kindling no more than ¾ inch wide by ¼ inch thick and 10 inches long. Don't pack it too tightly; leave room for air.

4. Place two split logs on top of the newspaper and kindling. The logs should be roughly parallel and at least 4 inches apart. Then place a third log diagonally across the first two.

5. Quick, check to make sure the flue is open so the room won't fill with smoke. Then light the newspaper in three places with a match and watch as the kindling catches fire.

6. A good fire is a well-tended fire. Add logs to the flames as the original fuel turns to hot coals. But don't smother the fire by adding too much wood at one time. Let your fire breathe.

Lose the Tie

A necktie is the article of men's clothing that women love most. The silk against her skin. The way it smells after being tied around your neck all day. Mmmm. So take it off and rub it against her skin, or, even better, use it to cover her eyes. She won't be able to anticipate where or when your next kiss or touch is coming, so every touch will feel more intense.

Use Code Words

Women are usually the better communicators but not necessarily in the bedroom. She might want to have sex but feel too shy to convey that to you. To find out if that's the case, wait until she's in a playful mood, then ask her to help you come up with a secret code word or phrase for sex. Creating your own language for sex helps intimacy and can get past her embarrassment.

Unhook a Bra with One Hand

This is a handy skill to have.

1. Find the clasp at the back (there may be more than one if she's well endowed, you dog). It's a hook-and-eye gizmo held together by the force of the elastic back strap pulling the hook into the eye. Slip your thumb under the back strap just to the right (your right) of

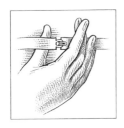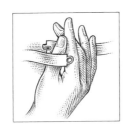

the clasp. Pull it away from her back about a half-inch.

2. With your middle finger, press against the back strap on the opposite side of the clasp from your thumb. Your thumb should be stretching the strap away from her back as your middle finger is pressing it in, toward her skin.

3. Turn your wrist slightly so the middle finger comes nearly under the thumb, thus transferring the stress on the strap to your finger and thumb. This will allow the hook to freely escape the eye and the strap to come apart.

Find Her Hidden Pleasure Zones

The sensitivity of a woman's entire body is tough to overemphasize. While the key to your sexual pleasure lies between your legs, women are less focused on the genitals and more aware of other parts of their bodies. The late sex researcher Alfred Kinsey found some women who were capable of reaching orgasm simply by having their eyebrows stroked, their earlobes kissed, or some pressure applied to their teeth. Find your partner's erogenous zones.

Worship Her Temple

Touch your partner's temples, and you'll feel veins throbbing with tension and stress. Use your forefinger and index finger to massage the temples in gentle circular motions. She'll melt into a state of blissful relaxation.

Give Her an Electric Kiss

Have you ever kissed someone and made sparks fly? The legendary "electric kiss" can be achieved by rubbing your stocking feet on a rug to create an excess of negative electric particles. Then move within a fraction of an inch of your partner's lips, and a tiny electric spark should jump from your lips to hers.

Discover What Your Kissing is Missing

Some guys approach a kiss like it's an invasion. It's not erotic when you try to annex her tonsils with your tongue. In fact, keep your tongue in your mouth until she wants it in hers. (Don't worry—she'll let you know.)

Another common complaint is that guys are only interested in kissing during the 5 minutes before they start removing a woman's clothing. If this sounds familiar, you'll enjoy kissing more if you try varying the speed (shorter and longer kisses) and pressure (softer and harder). Throw a few timid, tender kisses in with the brazen, forceful ones.

Remember that there's plenty of other stuff you can kiss. Slide your lips down her body, stopping at her throat, her fingers, the nape of her neck . . . you get the idea. Expand your repertoire by occasionally sucking on her earlobe and neck. If she likes it, move on to soft biting, paying particular attention to any move that elicits happy noises—from her, not you.

GIVE HER A BREAST ORGASM

Some women can climax just by having their breasts fondled. Here's how to do it:

1. Cup her breasts and gently lift them so they feel slightly supported.

2. Kiss and stroke the lower area of her breasts first, under the areolae.

3. Now move up. Don't focus on her nipples

4. Gently push her breasts together and kiss the center of her chest, along her breastbone. At the same time, softly squeeze her breasts to help make them more sensitive. By the way, leave the lights on while you're doing all this. Watching you at work will arouse her, too.

Be a Breast Magician

Guess what? Breasts change size when they're having fun, too. When they're kissed or stroked, blood flows in and dilates the arteries, causing the breasts to grow up to 25 percent. Watch her go from a B cup to a C in mere minutes!

Warm Her Up This Long

The average woman need about 15 minutes of foreplay. For goodness sake, don't look at your watch, but here's a guide.

Zero to minute 3: Mute the TV and get rid of the nachos. Kiss her like she's the only thing in the world that exists right now.

Minute 4 to minute 6: Kiss her some more. But while you're doing it, begin to touch her all over. Not like that. Like this: Gently, as if it's something you've never felt before. Then let her touch you.

Minute 7 to minute 12: Very slowly take off her clothes. Start to take off yours and let her finish for you. Do not fold anything.

Minute 13 to minute 15: Use your mouth. Nibble, lick, bite. A little roughly on ordinary skin; a little more gently elsewhere.

There, that wasn't so bad, was it?

Delight Her Secret Spot

The tender flesh behind the knee is good for both a tickle and a turn-on. Make sure your partner's leg is fully extended, then gently trace a figure eight on the back of the knee with your fingertips or the tip of your tongue.

Make Her Orgasm by Rubbing Her Feet

Some women can have an orgasm just from having their feet rubbed. To discover if she's one of them, do this: Using a dab of lotion, very slowly stroke the arch of her foot, back and forth from the ball to the heel. Pay special attention to the middle toe—in some people this digit has a direct nerve connection to the genitals. Apply moderate pressure—not so hard as to cause pain or so light as to tickle.

Pretend It's Too Hot to Handle

Don't rush to your partner's crotch during foreplay. Instead pretend that it's too hot to handle, that if you touch it for more than a second, you'll be burned. Don't rip off her panties. Slowly start to pull them down, then pull them back up and devote more attention elsewhere. It'll drive her wild.

Respect Her Little Pink Pea

While it's true that direct stimulation of the clitoris—the little pink pea above the woman's vagina—is the key to most women's climaxing, don't pounce too quickly. As a woman becomes more and more aroused, the clitoris will swell, producing a sort of erection. But her erection takes longer than yours does to develop, and any direct contact before that point can be painful.

Find Her G-Spot

The G-spot is located inside the vagina on the upper wall (toward the navel). When stimulated, the G-spot swells to about the size of a half dollar, and has the puffy consistency of a marshmallow. To find it, insert a finger and curl it toward you, in a kind of "come hither" motion.

Do It Like She Does

When a woman masturbates, she often rests her wrist on her lower abdomen and above the pubic bone. When touching her, try to do the same.

Lick, Then Blow

By licking her nipples, private parts, and neck, then blowing on the wet patch, you can create a sexy tingle that'll drive her wild. To make her head spin even more, use alcohol. It evaporates more quickly than water or saliva, thereby creating a greater cooling effect when you blow on it. So bring that glass of wine into the bedroom. Swish some around in your mouth and lick a choice spot. (Try her breasts first.) Then blow gently, give it a second, and take a long, slow lick. Repeat as necessary.

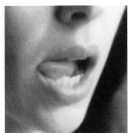

Put Your Honey Where Your Mouth Is

Here are a few new ways to use your kisser—straight from women's lips.

"Sometimes my boyfriend cuts a straw in half and blows and sucks through it on different parts of my body. The rush of warm breath drives me crazy." —Samantha, 26

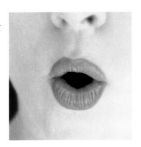

"I love when my boyfriend licks his hands and then touches my nipples, and then blows on them. A few minutes of that and I'm ready." —Debbie, 36

"My husband leaves messages on my voice mail when I'm at work, telling me how he's counting the time until we're home and he can have me all to himself. It's better than an e-mail because I can hear the urgency in his voice." —Amanda, 30

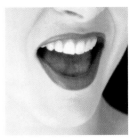

"Receiving oral sex from a guy with razor stubble is very cool. The rough hair and the softness of his tongue put me over the edge." —Jessica, 27

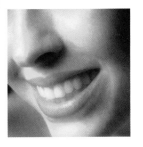

COVER HER WITH ROSES

Take fresh petals from a long-stemmed red rose and scatter them over the body of your lover just prior to engaging in intercourse. Kissing and licking around the rose petals on the stomach, breasts, nipples and thighs adds a new dimension to the experience. Finally, intercourse with rose petals between lovers provides a very sensuous addition to sex—the petals cling to both bodies because of the sweat generated and leave interesting patterns when sex is over.

Line Up for Pleasure

Men have three hot spots. One area is the small, triangular region on the underside of the head of the penis where a thin strip of skin, the frenulum, runs from the head to the shaft. The other area follows the raphe, the line you can see and feel that runs along the center of the scrotum. Ask your partner to trace a finger along this line, from behind the scrotum to the front, then up the penis. Hang on.

Most men don't know that the fleshy island between the scrotum and anus (called the perineum) even exists. Have your partner lift your testicles with one hand and use the forefinger of the other to massage this spot with deep circular strokes. The pleasure comes not from the proximity to the penis, but from the prostate gland, which lies just inside the lower pelvic cavity. Stroking the perineum stimulates the gland, a major hidden hot zone.

Don't Overlook Your Nipples

Men's breasts have the same potential for erotic pleasure as women's breasts. In both sexes, the breasts are richly supplied with nerve endings, especially in the nipple area.

Be Patient, Oh Semi-Erect One

Any time you're trying to penetrate or thrust with a penis that's not fully erect, you're susceptible to bending and buckling injuries. You can actually damage the structures inside your penis that fill with blood when you get an erection. The result? A penis that permanently bends, sometimes painfully, in one direction or the other. If penetration is difficult, then it's also dangerous. Try giving something your partner probably wants more of anyway: foreplay.

Seduce Her with Your Fingertips

Anticipation is a huge part of what turns women on. So help her undress. Then once she's naked, take her hand and stand facing her. Brush her hair back and let your fingertips hover over the surface of her skin. You're where you should be if the fat part of your finger pads are touching her skin ever so slightly. Now go ahead and run your pads over her arms, breasts, belly, and thighs. You'll be creating a delightful shiver up her spine—and making her feel as though you appreciate every inch of her body.

Touch Her in Waves

When you're stroking your partner, don't move up and down her body in straight lines. When you use a straight stroke, the nerves in the skin aren't surprised when they're touched. However, when you use wavy lines and the stroke is irregular, the nerves have no idea what's next, and they become that much more excited. Pick areas that aren't generally exposed to light. Parts like the back of her arms are only accustomed to feeling the pressure of clothing, so they're much more sensitive than other parts of her body—and easier to stimulate.

Look Her in the Eye

There's a reason they call them *bedroom* eyes. If her pupils are dilated, that could be a sign of sexual readiness. (It could also be a sign that you're in a dark bedroom, Sherlock. Light a candle.)

Monitor Her Breathing

How much foreplay is enough? Lubrication, or lack thereof, doesn't necessarily indicate readiness (especially in women approaching menopause, whose bodies have trouble creating proper lubrication). The best way to tell when she's ready is to listen closely. One of the best clues to a woman's level of arousal is her breathing. When your partner's approaching orgasm, she'll probably start to breathe hot and heavy, but at an early stage of the game, you want to listen for heavy, slow breathing. A transition from normal breathing to a deep, relaxed pattern should indicate that she's ready for intercourse. Either that or you put her to sleep.

Tease Her with Your Penis

Many women find it very erotic to be teased at the opening of the vagina. Grasp the base of your penis with your hand and gently make circles around the clitoris or run the underside of the shaft along her inner lips. Don't fully penetrate. Pull out before you're halfway in.

Focus on Insertion

Penetrate slowly, then withdraw completely. Wait a second and start over. Do this 10 times. Insertion is everyone's favorite part of intercourse. Repeating it will help make sex even better.

Put Petite Women on Top

The best position for sex if you're significantly taller than your partner is the woman-on-top position. So arranged, height makes no difference. Plus, it puts her in charge of the timing and depth of penetration, so she can stay comfortable.

Wake the Neighbors

Women love to hear sounds of pleasure, and most men dramatically underdo them. Go ahead and moan, groan, sigh, and scream.

Fit Together Perfectly

Think back on the last couple of times you and your partner made love. Try to remember if you felt the tip of your penis bump into something at the maximum thrust point. If it did, then you probably hit her cervix (or the diaphragm covering her cervix) and you're long enough to hit hot spots. If you hit it so hard she complained, you're probably a little on the long side. That takes some adjusting. In this situation, the missionary position works best because that's where you tend to get the least depth penetration. You might also want to try woman-on-top positions where the woman is facing you: These can minimize length while maximizing upper-wall stimulation. On the other hand, if you have never felt some type of resistance when thrusting, you may be a little on the short side compared to her anatomy. No problem. If you're using the missionary position, have her elevate her legs and bring them toward her chest. This shortens the vaginal canal. If you're kneeling in front of her, try to get your pelvis as close to hers as possible. This position maximizes your length.

SURF HER SEXUAL CHANNELS

The longer you spend in one position, the less control you'll have over ejaculation. Try switching from position to position—sort of like sexual channel surfing. Return to your favorites, but don't spend more than about 30 thrusts in each. Chances are, you'll be able to last two or three times longer than normal.

Try the CAT

The coital alignment technique, or CAT, reportedly intensifies female orgasms. Here's how to do it: Start in the missionary position, with your weight on your elbows and her knees slightly bent and raised. Now slide your entire body up, so that your pelvis is slightly above hers. In this position, the base of your ardent manhood is rubbing directly on her white-hot passionflower. (We write adult greeting cards on the side.) Relax your upper body and allow her to bear your weight. Now have her press her pelvis into yours; you respond in kind. Allow her to set a rhythm that feels right, and keep up the tango until the ceiling collapses.

Turn Her Upside-Down

Here's a new position for sex that'll blow her mind, literally: Have her lie on her back across the bed, with her head and shoulders dangling over the edge. (Make sure she keeps as much of her lower back on the mattress as possible, and stop if she gets too light-headed.) Enter her slowly, and show some restraint when you thrust—you don't want to knock her onto the floor. Any time you turn your head upside-down, you'll feel a rush as blood pours in. This head rush, combined with physical pleasure, can heighten orgasm for some women.

Do It on a Swiss Ball

Our vote for the most sexual piece of fitness equipment is a large Swiss ball. Why? The ball can actually help improve your depth of penetration, if you're in the right position. Try this:

BE CAREFUL, COWBOY

Penile fracture is almost always caused by an accident during intercourse, when the penis is jammed against an immovable object, such as her pelvic bone. These accidents are most common during "rodeo sex," when your partner is bouncing around on top of you. To protect yourself, make sure that if she's on top, she doesn't lift more than an inch or two off you on the upstroke. And tell her never to lean back against the direction of your erection while you're inserted. Also, be careful when changing positions; it's usually better to withdraw before you pick her up or flip her over. (Yee ha!) If you do fracture yourself, you'll know. Your penis will turn purple and swell up like an eggplant. Don't dawdle: Go quickly to an ER.

Sit on the ball and have her straddle you, facing away from you. Hold her hips for balance, and use the rocking motion of the ball to thrust in and out of her from behind. Do one set of at least 50 repetitions.

Make Circles

Men who thrust in a circular motion—rather than straight in and out—have greater ejaculatory control.

Hold the Boys Down

During sexual arousal, the scrotal sac tightens and lifts the testicles up against the body. You can't ejaculate unless they're in that position. So, to postpone ejaculation, you can pull the scrotum down manually, keeping the testicles down far enough to keep them from assuming the position that will make ejaculation inevitable. Some men do this by holding their testicles between their legs as they masturbate, and sometimes even while they have intercourse. Your partner can do it for you, too.

Go Down in the Basement

We like having sex in the basement—not only because it keeps us close to the Foosball table and the fuse box, but also because of the dark stairwell. Try a doggie-style position with her a few steps above you. Her skin and breasts will brush against the carpeted steps (she'll like that). You'll like the strong upward thrusts you have to make to stay connected.

Have Sex at Victoria's Secret

The best dressing rooms for sex are at Victoria's Secret. They have love seats in there. Ask the saleswoman if you can go in to make sure you like what your girlfriend is trying on.

Have Beanbag Sex

A beanbag chair is great for sex. You can contour it to any shape, and it's almost like being in water—it'll support you in ways you're not accustomed to. Doggie-style sex works great when she's on her belly, draped over the amorphous blob (the chair, not you). So does the missionary position. Stick a couple of thick books under the bag to keep her from sinking in too far.

Try the Cowgirl Position

How to do it: You lean back with your shoulders against the foot of the bed and your feet on the floor, supporting the bulk of your weight. She straddles your midsection and uses her legs to thrust.

Difficulty: Moderate

Payoff: Extreme

Even if she's never been the jockey type, she'll have a hard time resisting this invitation to ride. Not only does she control the angle, speed, depth and rhythm of the thrusts, but because she supports her own weight, she also has complete freedom of movement. This is as close as you can get to having sex in a swing set without having to install hardware in your bedroom. Your mate doesn't have to rely on your figuring out where she likes to be touched—she can stimulate whatever needs it on her own. One caution: Some women tend to get weak in the knees during orgasm, so brace yourself for a little extra weight once she peaks.

Have Sex on the Washer

Your washing machine produces more vibration than any other appliance in your home. Problem is, most people don't use it right. *You* should be the one with your butt on the lid. The motion will be transmitted through your pelvis, essentially turning your member into a life-size vibrator. Run a warm-water load so the top won't be cold.

Make a Hole-in-One

If you're considering having sex on a golf course, head for hole 5, 6, 13, or 14. They're the farthest from the clubhouse, which reduces your risk of being caught by the grounds crew. The greens are the softest places, but you'll want to use a blanket because courses are usually smothered with pesticides. Try explaining that to your urologist.

MAKE SEX TWICE AS GOOD

Want to drive her wild with desire? Look her straight in the eye during sex instead of burying your head in the goose down. Add in a little play-by-play of the action, and solicit her opinion, too. The combination of eye contact and dialogue—that direct connection during sex—is an incredible turn-on for women.

Coordinate Your Breathing

For heightened sexual pleasure, breathe together. During intercourse, exhale when you thrust toward your partner and inhale when you pull back. Have her do the same. This raises the physical sensations of sex and deepens the amount of stimulation you can tolerate before ejaculating. It also connects partners in a very special physical and emotional way.

Defy Gravity with Your Genitals

Just before ejaculation, your testicles ascend like an aircraft's landing gear to provide more power to your takeoff. To give your equipment an even bigger boost, have your partner give you a hand—literally. Ask her to gently press upward on your testicles with the palm of her hand just before you ejaculate. This will heighten your arousal and add intensity to your orgasm.

Become Multi-Orgasmic

For most men there is a period after the point of ejaculatory inevitability and before ejaculation that is intensely pleasurable. It lasts for about 5 seconds, and then the semen is expelled. To become multi-orgasmic, you want to come as close to that point as possible. Once you find it, you'll cut off the flow of semen, but not the sensation. To do so, use the "squeeze technique." Each time you feel ejaculation coming on, squeeze the head of the penis for 15 seconds.

Tell If She's Faking

The most important thing to know about a woman's orgasm is this: If she screams during the middle of it, she's faking. Here's why: While climaxing, it's nearly impossible to exhale. The female orgasm is not an explosion of endorphins and genital juices. It's an implosion. She'll draw her breath, tighten her muscles, suck every scrap of energy and sensation into the tiny nut core of her being and then give way exquisitely, the flow of goodness spreading up her chest and down her legs like someone's kicked over a can of red paint. Afterward, she might sigh, pant, or moan. But scream? Never.

Stop Her from Faking

If you suspect that your partner is regularly faking orgasm for your benefit, then you need to remove the pressure she's evidently feeling to validate you. First, tell her that you won't be offended if she doesn't climax. Then emphasize that an honest, open, loving relationship is what's most important to you. Say it this way: "If there's something I can be doing differently, anything that would help you respond the way you want to, I want to know."

Save Her Life with Fellatio

Gynecologists have found that women who frequently performed oral sex on their partners had about a 50 percent lower risk of developing preeclampsia, a potentially fatal complication of pregnancy.

Sweeten Your Semen

If your partner objects to giving you oral sex because, well, it just plain tastes bad, an apple a day might help. High in natural sugars, fruits reportedly bless men with sweeter seminal fluids.

ACE THE ORAL

All women have different preferences during oral sex, so the best advice is to experiment: Use both sides of your tongue, for example, or let your tongue go soft in such a way that you'd slur your words if you tried to speak. While you work through the lineup, ask her to provide a play-by-play of what she's feeling. When she can no longer speak, it's because her loins are screaming the equivalent of *"The Giants win the pennant! The Giants win the pennant!"*

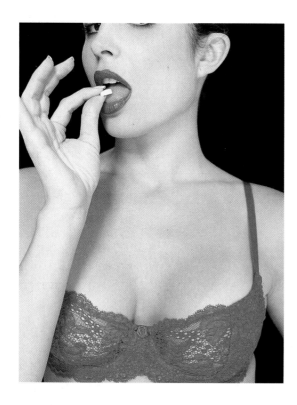

Suck on This

If your partner sucks on a breath mint before giving you oral sex, it'll be more pleasurable for you. The peppermint oil in some mints can cause a mild irritation that brings a flushed, warm sensation to the skin—especially the thin skin of the penis or vagina. If a strong mint is too much to swallow before sex, a menthol throat lozenge such as Halls Mentho-Lyptus also works.

Hum during Oral Sex

Any time you touch the skin with something vibrating, you transmit sensation to a wider area than you would through simple stroking. So relax your lips (think Mick Jagger) and hum a tune (maybe "Brown Sugar"). Bring the outermost portion of your kisser in contact with the outside of her clitoris (the hood that covers the little nub) and her vaginal lips. Move your mouth around her clitoris—very slowly. When she can't take any more, tap gently and in a circular motion with your fingertips on the swollen nub of the clitoris, or give it a few long, languid licks, staying in contact the whole time.

Play the Alphabet Game

Make capital letters with your tongue very slowly on her clitoris. See if you can make it to M.

Make Her Quiver, Not Shiver

When you're giving her oral sex, think about the back of your neck: A soft touch can make you shiver, but a more substantial caress doesn't. Her clitoris reacts to stimulation in the same way. Put your whole hand there for several minutes to build up her arousal. Then add your mouth, but keep using your hand, too; this will help her become accustomed to the feel of your tongue. Press firmly with the flat side of your tongue (don't flick with the tip), and use plenty of saliva. If she enjoys the sensation, you can also insert a finger into her vagina. Many women find the sensation of simultaneous internal and external stimulation very arousing.

Leave Her Panties On

Next time, try giving her oral sex through her panties. She'll like the way the damp cotton feels against her.

Give Her the After-Sex Test

You can tell if the girl you're dating is worthwhile if you really enjoy talking to her *after* you have sex.

Smell Swell at Sunrise

Don't let morning breath (yours) ruin her memories. Put an orange by your bedside before the nighttime nuzzling begins. Next morning, moisten your mouth with the citrus juice. Feed her a wedge or two.

Keep It under 10, Will Ya?

For some reason, many men think they have to last longer than the New York run of *Cats*. Relax. That just ain't the case. The truth is, if this goes on for too long, women get tired and their minds start to wander. After 10 minutes they get impatient. After 20, they're making shopping lists.

Get Back in the Sack

Clearly, this will not come as a surprise—sex is good for you. In particular, sex is great for your back. If all the world's orthopedic specialists convened to formulate the best single exercise for releasing muscular constriction, toning back muscles, and relaxing the nervous system, making love would be that exercise. Scientifically, it has been demonstrated that orgasm has 10 times the effect of Valium. Tell that to your chiropractor.

BY THE NUMBERS

GET IT UP AGAIN AND AGAIN

Here's your six-step plan.

1. Don't masturbate for several days beforehand. The more you ejaculate, the longer your refractory periods.

2. Skip the post-romp cigarette. Nicotine kills erections faster than reruns of *The Golden Girls*.

3. After sex, trade massages. Relieving tension in any of your muscles decreases anxiety, a factor in secondary erections.

4. Alcohol in low doses increases the arousal signals from your brain to your penile tissue. Your inhibitions are down, so you're more easily excited than if you were completely sober. But stop at two drinks. Anything more will inhibit performance.

5. Good circulation is also important for maintaining strong erections. Improve yours by simply standing up and moving around a bit.

6. Finally, change the stimuli. No, not your partner, but rather the surroundings, the erotic video in the VCR, the toys on the nightstand, her outfit, positions, etc.

UNCOMMON KNOWLEDGE

TELL HER WHAT SHE WANTS TO HEAR

The top three things women like to hear most from men are:

1. "I can't wait to see you."
2. "I love waking up with you."
3. "I brought you something."

Compute Your Calorie Burn during Sex

We wish we could say it's true, but heart rates raised in passion are not the same as those raised in exercise. Sex is a moderate activity—on a par with playing table tennis, weeding a garden, or walking slowly. It burns only about 5.25 calories per minute for someone weighing 160 to 170 pounds. Running at a $7\frac{1}{2}$ minute-per-mile pace burns more than twice as many. But orgasm is another story. When you climax, you burn calories at the glorious rate of 400 per hour. The catch, of course, is that orgasms last about 15 seconds, for a grand total of 1.6 calories.

Cure Hiccups with Sex

When you get the hiccups, don't breathe into a paper bag. Have sex. A 40-year-old Israeli man with chronic hiccups tried everything to stop the annoyance. Then his doctor suggested he try intercourse. The hiccups suddenly stopped right after he ejaculated—and they haven't been back for more than a year. The sexual stimulation may have had just the right effect on the reflex that causes hiccups.

Eat More Soy, Have More Joy

Want to boost your sexual health? One of the world's greatest sex foods is soy. Yes, we know: Tofu is the white noise of the food world. But consider the benefits. More than 200 studies have found that genistein—a crystalline compound found only in soy—wards off prostate cancer, shrinks enlarged prostates, and increases fertility. It also promotes firmer erections by lowering cholesterol levels and clearing your arteries. So find a way to work it in, okay?

Lower Your Cholesterol, Raise Your Erection

Your annual cholesterol test isn't just a measure of heart-disease risk, it's a gauge of your sexual potency. One of the biggest erection facilitators is a chemical called nitric oxide. It's a vasodilator, which means it helps trigger blood flow to the penis (and, thereby, harden it). Having lots of cholesterol in your circulatory system restricts blood flow to the penis and inhibits nitric oxide production, which makes Willy flounder.

Stay Happy, Healthy, and Hard

About 37 percent of men taking antidepressants will experience some form of sexual dysfunction. However, there are some things you can do to avoid becoming a limp statistic. Try taking the pill early in the morning. Some medicines will wear out by nighttime and won't affect your sexual function as much. You can also ask your doctor about Wellbutrin or Serzone. These two antidepressants affect the brain differently and trigger fewer sexual side effects.

Don't Let Your Penis Get Drunk

Alcohol impairs your ability to get an erection the same way it impairs your ability to drive and walk. It dulls the nerves that transmit sensation between your penis and brain. If you're looking to perform later in the evening, tell the bartender to cut you off after three drinks.

Lick Erection Problems

A healthy man normally has from four to seven erections while sleeping, though these decrease in frequency after age 50 or so. Presumably, all the psychological and emotional stresses surrounding sex are absent when you're asleep. So if you're getting good nocturnal erections, any performance problems you're having are psychological. To run a system's check on your equipment, wrap postage stamps around the base of your penis, and secure the ends together. If the stamps are torn along a perforation the next morning, everything is working correctly.

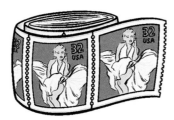

Watch Your Erection Go Up in Smoke

Smoking constricts the blood vessels and can interfere with your love life. A surprisingly large number of impotent men are smokers, but their condition often improves once they quit.

Yawn Yourself Hard

As far as your body is concerned, yawning and getting an erection are practically the same thing. They're both controlled by a chemical called nitric oxide. Released in the brain, it can either travel to the neurons that control mouth opening and breathing, or go down the spinal cord to the blood vessels that feed the penis. Sometimes it does both (that's why a big yawn can cause a tremor down under). Allowing yourself to yawn now and then throughout the day may help prime the neurochemical pathways that lead to good, sturdy erections.

Fire Your Mistress

It's common for men who start having affairs to stop having erections with their wives—so common, in fact, that doctors who treat erectile dysfunction often ask their patient if they're getting any action on the side. Guilt can turn to anxiety, and that can kill an erection.

Don't Be a Sore Loser

If your partner has a cold sore on her upper lip, rethink her suggestion of oral sex. It's possible that a cold sore can transmit the herpes virus to your penis, where it will live unhappily ever after.

DO THIS WHEN YOUR RUBBER HITS THE ROAD

Every night about 27,000 American couples experience a condom break or slip. Here's what to do if it happens to you:

1. Wash immediately. Wash yourself with soap and water. No studies have shown that soap destroys STDs, but it won't do any harm, and it might do some good.

2. Show concern. Gently ask her to a) inspect herself for condom bits, b) refrain from douching, as that can push in microbes, and c) see her doctor fast to inquire about the "morning-after pill," which is a concentrated dose of birth-control drugs that can reduce the risk of pregnancy by 75 percent.

3. Rehash histories. When she is infected, your risk for contracting an STD ranges from 50 percent for gonorrhea to 0.2 percent for HIV. Have another chat about previous sex partners and diseases. If you're concerned about STDs, see your doctor and get tested within a few days.

4. Troubleshoot. Did you use an expired condom or an oil-based lubricant? Maybe you nicked the condom with a fingernail while putting it on. Whatever the cause, eliminate it.

Avoid Dying during Sex

Don't have sex shortly after waking up—at least if you've had heart surgery. Researchers found that sex can trigger a sudden cardiac episode, and it's more likely to happen first thing in the morning.

Don't Take Viagra with a Big Meal

To avoid turning your Viagra pill into an expensive LifeSaver, wait at least 90 minutes after a lavish dinner to take it. High-fat foods prevent you from fully absorbing Viagra. Guys who complain that Viagra didn't work for them usually took it soon after a fatty meal.

Use Viagra for Insurance

Turns out the little blue pill may be able to prevent, as well as treat, erectile dysfunction. Taking half a tablet a week, especially for guys whose erections aren't always fully rigid, can stimulate blood flow and cause nighttime erections. Typical candidates for using Viagra preventively include men with impotence risk factors such as a history of smoking, high stress levels, or diabetes. Your urologist can assess whether it's right for you.

Masturbate before Sex

If premature ejaculation is a problem, try masturbating an hour or two before you plan to have sex with your partner. This trick may cause you to lose some of the immediate passion of sex, but it will help slow both the pace at which you become aroused *and* the speed of your climax.

Have Erections Often

In the flaccid state, the penis receives less than 0.1 percent of the blood circulating through the body. That's lower than virtually every other organ. Its oxygen level is also very low, 35 millimeters of mercury compared to 55 to 60 in most organs. The only time the penis gets a lot of blood and oxygen is during erections. Hence the saying, "use it or lose it." Erections recharge your batteries.

Toss an Inside-Out Condom

If you accidentally put a condom on inside-out, don't take it off and turn it around. If you've touched the condom to your penis, you should consider it ruined. (The condom, that is!) Your erect penis has probably already released a small amount of semen, which you've now placed at the tip of your sheathed erection, and this can be enough to get your lady friend pregnant. Although some condoms are treated with spermicide, this is still no guarantee. Grab another and start over.

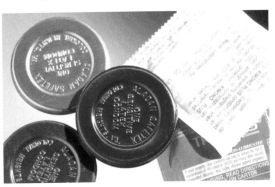

NUMB YOUR PENIS

If you ejaculate sooner than you'd like during sex, try Trojan's Extended Pleasure condom. The inside is coated with benzocaine, which briefly dulls the nerves in your penis, keeping you from getting too excited. It could help your staying power, but expect some trade off in sensation.

Measure Your Penis

The best way to gauge penis size is to measure yourself as a urologist would:

Flaccid length: Measure immediately after undressing, since a cold or warm room can cause shrinkage or expansion. Do it while standing, and use a flexible ruler. Position the tip of the ruler gently against the point where the shaft meets the abdomen. Then simply bend the ruler along the shaft and read the length. *Average: 3.43 inches*

Erect length: Immediately after you become fully hard, measure along the top of your erection from the base of the shaft to the tip. *Average: 5.03 inches*

Girth: While still erect, wrap a cloth tape measure around your penis at its base. *Average: 5.14 inches around; 1.67 inches in diameter*

Erection angle: Stand with your back against a wall and estimate your angle. A zero-degree erection (an oxymoron if we've ever heard one) would point at your feet; 90 degrees would point directly out in front; and 180 degrees would point up at your chin. *Average: 105.7 degrees*

Stop Worrying about Size

The mechanism of female orgasm has nothing to do with penis size. Nine out of 10 women have clitoral orgasms, caused by *external* stimulation to the clitoris. If you're physically fit and attractive and an adequate lover, even a 4-inch erection is long enough.

Add an Inch to Your Penis

In case you're not convinced that size doesn't matter, you can create the illusion

---

RATE YOUR CONDOM KNOWLEDGE

Take this quick quiz to rate your condom knowledge. Your life may depend on it.

1. The condoms that provide the most protection are made from:
   a. Natural animal membranes
   b. Latex rubber
   c. Silicone-coated linen
   d. Polyurethane
   e. Steel wool

2. Packaged condoms are good for approximately:
   a. 12 months
   b. 3 years
   c. 5 years
   d. 2 weeks at Club Med

3. Packaged condoms that are coated with a spermicide are good for approximately:
   a. 12 months
   b. 3 years
   c. 5 years
   d. 6 sex partners

4. Latex condoms should be stored:
   a. in the refrigerator
   b. in your wallet
   c. in a dry, cool place
   d. in a bedside drawer
   e. away from the cactus

5. The following should never be used as a lubricant with latex condoms:
   a. K-Y Jelly
   b. Vaseline
   c. Water
   d. Silicone gel

6. Carrying condoms in your wallet may:
   a. keep you prepared
   b. damage the condoms and the packaging
   c. wear off the expiration label
   d. make you feel really cool

7. Next to abstinence, the most effective protection against sexually transmitted diseases is proper condom use. Yet, some people still won't use condoms because:
   a. They're too embarrassed to buy them
   b. They trust their partner's health and assurances
   c. They do not take the risks seriously

8. The proper way to remove a latex condom from its package is:
   a. by tearing the packaging in half down the middle
   b. by opening it before you need it and placing it on a bedside table just in case

of length with a simple scissors. Simply trim back the pubic hair around the base of your penis. This exposes more of the shaft and can make you look an inch longer. Or, if you're feeling adventuresome, shave everything.

Stop Your Willy from Shrinking

The penis doesn't become significantly smaller with age, but it often looks that way. There's a pad of fat in front of the pubic bone, just above the base of the penis. It's there as a cushion for

c. by tearing off just the top of the foil package, being careful not to rip the condom

d. by using your teeth

9. The best way to put on a condom is:

a. place it on the head of the penis and unroll it all the way down to the base

b. remove it from the package, unroll it and pull it over the penis

c. remove it from package, inflate it and pull it over the penis like a sock

10. Next to a birth-control pill, the most effective means of preventing unwanted pregnancy is:

a. IUD

b. Sponge

c. Latex condom

d. Rhythm method

e. Hanging out with your grandparents

ANSWERS

1. (b) Latex condoms offer the best protection. Natural-membrane condoms, such as lambskin, are porous and may not stop sexually transmitted diseases.

2. (c) The shelf life of a properly stored, packaged condom is 5 years.

3. (b) The shelf life of a properly stored condom coated with spermicide is 3 years.

4. (c) Condoms should never be exposed to extreme heat or cold.

5. (b) Never use Vaseline or other oil-based lubricants, such as those that include petroleum jelly, mineral oil, vegetable oil, or cold cream. These can damage latex. Water or silicone-based lubricants are best.

6. (b) Carrying condoms in your wallet will damage them.

7. (c) Fifty-eight percent of respondents in a survey said they didn't believe they could be infected with HIV.

8. (c) The proper way to remove a condom from its package is to carefully tear off the top of the wrapper without damaging the condom.

9. (a) Place the condom on the head of the penis and gently roll it down the shaft. Do not pull it down tightly against the top of the penis. Leave a reservoir for semen.

10. (c) When properly used, especially in combination with a spermicide, condoms are 97 percent effective in preventing pregnancy.

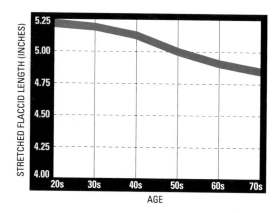

vigorous sex. But as you grow older and gain weight, this pad thickens from 1.8 centimeters to 3.1 centimeters. This can hide as much as 1.2 inches of the penis, making your onetime bratwurst look like a cocktail weenie. Unfortunately, sit-ups and crunches won't tighten the pad. The only defense is to stay lean.

Forget about Surgery

Unless you have a penis that's so short you have trouble urinating or inseminating a partner, you shouldn't even consider surgical, penis-lengthening procedures. We're talking about penises that are less than 3 inches long when erect.

Never Look Down

Looking down at your penis makes it seem smaller than it really is.

Exercise Control

Kegels are exercises that give some men stiffer erections and more control over ejaculation by strengthening the muscles of the pelvic floor. Here's the program: First, find the right muscles, the ones you use to stop your urine flow.

Then, squeeze and hold them tight. Half your contractions can be brief; hold the rest for 3 seconds. No one will now you're doing Kegels, so you can do them anywhere. Start with a few and work toward 200 a day. After doing Kegels for a few months, your pelvic muscles will be strong enough to prevent ejaculation if you squeeze them tight just before the urge to ejaculate reaches the point of no return.

Do Some Erector Sets

Here's a variation of the traditional Kegel exercise that's just as effective and a lot more fun. After your penis becomes erect, flex your pubococygeus (PC) muscles. You'll notice that your penis jumps slightly. Every time it does this, you're toning your PC muscles and improving your sex life. So why not build a few exercises around the jump? Have your partner hold a finger about an inch above the tip of your penis and try to flex hard enough to touch it 10 times. Or make your penis jump up and touch her nipples, clitoris, or tongue. Yachtsmen can attach a small flag and practice their semaphore. You can even do your Kegel lifts after you've entered your partner. Take it from us, women love it.

Switch If You Go Soft

Some prescription drugs, such as ulcer and blood-pressure medicines can cause temporary impotence. Even over-the-counter drugs such as Dramamine (for motion sickness) and Benadryl (for allergies) can have that unpleasant side effect. Sometimes it takes careful detective work to pinpoint the offending medication, but with the help of your doctor it's often possible to make substitutions.

Don't Do This One at the Gym

Move your hips around as if you were using a Hula-Hoop. We're serious. Do this for a few minutes each day, and you'll increase flexibility in your pelvis. You'll have more control over the thrusting of your penis during intercourse and improved circulation in the whole region. Ukulele and grass skirt optional.

Understand This

This is the paradox between sex and relationships: Men feel intimate as a result of being sexual; women feel sexual as a result of being intimate. It's the basis of the entire war between the sexes. If you can grasp the wisdom of these 18 words, you'll forever be blessed.

Remember You're in This Together

Couples who talked about themselves using the word "us" rather than "you" and "me" during the first year of their marriage had stronger, more satisfying unions when they were surveyed again in the third year.

Avoid a Valentine's Day Massacre

When it comes to buying Valentine's Day presents, most men think they know what they're doing, but you'd be surprised how easily Cupid's arrows can fall short of their mark. To help out, we've put together a little guide to February 14th gift giving:

Chocolate

What you see: A classic.

What she sees: A serious lack of imagination and 10 hours of aerobics.

Strategy: Skip it.

A professional massage

What you see: A way to pass the back-rub buck.

What she sees: A man who knows what a woman wants.

Strategy: Give it.

A romantic dinner for two at a French restaurant

What you see: $150 plus tax and tip.

What she sees: Candlelight, champagne, souffle . . . heaven.

Strategy: Charge it.

A slinky, red teddy from Victoria's Secret

What you see: The gift that keeps on giving.

What she sees: Soft. Silky. Just the right amount of sleaze.

Strategy: Get the right size.

Breakfast in bed

What you see: A dazzling display of your culinary prowess.

What she sees: Burnt toast.

Strategy: Cater it.

Those little candy hearts stamped with phrases like "Be mine" and "Luv you"

What you see: A boyish gesture of puppy love.

What she sees: Your love expressed on rock-hard lumps of corn syrup.

Strategy: Don't even think about it

A Hallmark card

What you see: A last-minute remedy for almost forgetting the holiday.

What she sees: Another guy.

Strategy: Don't bother.

A pair of tickets to the Knicks game

What you see: An offbeat present that she just might like.

What she sees: A thinly veiled attempt at giving yourself a present.

Strategy: Tape the game.

A dozen roses

What you see: An unoriginal gift that she'll love.

What she sees: An unoriginal gift that she loves.

Strategy: Buy two dozen.

Say This

The answer to the question "Am I getting too fat?" is always "No."

Keep Her Happy

It's really quite simple:

1. Stop watching the game.

2. Listen to what she's saying.

3. Repeat what she's just said.

4. Tell her that what she's said makes sense to you.

5. Resume watching the game.

Follow the Buddy Bylaw

Never screw a friend in order to screw a girl.

Be Her Best Friend

Concentrate as hard on the friendship part of your relationship as you do on the physical part. If you're intimate in conversation, you can bet she'll be intimate in bed.

Seduce Her with Clothes

Buying clothes for a woman is a classic win-win situation. Pick the right size and style and chances are she'll take you on the spot. If you're off by a bit, she'll reward you for your efforts tonight and return the outfit tomorrow.

Size her up: Rummage through her closet and find average sizes for her sweaters, belts, blouses, pants, and skirts. (Unlike with guys' clothes, these numbers have nothing to do with inches or other aspects of real life.) And look for brands. Women's clothing sizes vary depending on the manufacturer.

Spot the trends: List her favorite colors. Some women wear only neutrals—black, white, brown, khaki—while others prefer bright colors. Also, note if she prefers cotton, polyester/cotton blends, or silk.

Look for a personal shopper: Not in the closet, buddy, but once you get to the store if

---

REAL-LIFE SURVIVAL

SPOT A FAKE

Don't tell her you bought it from the street vendor. Just don't get ripped off.

Gold: Genuine 14-karat or 18-karat gold has a wheaty color, like your wedding ring or a Notre Dame football helmet. Bright yellow means gold-plated.

Watch: One way to tell a $1,500 Rolex from a $10 fake is to examine the second hand. It's genuine if it sweeps smoothly (like that of a classroom clock). Quartz impostors move incrementally.

you have her vital stats but you still need help. Most major department stores off the service free. Personal shoppers consider lifestyle, size, and color to make a sensible choice. Consider them your secret ally.

Buy Her Lingerie

The type of body your girl's got should dictate the kind of lingerie you're going to buy for her. In general:

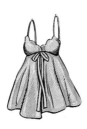

• A baby-doll nightie that comes down to just above the knee is good for all shapes.

• A bustier may be too much for a well-endowed woman: There's no need to gild the lily.

• A teddy is very difficult for most women to wear. If the woman in your life can audition to become a Spice Girl, go for it. Otherwise, buy one at your own risk or seek out some of the newer ones being made with stretchier laces and form-fitting microfibers.

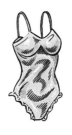

• Any woman looks good in a garter belt and stockings, because they really show off her stems. The question is, will she wear it? They tend to be uncomfortable for everyday use, so use them for show time only.

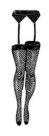

Create a Fantasy Box

Take an empty tissue box and make it your "fantasy box." Write five secret sexual desires on individual slips of paper, have your partner do the same, then deposit them in the box. (Hold off on the *ménage à trois* for a while.) Take turns drawing one whenever you make love.

Size Up Melons

What's a 36C? It's the average American bra size. Here's what it means: The number 36 refers to the bra's band size in inches. The letter C is how much breast fills the cup. To determine a bra size, find a tape measure, and then find a woman. Take the tape measure and put it directly above her bust at underarm level. If the result is an odd number, add an inch. That's the band size—the length of the strap that goes around the back. To figure the cup size, measure again, but this time right across the peaks. Subtract the band size from the new figure to get the difference in inches. Then consult this scale.

Difference in Inches	Cup Size	Produce Equivalent	Produce Weight
0	AAA	peanut	0 ounce
½	AA	kiwi	3 ounces
1	A	navel orange	7 ounces
2	B	mango	10 ounces
3	C	grapefruit	16 ounces
4	D	coconut	25 ounces
5	DD	cantaloupe	36 ounces

Mess with Her Head

The next time you hear "Not tonight, I have a headache," use your hands. No, not there. Give the poor woman a head and neck massage. By the time you've run through each step twice, she should feel better, and you should be able to reap the reward:

1. Have you partner lie with her head near the edge of the bed. You sit in a chair behind her. Gentle press your fingertips all over her scalp. This relaxes the muscles that contract during sleep.

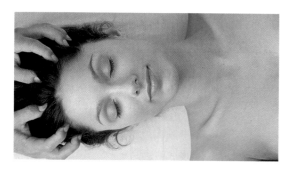

2. Have her turn her head to the left. While applying light pressure, slide your thumb down the right side of her neck from behind her ear to the tip of her shoulder. Then have her turn to the right and repeat this on her left side.

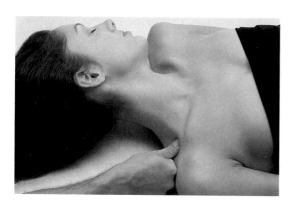

3. Pinch her upper right trapezius muscle (just above her shoulder, under her ear) with your thumb on top. Apply light pressure and gently pull the muscle toward you. Repeat on the left.

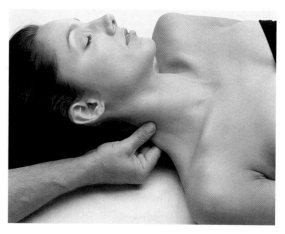

4. Have your partner turn her head to the right, and with your thumbs and forefinger gently knead the large muscle that runs down the side of her neck. (It's called the sternocleidomastoid, and it's worth 680 points in Scrabble.) Repeat this on the left side. You can also use this move to ease your own headache.

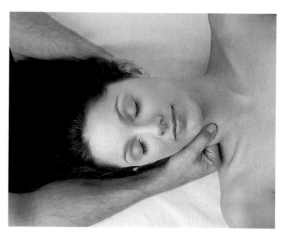

Rose to the Occasion

Men know flowers like women know brake fluid. That's why we're offering these bouquet-giving tips—so you don't put the wrong kind in her hands.

Situation	Best Flower		Why
First date	Sunflowers		They're informal, so she won't feel like you're putting a lot of pressure on her. Send them the morning after the first date.
A trip makes you miss something important like her birthday	Orchid plant		Women generally view long-lasting plants as thoughtful, which makes them a good comeback when she thinks you're not.
A milestone	Vase of Casablanca lilies		Women like them because they're one of the world's most impressive-looking flowers. Tip: Use a tissue to remove the rust-colored pistils; they'll stain your shirt or her dress.
After the fight	Anything but carnations		They're cheap, which is exactly the way you'll look if you try to make amends with these.
Secretary's Day	Potted African violet		A neutral plant expresses gratitude and accents her desk. Avoid roses, which roughly translate as "I want you right now, on the desk."
You pop the question	Red and white roses		She—and all of her friends—will admire the symbolism: red for love, white for eternity. Just like a Budweiser can.

BUILD HER A CASTLE

For sand castles of royal proportions, you have to dig deep. Most men use sand that's way too dry. So start by digging in the sand until you hit water. That's the stuff you want to work with.

Train for a Better Marriage

A relationship can be built just like a body in a gym. But it doesn't require that much sweat, specifically just 5 hours per week. Follow this training plan.

Exercise #1: Before saying goodbye to your partner in the morning, learn about one important thing that's happening in her life that day. This will break the "habit of inattention" that eventually turns couples into strangers. *Repetitions:* 2 minutes per day × 5 working days. *Time:* 10 minutes per week.

Exercise #2: Decompress after work by discussing the most stressful parts of your day. This will prevent job frustration from spilling over into your home life. When it's her turn to talk, resist the urge to give advice. Instead, be supportive and say you understand. *Repetitions:* 20 minutes per day × 5 working days. *Time:* 1 hour 40 minutes per week.

Exercise #3: Once a day, spontaneously tell your partner you appreciate something she's done or that you admire a certain quality in her. *Repetitions:* 5 minutes per day × 7 days. *Time:* 35 minutes per week.

Exercise #4: Show affection outside the bedroom by occasionally kissing or touching her. *Repetitions:* 5 minutes per day × 7 days. *Time:* 35 minutes per week.

Exercise #5: Plan a date once a week, just like when you were single. Go someplace, just the two of you, and get reacquainted with each other. *Repetitions/Time:* 2 hours, once a week.

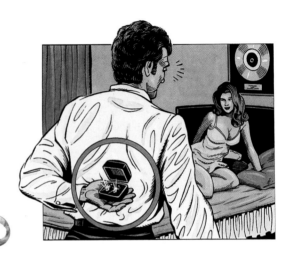

Give Her Presents of Mind

Earlier in the year, your wife might mention something she wants. Flip your calendar ahead to December and write down the gift idea. If you can remember to do this, you'll be sure to have a few presents come Christmas that will absolutely delight her.

Never Forget Your Anniversary

Have it engraved inside your wedding ring.

Buy a Great Last-Minute Gift

Here are some easy last-minute gifts.

• Stop at the drugstore. Buy a decorative gift bag and stuff it with as many bath products as you can find (bubble bath, sponge, shampoo, lotion). Attach a note that says, "Tonight, your body is in my hands." Flash your eyebrows, wink, and

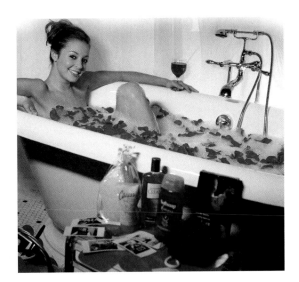

head for the bath. (She'll faint with pleasure, especially if you've cleaned the tub, too.)

• Go to the video store and rent the first movie you ever watched together in the theater. She'll be so touched you remember that she won't even notice that this gift cost you $2.99. Make popcorn, drink wine, and see if that old stretch-your-arm-around-her-shoulder trick still works.

• Pick her up after work, but don't tell her where you're going. Then take her on a tour of places that are special to the two of you—the bar where you had your first date, the park where you dropped the L-bomb, the parking lot where you dropped your virginity. At each spot, reminisce about your relationship. Memories are almost as good for her as ESPN Classics are for you.

Serve Her Breakfast in Bed

She was so very good to you last night. Thank her by rising early and preparing a memorable breakfast in bed.

• Comfort is most important. If possible, provide a shoulder bolster with armrests and a bed tray with legs. If not, use an ordinary serving tray (black provides a striking backdrop) and set it on a table at the side of the bed.

• Don't put flowers in a vase; it might spill. Instead, lay them flat on the tray: A single rose or a few wildflowers on sprigs of green will do.

• Use the best china and silver in the house (or a neighbor's house).

• Fold the newspaper and place it next to the tray.

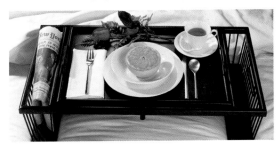

• Forget the bacon and eggs. It's ordinary, and you'll never keep it all warm. Halve a grapefruit and segment it with a knife so that the individual sections can easily be removed with a fork. Sprinkle with brown sugar. Broil for a few minutes to crystallize the top, and serve. It's deliciously sweet and sour.

• Coffee or tea? Her preference. Choose an exotic flavor, and fill the cup only halfway to reduce the risk of spills.

Keep Your Relationship Fresh

To keep a relationship fresh, tell the truth. If you don't tell the truth, then past feelings don't get resolved. Then you're continuously dealing with the same thing. The relationship gets old and boring, and it dies.

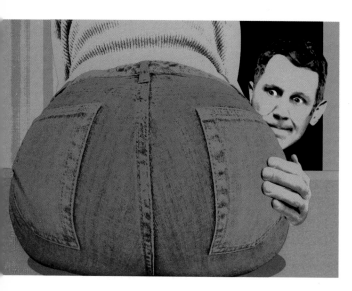

Get Her Rear in Gear

If your girl is putting on weight and it's changing her appearance, here's a relatively safe strategy: Say something like, "You know, honey, I'm gaining a few pounds, and I don't like how it looks. I'd like to start exercising more, and I'd like you to do it with me." Mind you, this flanking maneuver won't fool her one tiny bit, but it will help you look classy, supportive, and—most important—like you're not rejecting her. That way she's likely to get her backfield in motion.

Consult the *Men's Health* Baby Planner

Yes, the birth of a child is a wondrous thing. But so is the Indy 500. How do you make sure one joyous event doesn't prevent you from enjoying another? You have to plan, man. If you're hoping to have a child in the next year, here are some dates you should

heed. (To play it safe, give yourself a couple of weeks' leeway around each of these dates. Newborns don't always arrive on schedule.)

If you want to be free for next year's . . .	Don't have sex on or around . . .
Daytona 500	May 30
St. Patrick's Day	June 25
Final Four	July 9–11
Baseball opening day	July 11–17
Final round of the Masters	July 18
Indy 500	September 5
NBA Finals	September 12–18
World Series	January 23–February 5
Super Bowl	May 7

Get Out of Hot Water

The heat from a water bed can reduce your sperm count by 10 percent. That's not enough to affect the odds of conception for a man with a normal count. But if yours is already borderline (less than 20 million sperm per milliliter; a fertility specialist can test you), switch beds.

Beware the Accidental Vasectomy

Of the 250,000 men who undergo a hernia operation every year, 1,500 receive an unwanted bonus: a vasectomy. It's easy to harm small reproductive ducts or blood vessels while repairing a hernia near the spermatic cord. It's an even more frequent problem in children: Botched hernia operations sterilize about 5,000 boys every year. If you need a hernia repaired, choose a urological surgeon who regularly per-

RESCUE HER FROM A BURNING BUILDING

To save someone from a burning building, you'll have to master the "fireman's drag." Roll the victim onto her back. Next, get behind her, sit her up and cross her arms over her chest. Grabbing her right wrist with your left hand and her left wrist with your right, act like you're giving her a big hug—don't worry, she'll return it later—and lift her until she's a few feet off the floor. Now, drag her from the building. Doing it this way protects her head, neck, and spine.

forms hernia procedures, vasectomies, and vasectomy reversals. Tell your surgeon your concerns about fertility. If you had hernia surgery and you're having trouble getting your wife pregnant, see a urologist.

Check Your Fertility with a Mirror

The largest single cause of male infertility is easy to spot and easy to cure through microsurgery. Fifteen percent of all men—and about 30 percent of infertile men—suffer from *variocele,* or varicose veins of the testicles, a condition that elevates the temperature of the testes by as much as 4 degrees centigrade, an environment that makes sperms sluggish and misshapen. Inspect your scrotum with a mirror after a shower.

Be a Dad in 9 Months or Less

The best position for getting her pregnant is the modified missionary. Ready? You're on your knees, back upright; she's lying on her back, knees pulled to her chest, her hips nestled between your thighs. She can rest her feet on your chest. This not only allows for deep penetration, but her upward-turned vagina will also retain more sperm.

Drop Your Pants at Dawn

Your emotions make the timing highly individual, but technically, early morning is best. Male and female hormones peak between 5 and 9 A.M., maximizing both performance and pleasure. Incidentally, the best time to conceive a child is just before daylight when your testosterone levels are highest. This gives a boost to men with slow-moving sperm or low sperm counts.

Drive Away Fertility

A long commute may inhibit fertility. Researchers monitored scrotal temperatures (finally!) over the course of a long drive. After men had been behind the wheel for 2 hours, their scrotal temperatures had risen by 3 to 4 degrees. Higher temperatures often mean lower sperm counts. So if you're trying to become a dad, a warm welcome home from a long haul may not be your best shot.

DELIVER THE MALE

Want a baby boy? Try masturbating more often. Researchers found that Y-chromosome (male) sperm die after living in the testicles for more than a few days. If you don't release them regularly, more live X-chromosome (female) sperm will be waiting in your arsenal.

Have the Perfect Vasectomy

It's a seven-step process. Heed every single one.

1. Contemplate it. Talk it over with your mate for at least several months. Make certain this is what you want. Reversing the procedure is expensive, and even under the best of circumstances has only an 80 to 90 percent chance of success.

2. Find a smooth operator. Does your family doctor do vasectomies? If so, ask how many he does per year. Fifty or more is a good answer. Otherwise, ask him to suggest a urologist.

3. Inform your insurance company. Most will foot part of the bill.

4. Get cut on Friday. This way you can recuperate on the weekend.

5. Enlist a cheerleader. Ask if your partner can be in the operating room with you during the procedure. Hey, you were there when she gave birth, right?

6. Don't ignore complications. If you have swelling, bleeding, fever, or increasing pain, go back to the doctor immediately.

7. Practice safe sex. Use other means of birth control for at least the next 6 weeks, then take a semen sample to your doctor. Take in another a week later. If both are negative, you're sterile. Go home and go wild.

Don't Go Down If She's Pregnant

Expecting a child? If so, you may want to avoid performing oral sex on your wife until after she gives birth. Researchers discovered that streptococcus bacteria can be spread easily during sexual activity, particularly oral sex. While the bacteria is harmless to most adults, it can be deadly to infants—causing pneumonia, sepsis, and meningitis. It's still perfectly safe for her to satisfy you, however.

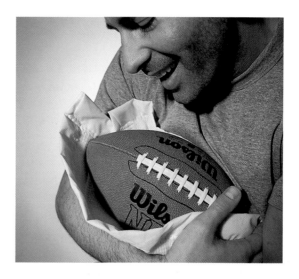

Score on Your Second Shot

Probably the biggest mistake couples trying to conceive make is to assume that a man's first ejaculation after abstaining from sex for a week or more is his best. Usually the *second* specimen is better, both in sperm count and motility. Make your first try 2 days before your partner starts ovulating and then go for the gold when she *is* ovulating.

Swear Off Intercourse

If you're unhappy with the quantity or quality of your sex life, make a rule: No intercourse for the next 4 to 8 weeks. But here's the thing: We're not saying no sex, we're saying no *intercourse*. No in-out, to use the technical term. That still leaves a vast array of erotic, sexual choices—from cuddling to cunnilingus—which the two of you can explore. You'll discover new ways to enjoy and give pleasure. Look out when the ban ends.

Get Your Touch Back

Married men tend to touch their wives only when they're looking for sex. That's a mistake. Men underestimate the power of nonsexual touch. Women who go to lawyers requesting divorce often talk about how their husbands no longer hold their hands or offer unsolicited kisses and back rubs—all the things that make women feel emotionally connected. Most of the marriages that fail could have been helped—if not saved—if the husbands had learned to be more affectionate.

Call a Bedroom Truce

Bed is the last place you should have prolonged conversations, sexual or otherwise, especially the airing of petty grievances. Some places must be sacred, safe spaces. You are never more naked or more vulnerable than when you're sleeping or making love. In fact, all financial, sexual, religious, or political discussions ought to take place elsewhere. Feelings, good or bad,

are often rooted strongly to a place, just as memories are to music. Let your bed be a vacation from conflict.

Save Your Marriage in 1 Week

It's simple. Just kiss your mate goodbye in the morning and hello at night. Therapists have seen patients make tremendous differences in their relationships in a short amount of time with simple gestures such as this.

Bring Home Flowers Every Wednesday

Couples fight most on Wednesdays and least on Thursdays. The reason: Wednesday is farthest from the weekend in both directions, making it the toughest day to get through. So Wednesday seems like an especially good day to leave job troubles at work and bring home flowers instead.

MAKE ANOTHER BRILLIANT SAVE

When your wife or girlfriend catches you staring at another woman, keep staring. Stare as if you're catatonic, and respond only when she pokes you in the shoulder three times. Act startled—like you've been awakened from a daydream—and say, "You know, I was just thinking about that wonderful weekend in the Poconos, and how much fun we had in that heart-shaped bathtub." Just like that, you'll be off the hook.

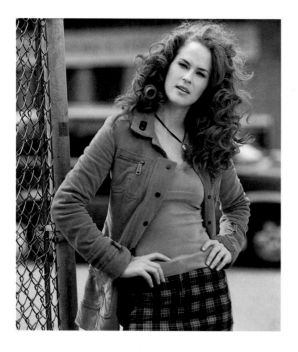

Stay Free of Her Wrath

If you're going to flirt with another woman, you'd be smart to wait until a couple of weeks after your wife's period. Women experience more intense feelings of jealousy during the first phase (day 1 to 14) of their menstrual cycles. So mentally consult her calendar before you grab lunch with Debra from data processing. If you make your wife crazy during her first phase, who knows what she'll do once PMS hits.

Teach Your Dog to Diffuse an Argument

Think of what you normally say to your wife when you're having a fight. Repeat this word or phrase every time you play ball with the dog. Eventually, when he hears it during an argument, he'll bring the ball and help defuse the altercation.

Never Try to Win an Argument

A common destroyer of marriages is seeing the relationship as a competition rather than a cooperation. When people see themselves as opponents rather than partners they may fight unfairly with violence, insults, or withdrawal, or they may fight fairly with logic, emotions, or excessively good manners. But they're trying to win, to be the "good" partner and prove that the other person is unworthy of them. Learn to resist doing that and, most important, apologize.

Remember That Boredom Afflicts the Boring

Lots of guys who cheat on their wives plead sexual boredom at home. And, often enough, a good case can be made. But if your sex life isn't everything you dreamed, make sure that you've given it everything you've got. Ask yourself how much ingenuity, improvisation, energy, joy, and lust you bring to the sheets.

REAL-LIFE SURVIVAL

EASE HER PMS

Lavender-scented candles and peppermint tea have been shown to help improve mood and promote relaxation in women with PMS.

See If Your Marriage Will Last

Answer true or false for each, then score yourself at the conclusion. If you're feeling brave, have your partner take the same test and see how you compare.

	T	F
1. I can list my partner's major aspirations and hopes in life.	T	F
2. I know my partner's current major worries.	T	F
3. I know the three most special times in my spouse's life.	T	F
4. I can easily list the three things I most admire about my partner.	T	F
5. I often touch or kiss my spouse affectionately.	T	F
6. Our sex life is generally satisfying.	T	F
7. I look forward to spending my free time with my partner.	T	F
8. My partner is one of my best friends.	T	F
9. My partner tells me when he or she has had a bad day.	T	F
10. I am genuinely interested in my spouse's opinion.	T	F
11. I usually learn a lot from my spouse even when we disagree.	T	F
12. I feel I have an important say when we make a decision.	T	F
13. I can admit that I am wrong.	T	F
14. Even when we disagree, we can maintain a sense of humor.	T	F
15. My spouse is good at soothing me when I get upset.	T	F
16. My partner and I are a good team.	T	F
17. When we argue, winning isn't my objective.	T	F
18. I accept that there are issues we will never resolve.	T	F
19. We share many similar values in our roles as husband and wife.	T	F
20. We share many happy memories.	T	F

Scoring. *13 or more true answers:* You have a solid relationship that will probably endure until both of you are toothless and incontinent. Fortunately, you'll still be so in love that neither of you will notice.

7 to 12 true answers: This is a pivotal time in your relationship. There are many strengths you can build upon, but there are also some weaknesses that need tending. It's time to put down that remote and get away for the weekend.

6 or fewer true answers: You may be in danger of divorce. If this scares you, you probably still value the relationship enough to try to save it. Honest talk is needed. But if that's not possible, see a therapist.

N E V E R   A R G U E   A B O U T   M O N E Y   A G A I N

To avoid marital money problems, view yourself as a financial team. Decide what's important to both of you (home, kids, college, retirement), and open a joint account to manage these areas. Deposit 80 percent of both paychecks there. Then, to keep each of you happy and to prevent arguments about "frivolous" spending, open two individual accounts. Agree that the remaining 20 percent each of you deposits every month can be spent however the earner wants. No questions asked.

Apologize Like This

Sincere apologies are direct and unequivocal. Any apology that begins with a long oration on why you did what you did (the dog begged for it) or why you never showed up (the train missed the station) or what you really meant when you said she looked like she'd gained 30 pounds (you thought the weight looked good on her) is not an apology at all. It's a defense of yourself.

Run a Precheat Check

When you recognize you're interested in another woman, figure out why. What's attractive about her is probably what was attractive about your wife when you first met her. Get the missus to fill the void.

Predict If She'll Be True

If you want to see where a woman's head and heart are when it comes to adultery, ask her what she thought of the heroine in *The Bridges of Madison County*. If she loves the book or movie and feels the heroine was justified in cheating, you may want to start looking for another woman.

Let Her Be the Judge

If you're not sure whether something was cheating, ask your wife. If she thinks it's cheating, it's cheating. If the thought of telling her is enough to give you a slight facial tic, that alone should tell you that you crossed a line.

Find Out If She's Cheating

Here are six ways to tell:

• Watch for excessive mileage on her vehicle.

• Evaluate your sex life. (If she's no longer interested in it at home, she's probably getting it elsewhere.)

• Check her clothes and hair for the scent of male cologne.

• Monitor your credit-card accounts for unusual charges or purchases that never materialize at home.

• Look for excessive cell-phone charges. (It's the easiest way to make a clandestine call.)

• Send her flowers at work without your name on them and see if she mentions them to you. (If not, she probably has another beau.)

Assess Your Relationship

If you're in a bad relationship (but not married), ask yourself these three questions:

1. Is the sex good and plentiful?

2. Do you have similar values regarding money?

3. Could you handle her crazy mood swings for the rest of your life?

Two no's—say goodbye.

Work Your Wedding Band Free

Why you want to get it off is your business, but if it's stuck, the best time to disband is in the morning, when your body is most dehydrated. Start by lubricating your finger with olive oil, butter, or hand lotion. Don't tug on the ring or try to pry it off with your teeth. That only makes the skin bunch up at the knuckle. Pull your knuckle skin back and work the ring over the area a little at a time.

End a 1-Night Stand

Don't just grab your stuff and leave while she's still sleeping. A man faces the music, even if it's "Taps." Here's the proper way to split.

Let her speak first. You may like what you hear. There's a chance she thought of you as just a sex object, too. If that's the case, you're off the hook. Shake her hand and call it quits.

Listen. If you sense that there may be bad blood, let her vent. Listening shows her you're

---

DECIPHER YOUR SEX DREAMS
Skip the couch and psychologist. Check out our dream translator.

• *Cheating dreams.* Those that involve a woman other than your wife or steady girlfriend are no cause for guilt. They help you explore the consequences without having to make the mistakes.

• *Dreams about sex with an unattractive person.* This is a common dream for younger men. It's a way of exploring what the qualities of a proper mate are and whether you can relate to someone who looks unappealing.

• *Homosexual dreams.* Sexual encounters in dreams are often metaphors for unrelated feelings. If you've had recent difficulty in a relationship with a woman, for example, a homosexual dream may actually be a way of comforting yourself. You, as a man, understand how guys think.

• *Frustration dreams.* Dreams in which sex is imminent but you never quite close the deal are often about other frustrating aspects of your life. Anxieties about not getting a new work project off the ground can manifest themselves this way.

• *Incestuous dreams.* They don't represent some deep-seated perversion. These dreams can occur when you're not doing well in dating or your relationships. By seeking out a family member, you're finding comfort in someone with whom there's no fear of rejection.

GET RID OF A LIPSTICK STAIN

If you get lipstick on your collar and it's not your wife's shade, spray the spot with hair spray or dab it with rubbing alcohol. Let it sit for a minute or two, then wipe it carefully with a cloth. Or place a piece of masking tape over the stain, then yank it off. If that doesn't work, put the tape over your chest hair and do the same thing—maybe then you'll wise up.

willing to take responsibility for last night. She wants to leave the situation feeling good about herself, so be honest about both the pleasures and the limitations of what you shared, so she can, too.

Be honest. An out-the-door "I'll call you" may get you home quicker, but if you don't mean it, you just prolong her anxiety. Be gracious and complimentary, but be assertive that there is no relationship and therefore no "next time" to discuss. That means not taking her number (or proffering yours), and saying this: "I had a nice time, but you and I will not work out." Giving her the truth may be tough, but if you can't handle it, you shouldn't have been handling her.

End a Relationship Like a Man

Unless absolutely necessary, never end a relationship over the phone. (Faxes, letters, and e-mails are also for cowards.) Be a man and tell her eye-to-eye. But if she might claw out that eye, break up in a public place—say, a Mexican restaurant during Cinco de Mayo. It's far from perfect, but it should help stifle her reaction.

Move Up If You Split Up

After a divorce, avoid the temptation to economize by moving into a cheap apartment. In fact, if it's at all possible, keep the same quality of housing you've been accustomed to or improve it a bit. Research shows that men who remain home-owners or who at least maintain an equivalent residence after a breakup feel less stressed and depressed than recently divorced men who "moved down" from a good-size house to a rented apartment or to a lower-quality neighborhood.

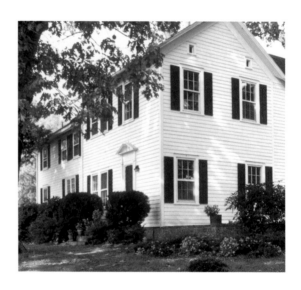

Hire a Mediator Instead of a Lawyer

If you're getting divorced, we're sorry she betrayed you. But if you can convince your soon-to-be ex to agree to use a mediator instead of a lawyer to work out the details, you'll save at least $5,000 and lots of suffering. Look in the yellow pages under "Divorce mediation" or contact the local bar association. And once the nice, civil discussions begin, float the idea of having most of any payments you'll make take the form of alimony, which is tax deductible, rather than child support, which isn't.

Know the 5 Stages of Divorce

There are five stages that men go through when dealing with divorce. The first stage is *denial/shock*. You find men saying, "No, this isn't really happening, we're going to get back together"—even if they initiated the divorce. The next phase is *anger*. Men displace anger in every direction: at their ex-wives, the legal system, friends. They've been operating all these years under the illusion that they are in control, the head of the household, and all of a sudden they're not. Following anger comes the *bargaining* phase, where the man tries to negotiate with whoever has the power—usually the ex-wife. Then comes the *depression* phase. This is usually a time when all the emotional and physical symptoms of divorce come home to roost. There's a lot of grief, sadness, and loneliness. But what a lot of men don't realize is that this ruminating, this depression over the loss of the relationship, is all part of the grieving process—it needs to happen. Only then will the last phase occur: *acceptance*. During this period, the man's focus shifts from looking back at the past to looking forward—he realizes there is life after divorce, and he starts socializing once again.

4

EXERCISE

and

FITNESS

As you're reading this, millions of Americans are sweating on treadmills, pedaling circles around neighborhoods, grunting out situps, or doing a multitude of other tortuous things to get in shape. We should honor them—our poor bastard brothers—with a moment of silence, because the majority are destined to fail. Like Blockbuster, gyms make most of their money not on what they actually rent, but on their members not being diligent about returns. There has never been more knowledge about fitness, more incentive to practice it, more alternatives for doing it, yet our society continues to grow more out of breath.

Here's the predicament: We're a get-things-done culture. Whether it's work or working out, we want to get in and get out. We want the express lane to everything. But fitness isn't like that. If you're going to be successful at it, you have to make fitness a part of your life rather than an interruption to it. For example, one of the most popular gyms in our area is located in a huge shopping mall. The other day we watched a guy circle the parking lot for 5 entire minutes—we know, we timed him—searching for a nearby spot. Even though he could have easily parked farther away and walked, he never thought to do it. Being active isn't a part of his life; it's an interruption to it. And as a result, we'd be willing to wager his membership will eventually lapse.

Another thing: Somewhere along the way what all of us used to do naturally as kids somehow got twisted. Play became working out. Games became competitions. Running and biking and swimming became training. Sweatshirts became high-performance wicking mid-layers. Sneakers became $175 Nike Air Jordan XVIII. Timelessness became sports watches, heart-rate monitors, and calorie counters. Coaches became exercise physiologists. Smiles became grimaces. And fun? Well, fun is still struggling to make the transition. And that's the other part of the problem. The next time you're at a gym or in the park, count the number of smiles on faces of the people you see exercising. We bet it'll be less than 10 percent.

Whether you're currently in an exercise program or considering starting one, it's time to revaluate just what the hell you're doing. First, if you're going to get it right this time, you need to approach this with a child's mind. Pick an activity

you really enjoy, something you can lose yourself in, an adult form of play. Then make it your chief way of getting in shape. Second, strive to become more active rather than more fit. It's a subtle yet startling mind shift that's less intimidating, more achievable, and even less stressful. Park in the far spot, take the stairs, ride your bike to work, and cut the grass instead of hiring a service. Get the idea?

Then, finally, peruse the 234 tips on the following pages. They were plucked from the *Men's Health* knowledge vault because each one is especially creative, motivational, and effective. Everything you need to get in shape is right here.

Now who wants to go play?

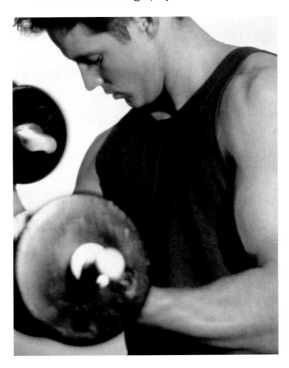

Put It in Perspective

If you are currently sedentary and begin a regular exercise program, you'll do as much good for your heart as a smoker who quits a pack-a-day habit.

Exercise Yourself into Bed

The more fit you become as a result of exercise, the more sex you'll have and the better it will be.

Ask Your Wife to Join You

Exercise programs are better followed when working out with your spouse. Nearly half of men who exercise alone quit their programs after one year, but two-thirds of those who exercise with their wives stick it out.

Make Exercise a Habit

Try to work out on the same days, at the same time. That will solidify your sense that this is a firmly scheduled activity, not an option. Eventually, the routine will become ingrained and if you skip it, you just won't feel right.

Tell Everyone You're Training

Nothing firms up a commitment like going public. Tell everyone at work that you're going to go to the gym every lunch hour. If you don't go, you'll lose face. Plus, everyone will ask you how the workouts are going. It's positive reinforcement.

Test Yourself Often

Every 4 weeks, measure a variable—waist size, body fat, bench press—that equates to your end goal. It'll show you the tangible results of your training. And that translates into motivation.

Measure Your Body Fat

You can get a rough estimate of your body fat level by giving yourself a skin-fold test. It won't be as accurate as having the measurement done by a professional, but it'll tell you if your fat level is higher than it should be. Here's what to do:

1. Find a millimeter ruler, and take off your shirt.

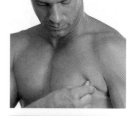

2. Pinch a diagonal fold of skin at your chest, halfway between your shoulder crease and nipple. Measure the thickness of the fold in millimeters.

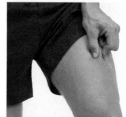

3. Pinch a vertical fold of skin at the front of your thigh, halfway between your hip and knee, and measure that one, too.

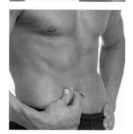

4. Pinch a vertical fold of skin at your abdomen, about an inch to the side of your belly button, and measure that.

5. Add all three measurements together and see the adjacent chart. A measurement of more than 20 percent could indicate an elevated health risk.

Total (mm)	Body Fat (%)
8–19	2–4
20–34	5–9
35–67	10–20
68–85	21–24
86–100	25–28

Join a Nearby Gym

If you're looking to join a gym, find one within 15 minutes of home. Any farther away than that and your chance of sticking to an exercise routine slides considerably. It'll be just too much of a hassle to visit.

Forget Something at the Gym

Make it a point to leave something in your locker or with your gym partner that you can't be without for long. This forces you to go to the gym whether you feel like exercising or not. Once there, you'll be more inclined to work out.

Exercise in the A.M.

Most people are so busy that if they don't exercise in the morning, before their day begins, they don't exercise at all. Make an extra effort to get out of a bed early enough to get a workout in.

Work Out at This Time

If you're able to discipline yourself to do it, physically the best time for exercise is 4 to 5 P.M. Think of it as your power hour. Not only do people generally feel good at this time of day, but body temperature also peaks. Even you handshake is firmest. Muscles are warm and, since they've had a full day to stretch after lying inert all night, flexible. Fine motor skills are high, too.

Schedule an Exercise Meeting

If you're so busy with work that you have trouble finding time to train, schedule exercise meetings. Arrange workout sessions with fellow employees or clients, when possible, in place of normal meetings and business lunches. It's a smart way to multitask.

Never Miss Another Workout

A trainer will charge you for an exercise session if you cancel without notice. Treat yourself the same way. Pay a spouse or friend $5 if you miss a scheduled workout. Or take the opposite tack: Pay yourself for every session you attend. Put the money in a fund for a new set of golf clubs, say, or those calf implants you've been eyeing.

Use a Point System

Track your exercise by assigning a point value to every fitness activity—for example, 1 point for running 1 mile, biking 3 miles, swimming 1/4 mile, or lifting weights for 10 minutes. Set a weekly and monthly point total goal. Keeping track of exercise this way makes it easier to recognize when you're falling short of your goals.

Work Out the Fatigue

No matter how tired you are, exercise will make you feel better. Taking those first few steps after a grueling day is tough, but study after study has shown that working out raises your energy level rather than depletes it.

Baby Your Muscles

Fathers often use their newborns as an excuse for exercising less. But you can use your baby in playful, creative ways that'll help you exercise more. For instance, hold the kid while doing squats, put him on your chest for crunches, and carry him on your back while hiking and doing pushups. It's a natural form of progressive resistance training that'll make you stronger as junior grows. Plus, the baby will love it.

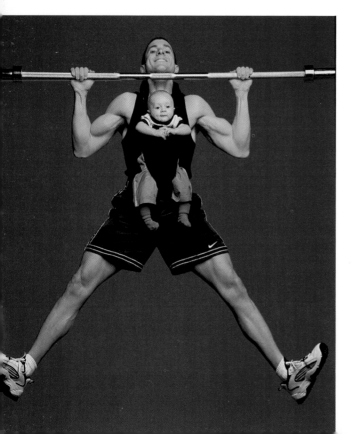

Sweat Profusely, Sweat Proudly

How easily you sweat is a good indication of how fit you are. Regular exercise teaches the body to drench itself easily and early for purposes of cooling. It's the guy with the red face and the dry body who has some more conditioning to do.

Step on the Sweat Scale

To calculate how much fluid you've lost while training, weigh yourself before and after a workout. Every pound you lose is a pint of water you need to replace.

Exercise Your Mind First

The technique is called visualization. When you imagine yourself exercising before you actually begin working out, you get tangible muscle-building benefits as well as better performance. There's evidence that this type of mental preparation may have some direct impact on the nerves, effectively priming the muscles needed for a specific task. Some studies have measured a 30 percent contraction in the biceps of test subjects who simply envisioned flexing the muscles.

Buy the Treadmill When . . .

Too many guys buy exercise equipment for the wrong reason. They decide they need to start working out then purchase an expensive gizmo. That's backward—like buying a car because you want to learn to drive. If you're pondering such a purchase, ask yourself this question. Do I exercise now? If the answer is no, start exercising first—walking, running, or cycling. A

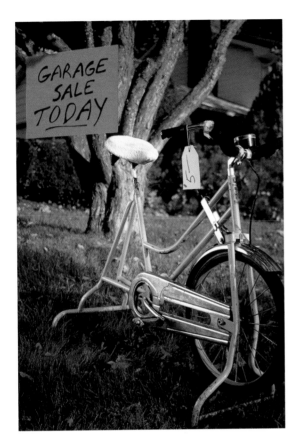

home-exercise machine should be a complement to your regimen, never the focus of it.
Otherwise, you'll be on the treadmill to
boredom and frustration.

Switch Sports in Winter

Because of the weather, the holidays, and reduced daylight, winter is the most challenging
time of year to maintain an exercise program. So
quit. If you've been running or cycling all
summer, switch to a different activity, like weight
training, swimming, or even a martial art. The
change of pace will renew your commitment and
help make exercise fresh and fun again.

Take Honey before a Workout

Honey is a cheap alternative to pre-exercise
sports drinks and carbohydrate gels. Researchers gave people about 3 tablespoons of
honey just before their workouts. Turns out
that nature's carbohydrate gel was just as good
a source of energy as commercially available
gels and sports drinks. You'd have to slug
about a liter of a sports drink to get the same
effect you get with the honey.

Mint Some New Muscle

Smelling peppermint boosts exercise performance levels. The scent alters your perception
of how hard you're working, which makes
workouts seem less strenuous, slower-paced
and easier to complete. Any minty smell should
work, including the scent of gum.

Kick In Those After-Burners

For a jolt of energy late in an event, carry a small
water bottle or plastic flask with defizzed Coke or
strong, sweet coffee. The sugar and caffeine will
give you a rocket-like lift when you need it most.

Get a Boost from Joe

Caffeine boosts endurance by delaying fatigue.
Research shows that when consumed an hour before an endurance event, three or four cups of
coffee (about 400 milligrams of caffeine) can help
athletes run or cycle up to 20 minutes longer than
their caffeine-free competitors. Daily caffeine
users should abstain from caffeine for 4 days
prior to the athletic event to get the same kick.

If you're not a regular coffee-drinker, be
careful, it could upset your stomach. Experiment in training first.

Drink before You're Thirsty

Once you feel thirsty, you've already lost 1 to 2 percent of the fluid in your body. When you hit the 3 percent mark, you'll start to notice a decline in physical performance.

Shower before Working Out

Hot water warms up your muscles enough to loosen them for exercise.

Put Sex before Sports

As long as it doesn't keep you up all night, there's a tremendous benefit to sex before an athletic event. There's probably no better natural anti-anxiety drug available.

Two-Time Your Workouts

If you can spare the time, do two shorter workouts rather than one longer one. Splitting your exercise session like this enhances what's known as the "afterburn effect." You already know that you burn calories when exercising, but what you might not realize is that exercise stimulates the body to continue burning calories for several hours afterward. Whether you're back at your desk or flat on your couch, you're combusting more calories at that moment than you would have if you hadn't exercised. Doing a second exercise session later gives you this afterburn effect twice in one day.

Know the Better Sequence

One of the oldest debates in the gym—right up there with whether women wear those thongs for personal pleasure or for athletic function—is the question of whether you should do your aerobic exercise before or after you do your weight lifting.

To find an answer, we hooked a fit, healthy guy up to equipment that measures calorie expenditure and reveals how many of those calories come from fat. We had him do identical combinations of aerobics and strength training on two different days, once doing aerobics first, once hitting the weights first. The weight

---

WIN AT ARM WRESTLING

1. *Grip high.* By getting a high grip on your opponent's thumb, you automatically increase your leverage and your chances of winning.

2. *Stay close.* Always keep the distance between your hand and body as short as possible, because the closer you are, the more leverage you get.

3. *Start fast.* Most arm-wrestling matches are over in less than 10 seconds, and usually the one who makes the first strong move wins. So hit hard and keep pulling.

BE A BETTER DART-THROWER

1. *Loosen your grip.* Hold the dart like you would hold a small bird.

2. *Keep both eyes open.* Closing one eye will throw off your depth perception.

3. *Push, don't throw.* Start with the dart at the side of your head just in front of your eye, then moving only your elbow, push it toward the board. Never pull the dart back behind your field of vision. You should be able to see the dart at all times.

workout consisted of 15 sets; the aerobic workout was 20 minutes.

Here are the results:

Sequence	Total Calories Burned	Fat Calories Burned
Weights, then aerobics	371	107
Aerobics, then weights	346	66

Pump It Out to Pump It Up

You can increase the strength of your heart with activities that force it to pump blood to distant parts of the body (and no, sex is not one of them). For example, cycling is considered a good "heart sport" because vast amounts of oxygenated blood are required to fuel the large muscles of the legs and buttocks. Cross-country skiing and rowing demand constant delivery of fresh blood to working muscles in the legs *and* arms.

Forget about These Exercise Myths

They're old, they're pervasive, and they're wrong. Here's why:

1. *It's supposed to be fun.* Sometimes it is, sometimes it isn't. Fun really isn't the point. The point is how good you feel *after* you've put your body through its paces.

2. *Crunches flatten your belly.* They'll tone your stomach muscles, but they won't do much to reduce any fat that covers those muscles. You can't spot-reduce with exercise; if you could, people who chew gum a lot would have thin faces.

3. *You'll lose weight.* The scale is not a good measure of how well your exercise program is working. If you lift weights, for example, you'll lose flab; but because you're losing fat tissue and replacing it with denser, heavier muscle tissue, your weight may stay the same. The important thing is, you'll look better.

4. *When you stop, muscle turns to fat.* Hard muscles may degenerate into soft muscles, but they won't turn into fat. Muscle cells and fat cells are two completely different tissues and neither can ever turn into the other.

5. *No pain, no gain.* The reality is: ignore pain, no brain. You can get very fit without feeling

any serious discomfort, so don't strain when you train. If it hurts, stop it.

Get Older, Get Stronger

The closer you get to the half-century mark, the more your focus should shift toward strength training. If you don't do any resistance exercise, you'll lose about 10 percent of your muscle mass between ages 25 and 50. Between 50 and 80, you lose another 35 percent. Everyone should be lifting weights by midlife. However, don't stop your cardiovascular exercise, because that will help ward off heart disease.

Ditch the Weight Belt

Don't train with a weight belt. Over time, regular training in a weight belt actually weakens your abdominal and lower-back muscles. Wear it only when attempting maximal lifts in such exercises as squats, deadlifts, and overhead presses.

Multiply Your Muscles

Follow this simple formula to build more muscle: Multiply the amount of weight you lift for a particular exercise by the total number of times you lift it. Try to increase that number every workout by lifting heavier weights, increasing your repetitions, or doing more sets.

Extend Your Strength Range

When weight lifting, most guys have too short a strength range. They might do a set of bench presses at 135 pounds, a second set at 145, and a final set at 155. For a greater challenge—and faster strength gains—start with a very light set—say, 115 pounds—followed by a moderate set (145) and a very challenging set (175). This loads the muscle more efficiently; yet since you're starting light, you're less likely to be injured.

Calculate Your Max

To tell how much weight you can lift in any one exercise without herniating yourself, use some math. Add 33 percent to the weight you can do for 10 repetitions. If you consistently bench 150 pounds, for instance, your max should be about 200.

Get a Total Body Workout in 10 Minutes

The "four-count squat thrust" works many major muscle groups at the same time. To do it, stand with your feet shoulder-width apart. Quickly drop to a squat, putting your hands on the floor in front of you so that your knees are touching your chest (count one). With your hands still on the floor, shoot your legs to the rear so you're in a pushup position (count two). Draw your knees back to your chest (count three), then explosively push off (count four). Perform with continuous motion, each step leading directly into the next. Three sets of 20 will wind you. This move works the chest, shoulders, arms, legs, buttocks and lower back.

ASK SOMEONE TO SCREAM AT YOU

You'll be able to lift 5 to 8 percent more weight if you receive verbal encouragement from a spotter. That could be the difference between nailing a 200-pound and a 215-pound bench press.

Be a Disc Jockey

The simple backhand delivery—the way we all learned to throw a Frisbee—is for amateurs. If you want to throw like a pro, with lots of power, you have to learn the sidearm delivery.

1. Place your index and middle fingers on the underside of the disc against the rim, thumb on top. This is the two-finger grip.

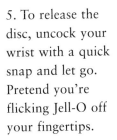

2. Make sure the rim of the disc makes contact with the web of skin between your thumb and index finger. Press down with

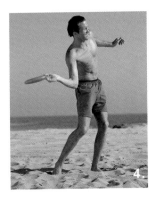

your thumb so the grip is firm, but comfortable. Curl your last two fingers against your palm.

3. Stand with your feet shoulder-width apart. Your body should be perpendicular to your target. As you bring back your throwing arm, shift most of your weight to your rear foot. Cock your wrist with the disc high behind you.

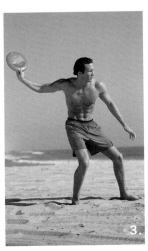

4. Begin to shift your weight to your front foot, turning your hips and then upper body. Swing your throwing arm forward. Keep your elbow close to your body throughout the delivery.

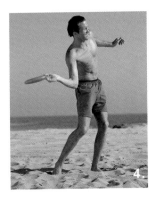

5. To release the disc, uncock your wrist with a quick snap and let go. Pretend you're flicking Jell-O off your fingertips.

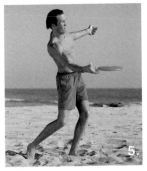

6. For a cool catch, as the disc descends, tip it to make it spin flat, then let it settle on your fingernail. Move your hand in slow circles in the direction of the spin to keep it centered.

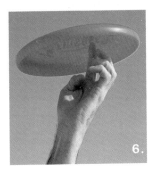

Count Backward

Here's a trick to make your workout feel faster. When counting repetitions, start at the target number and work backward. When you near the end of the set, you'll be thinking about how many you have left instead of how many you've done.

Burn Yourself Completely Out

Partial repetitions or "burns" consist of pressing a weight only halfway up. You do them at the end of your usual set when you'd ordinarily be too tired to do any additional full reps. Burns allow you to go beyond what you would normally do and place a little more overload on the muscles. Here's how to do them:

Let's say you've bench-pressed a weight 10 times, and you can't do it even one more time. Instead of simply letting the weight down and moving on to the next exercise, slowly lower it just a few inches. Then raise it back up to the fully extended position. Often you can squeeze out two or three additional half-reps before your muscles are completely fatigued.

BLOW THE WEIGHT UP

One of the biggest mistakes guys make when they're lifting weight is not breathing. As a rule, exhale during the strenuous parts of each lift and inhale through your nose as you lower the weight. You won't be as red-faced.

Shore Up Your Weak Side

Training the weaker side of your body to carry its share of the weight is one of the most effective ways to increase overall strength. To see how your left and right sides compare, test yourself with exercises that work each side individually: biceps curls, single-arm rows for the back, incline dumbbell bench presses for the chest, and overhead presses for the shoulders. For the lower-body, try single leg-presses, leg curls, and leg extensions. Do each exercise with a moderate weight and compare how many repetitions it takes each side to reach fatigue. Then use these exercises in your regular workout and load up your weak side. If your weak side is only a few reps short, add reps to that side's set. But if it's 8 to 10 reps short, do the same number of repetitions but use 5 to 10 pounds more weight on the weak side.

Make a One-Sided Agreement

When you're lifting weights and you're not getting results as fast as you'd like, give one of your arms a rest. Using a trick that rehabilitation specialists call "cross-education," you may be able to build bigger muscles quicker by lifting with one side of your body one day and the other side the next. More than a century ago, Yale researchers found that if you exercised, say, your right index finger, your left one would also get stronger. They don't exactly know what causes the muscle growth, but they found that cross-education exploits the spinal-cord reflex and leads to faster strength gains than conventional training. By exercising alternating sides, you can lift every day without taking a day off to rest. Using dumbbells and machines, follow your routine using only your right arm and right leg. Next day, repeat using your left side, and so on. Be sure to use lighter than normal weights so you're not lifting off balance.

Leave Your Glasses in the Locker

If you find yourself wasting a lot of time at the gym—sitting around enjoying the sights rather than working out—then here's a simple way to minimize the distractions: Don't wear your glasses or contacts. If you're not too blind without them, it'll do wonders for your work ethic.

Surf Past the Gadgets

Don't buy fitness equipment advertised on TV. Virtually every infomercial gadget that the editors of *Men's Health* have checked out over the years is worthless. Buy free weights or good running shoes. And use them.

Make Quality the Goal

The main reason people in their 40s and 50s should train isn't to increase the *length* of their lives, but rather to increase the *quality* of their lives.

Do the Full-Body Dumbbell Workout

There are more than 200 exercises you can do with dumbbells. We asked our fitness experts to help us select the 12 exercises that do the most good. Here's an at-home muscle-building plan for every part of you:

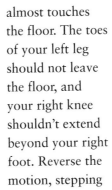

Quadriceps/Hamstrings: *Lunge.* Standing with your back and neck straight and your feet 9 inches apart, grasp a dumbbell in each hand with your palms facing in. Keeping the weights at your sides, take a large step forward with your right foot, then bring your left knee down until it

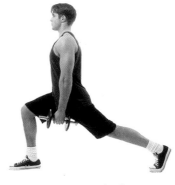

almost touches the floor. The toes of your left leg should not leave the floor, and your right knee shouldn't extend beyond your right foot. Reverse the motion, stepping back to the starting position. Repeat the lunge with your left leg, inhaling as you lunge and exhaling as you return. Do 10 to 12 repetitions with each leg.

Calves: *Calf Raise.* Holding a dumbbell at your left side with your palm facing in, step up onto a secure platform high enough so that your heels hang off the edge and your weight is supported by the balls of your feet. Place your right hand against the wall or on a railing for support. Tuck your right foot behind your left heel. Now, with both your head and your back straight, inhale

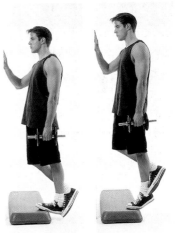

as you rise up on the toes of your left foot. Hold the position for a moment, then exhale as you return to the starting position. Do 15 repetitions, place the dumbbell at your right side, then perform the exercise using your right leg.

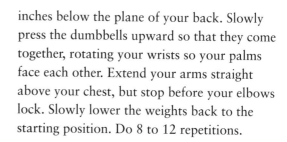

inches below the plane of your back. Slowly press the dumbbells upward so that they come together, rotating your wrists so your palms face each other. Extend your arms straight above your chest, but stop before your elbows lock. Slowly lower the weights back to the starting position. Do 8 to 12 repetitions.

Obliques: *Side Bend.* To work the muscles on the sides of your abdomen, stand with your back straight and your feet shoulder-width apart. Hold a dumbbell in your right hand and place your left hand on your waist. Now, slowly bend to the right as far as possible, return to the starting position, and then bend to the left. Do 20 repetitions before switching the weight to your left hand and re-peating. Once you're able to do this comfortably for two or three sets, add 5 pounds to the weight.

Chest: *Bench Press.* Lie face up on an exercise bench, knees bent and feet flat on the floor. Hold the dumbbells on each side of your chest, palms facing your feet. Your elbows should be pointing down, a few

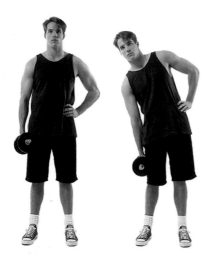

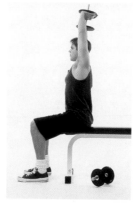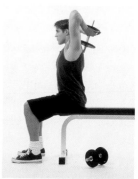

Triceps: *Seated Triceps Extension.* Sitting on a chair or an exercise bench with your back straight, place your feet firmly on the floor and grasp a single dumbbell with both hands. Raise the weight above your head, rotating it so it is vertical and the top plate rests comfortably on the palms of your hands, thumbs around the handle. This is the starting position. Now slowly lower the weight behind your head until your forearms touch your biceps. Return to the starting position. Do 8 to 12 repetitions.

Biceps: *Concentration Curl.* Sit on an exercise bench or a chair with your knees slightly wider than shoulder-width apart and your feet flat on the floor. Grasp a dumbbell with your right hand, palm up, and rest your upper right arm against your inner right thigh. Now, placing your left hand on your left knee for

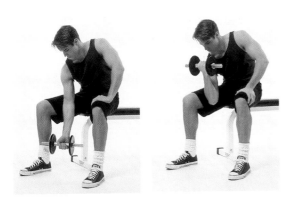

Shoulders/Neck/Back: *Standing Upright Row.* In a standing position, grasp a pair of dumbbells and hold them against the front of your legs with your thumbs pointing toward each other. Now lift the weights, keeping them close to your body, until they are just below your chin. Hold for 2 seconds, then slowly lower the weights back to the starting position. Perform 8 to 12 repetitions.

support, curl the dumbbell up toward your shoulder, keeping your upper right arm and elbow tucked against your inner thigh at all times. Do 8 to 12 repetitions, then switch to the opposite side and repeat the exercise with your left arm.

Buttocks/Thighs/Lower Back: *Deadlift.* Standing with your feet about 16 inches apart, place a dumbbell on the floor near the outside of each foot. Bend down and grab the dumbbells, palms facing in. Keep your knees bent, your back straight and your head up. With your elbows locked, inhale as your slowly straighten up. Exhale as your return the weights to the floor. Use light weights at first—10 to 20 pounds—and do 10 to 15 comfortable repetitions.

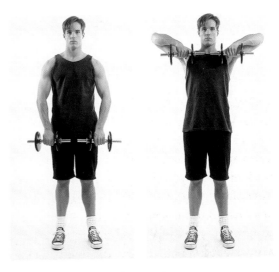

Back and Chest: *Pullover.* Lie face up on an exercise bench so the top half of your head extends past the end of the bench. Your feet should be flat on the floor. Hold a single dumbbell above your chest so it's vertical and the top plate rests comfortably on the palms of your hands, thumbs around the handle. This is the starting position. Slowly lower the weight behind your head in a semicircular motion, bringing it as far down as you can without strain. Hold for a second, then raise the weight to the starting position. Do 8 to 12 repetitions.

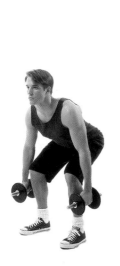
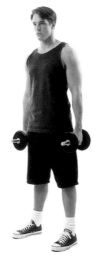

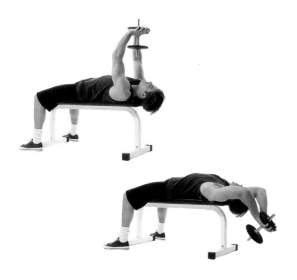

Abdominals: *Crunch*. Lie on your back on the floor with your knees bent and your calves draped over an exercise bench. Fold your arms comfortably across your chest, your fingertips lightly touching your shoulders and your elbows tucked against your body. Keeping your head tucked slightly in toward your chest, slowly curl your upper body up toward your legs until your shoulder blades come 4 to 6 inches off the floor. Hold this position for a couple of seconds before slowly returning to the starting position. Do 15 repetitions. When three sets come easily, you can try cradling a 5- to 25-pound weight plate across your chest.

Shoulders: *Military Press*. Sitting on a chair or exercise bench, with your feet firmly on the floor, grasp a pair of dumbbells with your palms facing in. Slowly raise the weights to shoulder height, rotating your palms forward as you go up. This is your starting position. Now press the weights straight above your head, stopping before you lock your elbows. At the top of the movement, the weights should be shoulder-width apart. Lower the weights to shoulder height. Do 8 to 12 repetitions.

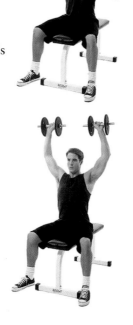

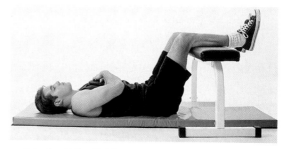

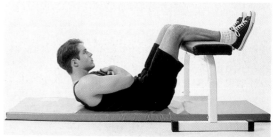

Forearms: *Wrist Curl*. Sit on an exercise bench or a chair with your knees about 8 to 12 inches apart and your feet flat on the floor. With a dumbbell in each hand, palms up, lean forward and place your forearms on your upper thighs so the wrists are hanging over.

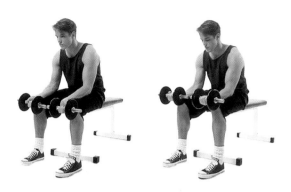

Slowly bend both wrists back as far as your can. Then, using only your wrists, curl the weights up as high as possible. Do 12 to 15 repetitions with both arms for two sets to work the inner forearm muscles, then perform two sets with your palms facing downward to pump up your outer forearms.

Get Huge by Deadlifting

If you want to get really, really big, do the exercises that are most likely to put on muscle where you don't have it. On most men, this means the muscles on the back of your body. The deadlift

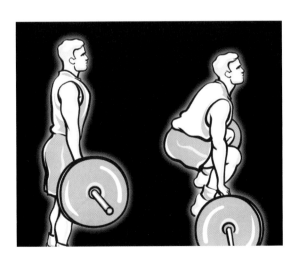

builds the hamstrings, gluteals, lower back, and middle trapezius. To do it, squat over the bar with your heels flat on the floor and the bar up against your shins. Your thighs should be parallel with the floor, your torso upright, and your eyes looking straight ahead. Grab the bar with an overhand grip just a little beyond shoulder-width. Squeeze your shoulder blades together in back, and stand with the bar, keeping it as close to your legs as possible. If you keep your shoulder blades pulled back, you'll build muscle in your middle back.

Improve Your Max

Before you try a maximal lift, load the bar with a weight that's 20 to 30 percent heavier than what you think you can handle. Then simply lift it off the rack, hold for 1 to 2 seconds, and put it back. Wait 3 to 4 minutes, then try your true max—the weight will feel noticeably lighter. Never attempt this without a spotter.

Push Up Your Performance

To improve your strength in throwing, shooting, serving, or spiking, build your serratus muscles, which extend from the bottoms of your shoulder blades through your armpits to the sides of your rib cage. Uneven pushups—where you put one hand on the floor and the other on a sturdy object about 4 inches high (such as a briefcase)—are the best way to do it.

Make Pushups Easier

As you're doing pushups, concentrate on your breathing. Inhale as you drop toward the floor, then exhale as you push back up. The rhythm focuses your energy, and all that fresh oxygen minimizes lactic-acid buildup, which is what causes the burning sensation in your shoulders, chest and triceps.

Blast Your Torso with Countdown Pushups

Take 1 second to push up, then count to 10 as you lower your body. That's right, 10. The second pushup is 1 second up and 9 down. The third is 8 seconds down, then 7, and so on, until you lower yourself in 1 second. This 10-pushup set should take you 65 seconds. If you want to make this drill even harder, put one foot on top of the other, so your body weight rests on three points instead of four. If you want to make it excruciatingly hard, elevate your feet.

Play Some Pushup Poker

Challenge a few studs. Take a deck of cards and flip one over. Do that number of pushups. Have the next guy pick a card and do that number. Jacks count for 11, queens for 12, kings for 13, and aces for 20. If you can't continue, you fold.

Do a One-Arm Pushup

Widen your feet and place your right hand on the floor beneath the middle of your chest. Tuck your left arm behind your back. As you lower yourself, you'll realize that this isn't a straight-up-and-down movement like a regular pushup. You'll twist on the ball of your left foot and untwist as you push yourself back up (if you can). You'll feel muscles working all up and down the right side of your body. Do an equal number with each

arm, and don't even try one-arm pushups unless you can bench-press your own body weight 8 to 10 times.

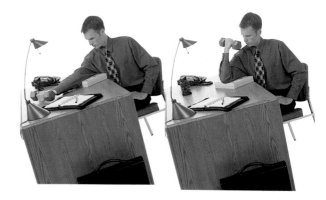

Get Big Guns at Work

Here's an exercise you can do in your office with a light pair of dumbbells. It's called the desk curl. Place a phone book on your desk. Grab a dumbbell (resist the urge to recruit your boss), sit down and lean forward so that your upper arm is resting on the phone book and the dumbbell is nearly touching the desk. Slowly curl the weight to your shoulder. Pause, and then slowly lower it back to the desk. Repeat 10 times and switch arms.

Build Big, Veiny Biceps

Do one to three sets of the one-and-a-quarter cable curl. Do four to six slow repetitions in each set. This exercise forces your biceps to contract twice on each rep, increasing their "peak."

Strength training also increases the amount of blood flow in your body, which makes veins bigger. So alternate these cable curls with sets of pushup to maximize your muscle bulk, and drop fat with aerobic exercise and a

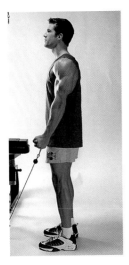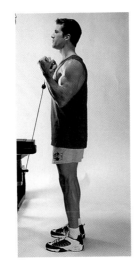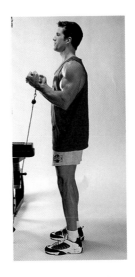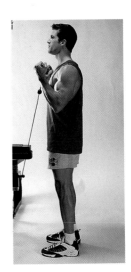

low-fat diet. Keep at it for a while and your veins will pop like bungee cords.

Curl Better for Bigger Arms

If your biceps aren't getting any bigger, even though you exercise them regularly, try a static-hold dumbbell curl. Grab a pair of dumbbells with an underhand grip and hold them at arm's

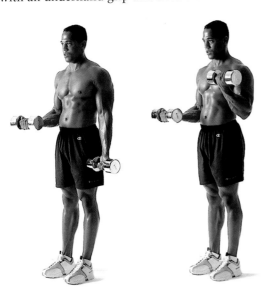

length in front of your upper thighs. Raise your right forearm so that your elbow is bent 90 degrees and hold it there. (This is the static-hold part.) Then curl the dumbbell in your left hand toward your chest as far as you can without moving your right arm. Continue holding your right arm at 90 degrees while you perform six to eight repetitions with your left arm. After you finish, switch arms so you're curling your right arm while performing the static hold with your left arm. Do two or three sets with each arm.

By holding your noncurling arm at a 90-degree angle, you'll keep the muscles under tension and improve your strength in the most difficult part of the lift.

Become a Bar Fly

Most men in the gym can't do a single pullup or chinup. Here's how to hoist yourself:

Reverse pushup: Set the bar of a Smith machine (the barbell-on-rails device) about 3 feet off the ground. Lie under the bar and grab it with an overhand grip, your hands a bit wider

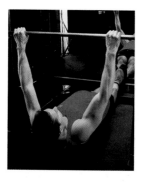

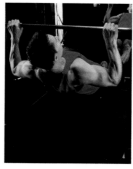

than shoulder-width apart. Your chest should be right under the bar, and only your heels should touch the floor. Pull up as high as you can, hold for 2 seconds, then slowly lower yourself. Do two or three sets of six to eight repetitions.

Negative pullup: Now set a box under the chinup bar and grab the bar with an underhand grip, your hands about shoulder-width apart. Jump up so your chin is over the bar. Take 6 to 10 seconds to lower yourself. Then jump back up and repeat. Do one set of four repetitions, and build up to two or three sets of three to five repetitions.

After 2 weeks, you should be able to do a couple of chinups. One trick is to avoid thinking about pulling yourself up. Instead, imagine pulling your elbows down. This will make it seem easier. Continue with the other exercises until your can do two or three sets of six to eight chinups. Then try pullups, which are the same exercise only with an overhand grip. You're really a stud when you can do wide-grip pullups—your hands about double shoulder-width apart—for six to eight repetitions per set.

Unwrap Your Thumbs

When doing lat pulldowns, don't wrap your thumb around the bar. Instead, place it on top, alongside your index finger. This decreases the involvement of your arm muscles, so you'll work your back harder. Works for pullups, too.

Establish Balance, Generate Power

If you have one handy, you can use a Swiss ball to strengthen your arms. The bonus is that when you balance on a Swiss ball, every muscle has to help. If your legs and torso muscles don't do their part, you'll fall off. Here are two exercises that work:

Swiss-ball pushup: Lean your entire torso against the ball and place your hands on the floor in front of it. Slowly walk yourself forward on your hands until your legs are up on the ball. How far forward you go is up to you. For an easier pushup, rest your thighs on the ball. For more of a challenge, rest your shins or just your feet on the ball. Tighten all your torso muscles (abdominals, lower back, chest, and upper back) to help stabilize your body. Slowly lower yourself until your upper arms

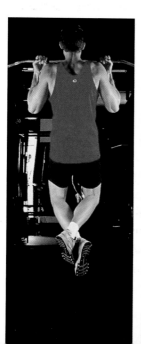

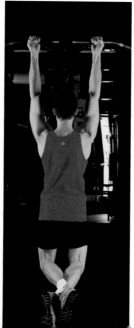

are parallel with the floor. Pause for 2 seconds, then push yourself back up until your arms are straight. Do three sets of 12 to 15 repetitions.

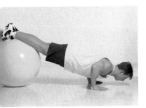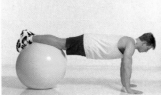

Unilateral dumbbell press: Grab a pair of dumbbells, lift them to your shoulders, and lie back on the ball so that your torso is parallel with the floor. Press the weight in your right hand straight up from your shoulder. Pause for a second at the top, then slowly lower the weight to your shoulder. Do the same with the weight in the left hand. That's one repetition. Perform two or three sets of six to eight repetitions.

Note: This exercise is much harder than it looks, so start with light weights.

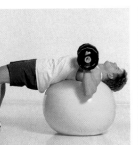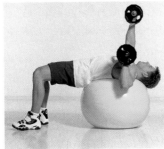

Get Popeye Forearms

Find a broomstick handle that's at least 8 inches long and drill a hole in the center of it. Thread a 3-foot-long rope through the hole and tie one end to the stick. Attach a 2½-pound barbell

plate to the other end. Now hold the stick at both ends, standing with your feet shoulder-width apart and your arms out in front of you. Your forearms should be parallel with the floor, palms down. Roll the stick so the rope wraps

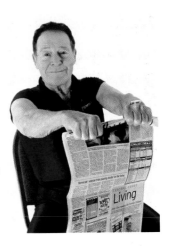

around it. Continue rolling until the weight reaches the stick. Now unroll counterclockwise until you're back where you started.

Do this exercise three times for a complete forearm workout, adding 1 pound each time the exercise becomes easy. Over time, this will give you more than just Popeye-like arms; you'll also get a firmer handshake and a distinct advantage in any sport in which you have to carry or hit a ball, such as tennis, golf, football, or baseball.

As an alternative, simply roll up a section of newspaper from top to bottom with your arms extended in front of you. You'll feel the burn in your forearms. Work up to the Sunday Times.

Don't Lock Out

To "lock out" means to fully extend your elbows (or knees) during a pushing exercise, such as a bench press, military press, or squat. When you lock out, you're giving your muscles a rest. By keeping a slight bend in the joints, you can work the muscles harder with less weight. Stop short of full extension, and you'll maintain maximum tension on the muscle.

Throw in the Towels

A strong grip can help you open a spaghetti-sauce jar, peel gym plates off a bar, or win a political campaign. This modification to the basic pull-up will get you a gorilla grip. First, loop two long, strong cotton towels over a chin-up bar. Space them a little wider than shoulder-width apart. Grab each towel firmly, and raise your feet so you're hanging in air. Keep your legs still and pull up until your chin is almost level with your hands. Then lower yourself. Even if you can easily whip off 15 regular pullups, three or four of these bears will make your forearms burn. Slowly work up to three sets of 10.

Never Arch Your Back

Arching your back to complete a bench press (like the guy is doing below) is one of the biggest mistakes you can make in the gym. Sure, it provides the extra leverage to finish the move, but it puts your back at risk and also gives an inaccurate measure of your progress.

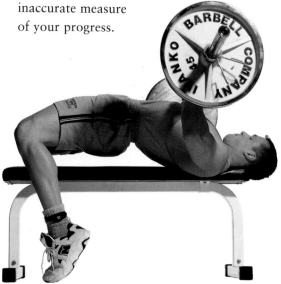

BECOME MORE DEXTEROUS

Place your hand palm-down on a table and spread your fingers as wide as possible. Hold the position for 10 seconds, relax and then repeat. Do five repetitions three times a day, and you'll increase your dexterity.

Incline to Define

A barbell bench press done on a slight incline will give your chest a great workout. Unlike a flat bench press, it stresses both the horizontal and vertical fibers of the pectoralis major—the chest's biggest muscle. Tilt that bench up a mere 15 to 20 degrees, not the 30 to 35 degrees most guys use. Now lie on your back and grip the bar with your hands slightly wider than shoulder-width apart. Press the bar toward the ceiling, hold for a moment, and return. As you raise and lower the bar, keep the movement as slow and controlled as possible.

Bench-Press with This Grip

The best grip to use for a bench press depends on the muscle groups you're trying to build. The wider your grip, the more chest involvement you're going to have. The narrower your grip, the more you'll work your triceps and shoulders.

Give Your Abs a Break

Don't work your abdominal muscles every day. Physiologically, your abs are like any other muscle in your body. They need rest to recover and grow. Train them only 2 or 3 days a week.

Believe in the Anticrunch

Lie on your back, with a rolled-up towel under the small of your back. Bend your knees and place two books between them. The heavier the books, the harder the exercise. Hold your feet slightly off the floor, and put your palms flat on the floor. Now pull your knees up toward your chest. Hold for a second, then lower them. Repeat until your midsection feels as if it's been beaten with a meat tenderizer.

Try the Tongue Trick

Press your tongue against the roof of your mouth while doing crunches. This keeps you from using your neck muscles to jerk yourself up. Keep your eyes focused on the ceiling to further isolate your stomach.

Paint the Gym Red

If you want to maximize your workout, exercise in red surroundings. Working out under red light increases the electrical activity of muscles. In nature, red spells danger and excites the central nervous system, resulting in greater muscle contractions. A red room may be especially helpful for weight lifters and other athletes who need short bursts of energy.

Build a Mighty Chest

Here's a secret about the bench press: Despite it's reputation as the King of All Chest Exercises, it doesn't really work the pectoral muscles through the full range of motion that nature designed for them. The cable fly movement trains them more completely. It's done on a cable machine at your local gym. Just remember to keep your wrists straight and your elbows high, so the movement looks like a giant crab grabbing for a piece of food.

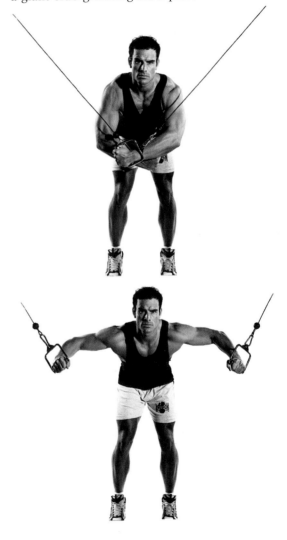

Try Negative Crunches

Over time your abdominal muscles adapt to the bash crunch motion, so the exercise grows less effective. To continue to build definition, you need to constantly shock and fatigue your stomach muscles in new ways. Try negative situps, in which you stress the *downward phase* of the movement. Lie faceup on a floor mat with your knees bent, your feet flat on the floor, and your hands behind your ears. Curl your body up until your torso is at a 45-degree angle to the floor. Now, clasp your fingers together facing your knees, and turn your palms out so you see the backs of your hands. Keep your hands clasped throughout the movement; they serve as a counterweight to ease the strain on your lower back. Keep your ab muscles tight, and slowly lower your torso while counting to 10; don't let your head touch the floor. Your shoulders should touch the mat by the time you say "10." Then raise your torso back to the 45-degree starting position and repeat the exercise. Go for 10 repetitions first, then 15 when you can handle the burn.

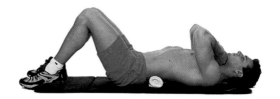

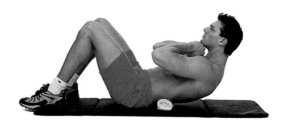

Make a Simple Exercise Much Harder

Wedge a rolled-up towel under your lower back when doing crunches. This gently curves your back, forcing your abdominal muscles to stretch a little farther at the starting position and contract to a greater degree when you crunch. Also, rest your hands comfortably under your chin as you crunch (placing your right fist inside your left hand, as shown). This little tricks stops you from jutting your head forward, which can cause pain in the neck. Adding the towel makes crunches harder, so start with two sets of 10.

Stay Away from the Slant Board

Don't do crunches on a slant board. When you lock your ankles under the board's support pads, you force your hip-flexor muscles to do more work than they would on any other ab exercise. This work tightens the hip flexors, which in turn can tilt your pelvis and strain your lower-back muscles.

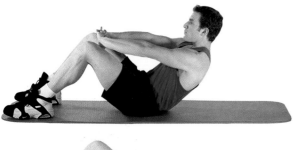

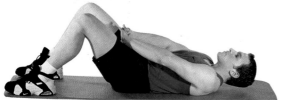

Try the Cross-Legged Crunch

Lie on your back on the floor with your lower legs crossed on the floor. Hold your hands behind your ears and pull your elbows back as far as possible. Now crunch your head and shoulders up

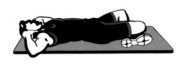
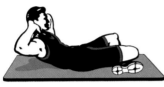

off the floor and hold the contraction; then slowly lower yourself. Do three sets of 10 to 15 repetitions. You'll have washboard abs in no time.

Learn the Standing Abdominal Twist

To do this gut-ripping exercise, hold a medicine ball or weight plate with both hands out in front of your chest, your arms slightly bent. Without moving your legs, rotate your torso 90 degrees to the right. (Don't go any farther—that would be too tough on your lower back.) Pause, then rotate back 180 degrees so you're

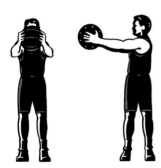
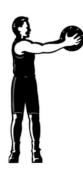

facing left. Pause and rotate right to the starting position. That's one repetition. Work up to three sets of 20 or more repetitions, beginning and ending each set with the weight in the middle.

Bust a Gut at Work

Here's a simple exercise you can use to work on your abdominals at the office, on the subway, or anywhere else, all without breaking a sweat.

Inhale and suck in your stomach until it feels small and tight. Pretend you want your belly button to touch your spine. Contract your stomach muscles and hold that tension for 5 seconds. Then exhale. Next, with your lungs just about empty, puff out your stomach and tense the muscles again. Hold that position for 5 seconds, then inhale. This exercise mainly strengthens the *transverse abdominus,* the deep-seated, cummerbund-like stomach muscle that holds your internal organs in place. Do it for just 2 minutes and we guarantee your stomach will feel tight and tender from the effort the next day.

Build Abs on a Stairclimber

Here's an exercise that'll fry your gut faster than a habanero pepper. Find a stairclimber. Enter a "fast" setting and a body weight of 50 pounds. Then get into a pushup position behind the machine. Place your hands on the pedals, with your shoulders over them. Keep your legs straight and your feet shoulder-width apart. Step with your hands to keep up with the quick-moving pedals. Your abdominal muscles will be

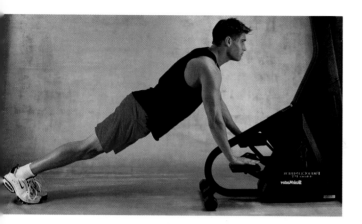

under constant strain while trying to keep your body balanced during the movement. Go 30 to 45 seconds (or as long as you can) then rest for a minute. Try to do three to five sets.

Do the Genie Test

To check the stability and flexibility of your "core"—your back, abdominal, and hip muscles that are so important to overall fitness—do this test. Stand beside a mirror with your legs shoulder-width apart, toes pointed out about 10 degrees from straight ahead, arms folded and held out parallel with the ground. (You're in genie mode.) Slowly lower yourself into a squat, keeping your weight on your heels. Stop when your thighs are parallel with the ground. If your back is vertical and your knees are just over your toes (no further, please) you get a green light for training. If your back looks hunched or round, your back muscles are probably out of shape. If you look knock-kneed (knees pointing inward), your hips are weak and tight. In either case, spend some time doing back extensions, abdominal work, and hip stretches to strengthen your core.

Build a Muscular Back

Seated cable rows can add girth to your upper back, making your shoulders appear broader. They also develop tremendous pulling power—a boon when your mower won't start or when your Rottweiler decides your neighbor is no longer amusing. When you perform two-handed cable rows, though, your two latissimus muscles (the broad bands that connect your shoulders to your spine) brace each other, and each receives less stress than if you trained one alone. That's why the one-armed variation is better. It requires more coordination and trains more muscle fibers.

Set the machine's resistance to a light weight (say, 20 pounds). With your feet in the foot platforms and your knees slightly bent, grip the edge of the seat with your right hand for support, and grasp the cable handle with your out-stretched left hand palm down. Slowly pull the handle inward to your left hip while turning your palm face up; the twist will also work your biceps. Don't bend at the waist as you pull, and *do not rotate your upper body*—that can strain your lower back. Hold for 1 second, then re-turn your left arm to the starting position. Perform 10-12 repetitions, then switch arms. Work up to three sets and gradually increase the weight.

Quiet Creaky Knees

A lot of the dull pain men feel in their knees stems from the fact that they sit around in office chairs all day, and the joint isn't being effectively lubricated. But there's a simple remedy—a 10-second exercise called quad pumps. Basically, they cause the cartilage to secrete a fluid that bathes the joint in nutrients. Here's how to do them:

1. Sit and extend your legs straight out so that your heels are resting on the floor.

2. Tighten your quadriceps, the thigh muscles just above your knees. Hold the contraction for two seconds, then release. Repeat five times. Then do another set.

Quad pumps will also keep your knees from cracking and creaking when walking up stairs.

Beat Back Pain

Back pain is like SPAM: No one's really sure where it comes from. One likely source, though, is a weak *quadratus lumborum* muscle

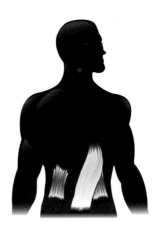

(shown in red here), which connects your ribs, pelvis, and lower spine. This muscle stabilizes your spine, especially during twisting sports movements and long periods of sitting. To prevent lower-back pain, you need to train the *quadratus lumborum* to stay tensed for longer periods. Here's an exercise that'll help:

Start by lying straight on your right side. Then lift your pelvis so your weight rests on your right forearm and feet, as shown below. Hold this pose for 8 seconds.

Roll over on your left side and do the move again. You should complete five repetitions per side, three times per week.

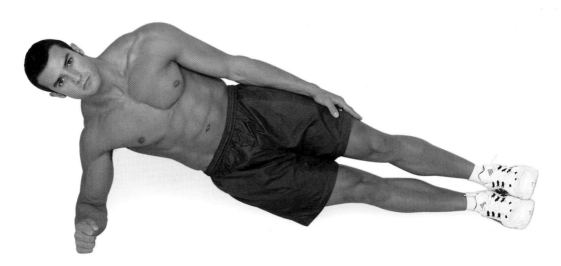

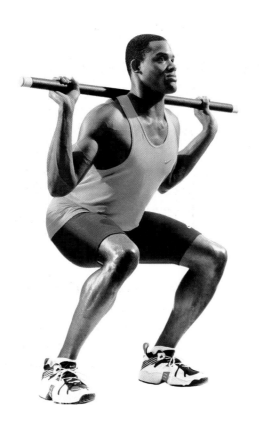

Get to Know Squat

You could use six to eight different lower-body machines in the gym, or you could basically cover all the same muscle groups with the squat. This one exercise works the "power zone"—your thighs, hips, butt, and lower back. For just about any sport, that's where your strength comes from. You'll tone up your calves, shins, and abdominals as well.

But play it safe. Use a power rack or squat safety rack. Start with one set of 8 to 12 repetitions and gradually add a set or two. It's important to always warm up with a light weight or even a barbell with no weight at all.

Sit Back, Squat More

Use a bench to squat with perfect form. That is, stand in front of the bench when you squat. Lower yourself as if you were sitting down. When your butt touches the bench, push yourself back up. Try it with a light bar or a broomstick first.

Let the Leg-Extension Machine Gather Dust

Don't use the leg-extension machine if you have gimpy knees. The leg extension is horrible if you have any kind of knee problem. The exercise places shearing forces on the knee, depending on the range of motion the machine allows and how quickly you do the movement. This can tear the cartilage around the kneecap.

Strengthen Your Ankle with Beans

If you're continually turning ankles, here's a simple exercise to help strengthen those weak ligaments. It's called the burrito lift. Head to the kitchen and grab a plastic grocery bag and two cans of refried beans—or any combination of cans that totals about a pound. Put the cans in the bag and sit on the edge of a table or stool that's high enough so your feet don't touch the floor. Hang the bag handle over the top of your left foot, close to your toes. Now, without moving your leg, raise your toes and point them at the ceiling. Hold that position for 10 seconds. Now slowly point your toes down (but no so far that the bag slips off). This exercise works the muscles on the front of the ankle and the shin. It also stretches the Achilles tendon. Repeat the move nine more times, then place the bag over your right foot. Do two sets of 10 with each foot, every other day.

Dress 10 Degrees Warmer

Should you decide to venture outside of the gym to work out, it's important to dress right. If it's cold outside, you should feel slightly chilled when you first start exercising. If you're cozy at the start, you're overdressed.

Buy Bigger Running Shoes

Your running shoes should be a bit larger than your dress shoes. You need to allow room in the toe area for your foot to swell as you run. In general, go for a fit that leaves about a thumbnail's distance between your big toe and the end of the shoe to allow for that expansion.

De-Stink Your Shoes

To keep your training shoes from smelling, take an old pair of tube socks (no holes please) and fill them with talcum powder. Then tie the open ends and stuff one into each shoe after your workout.

Write on Your Shoes

One of the leading causes of injuries in runners is worn-out shoes. To protect yourself, write an "expiration date" on your shoes as soon as you buy them. This will save you the hassle of tracking their mileage or the stress of wondering if they're shot yet. Because shoes should last about 500 miles, simply divide 500 by your average weekly mileage to determine how many weeks your shoes should last. One exception: If you're a big guy or have ankles that roll in or out too far, you may go through shoes faster—in as little as 350 miles.

BUY TWO PAIRS

If you end up ditching your athletic shoes because they smell so bad, buy two pairs the next time you go shopping. Wear them on alternating days. This will increase the life span of both pairs, because the insides will have a chance to dry out between wearings.

Cool Your Heels

Don't leave athletic shoes in your car or its trunk on sunny days or in hot weather. Heat and direct sunlight deform the leather and midsole material or even cause them to deteriorate. Temperatures in your car can exceed 120 degrees.

Compliment Your Way to Victory

In order to play a sport well, your actions must occur automatically. So the more you think about what you're doing, the more likely you are to lose control. One trick a lot of clever players use is called "complimenting the hot stroke." Your opponent compliments the mechanics of, say, your golf swing, tennis serve, or jump shot. He's not trying to be a good sport. He's trying to beat you. The compliment draws your attention to your stroke or shot; instantly you'll exaggerate whatever he's just noted, and you'll screw up. This offensive trick works in all sports that require high skills.

S T E P B Y S T E P

B R E A K I N A B A S E B A L L M I T T

A new baseball glove is like 3-day-old roadkill. Here's how to beat your glove into submission.

1. Massage the palm and ball pocket with shaving cream. Repeat this at midseason and twice a year thereafter (but no more) to keep the leather supple.

2. Stuff a ball in the glove and put it under the mattress for a few days. Always store your mitt with a ball in it so it keeps its shape.

Don't Choke

Next time you're facing a tough opponent in any sport, try this mental trick: Focus all your intensity on one aspect of your game. In practice, say to yourself "I will not double-fault" or "He's isn't going to beat me to my right." Achieving perfection in one aspect of your game will help you achieve it in everything.

Don't Reach for a Doughnut

Warming up for your turn at the plate by slipping a weighted doughnut onto your bat may not be such a good idea. Countering years of baseball tradition, a study found that players swung their bats fastest in a game following warm-up swings with bats of the same weight. Warming up with weighted bats or lighter-than-ordinary bats caused a *decrease* in bat velocity.

Catch a Major-League Foul Ball

If it's a line drive into the stands, never try to catch it. Instead, play it off the guy who's trying hardest to snag it. He'll muff it, and you'll be there for the carom.

See the Ball Better

When you step into the batter's box, first focus your eyes on the symbol on the pitcher's cap, then focus on a point in center field, then back to the pitcher's cap. Repeat as many times as you can before the first pitch. It gets the eyes ready to track the ball.

Never Boot a Grounder

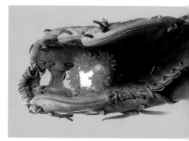

Hone your hand-eye coordination with these reaction drills: Practice snagging grounders using a smaller glove than you normally use and a baseball instead of a softball. Or go to a pet store and buy one of those spiked rubber balls for dogs, then practice catching bad hops.

Train Specifically

The best way to condition yourself for any activity is simple: Do it. You must condition your muscles in the specific way they'll be used. So if you want to get in shape to play basketball, pull on the baggy shorts twice a week and play basketball. If you want to run a half-marathon at a faster pace, don't fool yourself into thinking that more sets of leg lifts will help. The only solution is faster training runs.

Block a Runner's View

If the ball's hit to the outfield as you're covering third base and the runner is planning to tag up, stand between him and the outfielder while the ball's in the air. Because the runner can't see the ball, he may leave early, and be called out if it's caught—or break too late and be tagged out if it's not.

Survive Your Day on Court

Basketball mishaps cause about 653,000 injuries annually. Follow these tips to stay healthy:

• Stretch thoroughly first. Men who loosen up while they play go home on crutches. Do a few light calisthenics to warm cold muscles, then be like Michael Jordan and stretch everything from top to bottom.

• Play in slow motion first. Pivot, jump, twist, and fake left and right in slow motion, gradually speeding up as you go. This slowly conditions the knees, hips, and ankles.

• Wrap your assets. Protect your weak points—ankles, hamstrings, and lower back—with ankle braces, neoprene sleeves, and compression shorts.

• Land on both feet. If you spring off one foot, you risk coming down on the side of your other foot and twisting your ankle. Always jump and land with both feet shoulder-width apart.

Swipe Up Not Down

To make a steal in basketball, swipe up, not down. Refs and whiny opponents are just waiting for you to hack down on the ball. Flicking up is more subtle and surprising—and if you do poke the ball away, it'll be higher and easier to grab.

Sink Every Free Throw

The key is consistency—you need to grip and release the ball the same way every time you shoot. To hold the ball in the same place every time, put the middle finger of your shooting hand on the ball's black air valve, which is conveniently positioned in the middle of the ball. The fact that the valve is slightly raised above the surface of the ball will give your shot a little more spin, which helps those rim shots fall in. Use your other hand only as a guide.

WHEN ALL ELSE FAILS

DE-BUG YOUR LIFE

If bugs are bugging you when you're playing sports, or even when you're watching them, dab some vinegar on a cotton ball and rub it on your ears, face, or the bill of your cap to keep mosquitoes from buzzing around you.

SIZE A JUMP ROPE

Jumping rope is a great way to improve cardiovascular efficiency and coordination. But make sure the rope fits you. Stand on the rope with both feet; then pull up on the handles. The top of the handles should be level with your armpits. Shorten the rope by knotting it close to the handles.

Try a New One-on-One Game

Anybody can make shots in the comfort of their driveway. You have to be able to make shots at game speed. Here's how to develop that knack:

Stand beneath the basket with the ball. Your pal hangs out on the sideline with a stopwatch. After you make a quick lay-up, your partner sets his watch for one minute. You take two hard dribbles in any direction, square up to the basket, shoot and hustle for the rebound. Repeat this—two dribbles, shoot, rebound. Your goal is to hit as many as you can before your partner calls time. Then you collapse for a breather, and he's up. Each basket scores one point, and whoever scores the most in a minute wins.

Listen to Kareem

Jumping rope is one of the best things a basketball player can do. It not only conditions your legs, helping you to jump higher and more quickly, but it also provides a great cardiovascular workout. NBA Hall-of-Famer Kareem Abdul-Jabbar uses a weighted jump rope to make it a little more challenging. We're certainly not going to argue with him.

Be a Better Jumper

If you're a novice jumper, do as many jumps with the rope as you can, then swing the rope to the side and continue hopping up and down as long as you can. The motion will build endurance without the frustration of stumbling over the rope as you get tired.

Learn the Ropes

Jumping rope is a great way to burn a lot of calories, fast. Here are a few variations on the standard move:

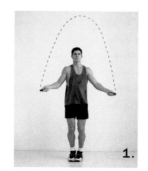 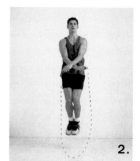

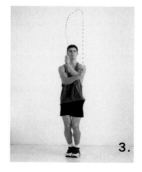 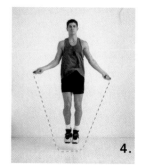

Classic Crossover: The classic crossover move that you marveled at in every Rocky film is actually easier to do than it looks. Start with the basic jump, then, when the rope is completely overhead and coming forward, cross your arms at waist level so your left hand is at your right hip, and vice versa. Keep your wrists straight so the handles are pointing out to the sides, not downward. As the rope comes down to your toes, hop over it. As it once again comes up overhead, uncross your arms. Your hands should be back at your sides in the starting position. Remember to keep your hands low and in: If you flail them out to the sides, you'll get tangled up. Try adding this variation to your normal routine once every 10 jumps. You should soon be able to cross and uncross your arms every other jump.

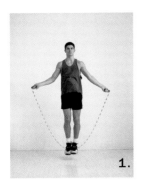

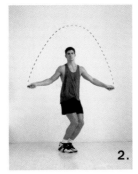

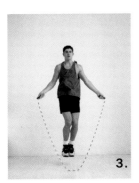

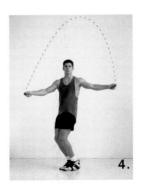

Jump and Twist: This time, as you jump straight up, twist at the waist, shifting your legs and feet to the left. When you land, your feet

will be pointing diagnoally out to the left instead of straight ahead. Concentrate on keeping your feet together through the exercise. At the next pass, twist back to the original, feet-forward position. For the next jump, twist so that your legs and feet are angled to the right as you land. Return to the starting position and continue to alternate left, center, right, and center.

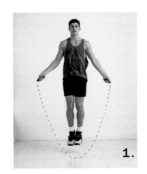

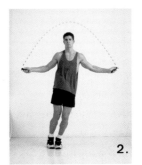

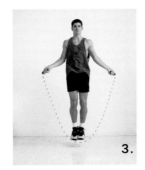

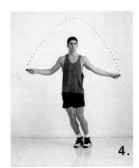

Ski Jumping: This variation mimics the movements of skiing. Instead of jumping straight up, hop about 6 inches to your right side as the rope passes underneath your feet. For the next pass, hop back into the original position. Now hop 6 inches to your left side as the rope comes around again. With the fourth and final pass, hop back to the starting position and continue to alternate right and left. Keep your feet together throughout the exercise.

Q U I C K E N   Y O U R   D R A W

Quickness is important in the game of life. Know who knows this better than anyone? Cops. Is that guy pulling out a gun or his driver's license? Some police departments have adapted drills to teach their officers how to think and react faster. Here's one that will work for you:

1. Get together a couple of buddies, two baseball caps, three foam balls (each one a different color), and a table.

2. Sit directly across the table from one friend. Both of you place your hands flat on the table. Each needs to wear a baseball cap. (No wearing it backwards.) Your second friend's job is to hold two of the three foam balls high above the table, out of your field of vision.

3. Without warning, the ball-holder should drop both balls while shouting which color ball you and your seated friend should grab. Both of you try to get that ball first.

This forces you to recognize the right object, then react to it. It will give you the mental and physical agility to make those saving grabs and instant decisions that can help keep you from landing in hot water—or hot coffee.

Develop Quick, Powerful Legs

To improve your agility, lateral movement, and jumping ability for sports such as basketball, do this drill: Place a shoe box on the ground and stand with your feet together next to it. Now jump sideways across the box. As soon as you touch down, jump back. Jump as high as you can. Do two sets of five, resting between sets. Each week, add five repetitions. This is one of the best exercises for building leg power.

Play Basketball Blind

To be quick on the basketball court, ball control is more crucial than running speed. You need to have a sense of where the ball is at all times. One way to work on this is a method called "blind dribbling." Start by walking and bouncing the ball up and down the court with your eyes closed. You'll begin to develop a sixth sense of where the ball is; soon you'll be able to change directions quickly and easily without losing the ball.

Likewise, shoot 5 or 10 free throws conventionally, then try shooting blindfolded. By practicing without the benefit of vision, you'll invariably learn the moves and feel for the sport more quickly, since you'll be forced to concentrate more intensely on those moves—and they'll be committed to memory much faster.

Check Peripheral Vision

If you're wondering why you always miss the open man while running the fast break, your peripheral vision may be to blame. Here's a way to test it: Stand up and point straight ahead with your right arm. Now close your left eye and, as you look forward, sweep your arm to the right. Assuming that straight ahead is 12 o'clock, you should be able to detect your fingers (even if you have to wiggle them) using your peripheral vision until they reach 3 o'clock. Next, sweep your arm to the left. You shouldn't lose sight of your fingers until 10 o'clock. Switch arms and repeat with your right eye closed. If your peripheral vision is poor, see your eye doctor.

Also, try this trick for improvement from Senator Bill Bradley, the former Knicks star: As you walk down the street, keep your eyes looking straight ahead. Now rattle off the objects you can see at the very edges of your vision. Bradley claims this exercise helped him develop the kind of basketball skills that other athletes believed were God-given.

Buckle Down

Your helmet needs to be on correctly to work properly. Head off cycling and in-line skating injuries by adjusting the helmet's side straps so they meet in a V just below your ears. Make sure the helmet is level, touching the front, sides, and back of your head evenly. It shouldn't shift when you shake your head up and down.

Control Your Wind

When cycling, running, or whatever your outdoor winter activity, try to head into the wind on your way out so you'll have it at your back on your way home. A tailwind supplies a subtle push when you're tired, thereby preventing you from slowing down and getting chilled.

Ride Tall in the Saddle

To get the most benefit from cycling, you need to set your seat to the proper height. If it's too high, your hips and knees are strained beyond their normal range of motion. If it's too low (like this guy), the knees can't fully unbend. That stresses them and can leave you hobbling after long rides. For perfect cycling form, make sure that when the pedal is at its lowest point, your leg is almost, but not completely, straight.

Ride Cross Country on a Stationary Bike

Here's a simple game that will keep you motivated for indoor riding. Hang a map of the United States on your wall and, after every workout, plot your mileage across it. Challenge a buddy to race across America or around Lake

Michigan. The same technique works with treadmills, cross-country ski machines, rowers (the length of the Mississippi?), and stair climbers (first one to the top of Everest wins).

Turn Off the Tube

Watching the news while pedaling a stationary bike may prevent boredom, but it could also be preventing a complete workout. Researchers found that subjects who were allowed to watch television worked at a lower intensity level than those who weren't. Reading material can have the same effect. To get the best results, focus on the exercise.

Pedal in Circles

If you want to cycle faster and farther with less effort, learn how to pedal in circles. Push down from the top of the stroke (a) until the crankarm is horizontal (b). Now pretend you're scraping mud off the bottom of your shoes from this point until the next time the crankarm is hori-

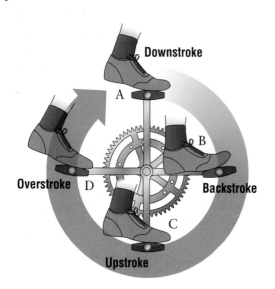

zontal (d), and continue to exert force by pulling across the bottom of the stroke (c). Finish by pulling up on the pedal to the top of the stroke (a).

This trick works whether you're cycling indoors or outside, although you will need toe straps or clipless pedals to anchor your feet. To learn the technique faster, just keep thinking "circles" as you're pedaling.

Cycle with One Leg

Practice cycling one-legged to ride more efficiently. This forces you to concentrate on pulling up at the bottom of the stroke, which better distributes the work among the major leg muscles. Lock both feet on your pedals, but let your left leg go limp while you do all the work with your right leg. Do this for 30 seconds, then switch legs. Ride normally for 5 minutes, then repeat the drill. Continue this way for a 20- to 30-minute ride.

Be a Roll Model

Instead of struggling to break away from the office or your family to spend time in the gym, try commuting to work by bicycle. You'll save time by exercising when you'd normally be trapped in traffic. Here are a few suggestions to get you going:

• Map out a quiet, indirect route. If it looks too far, drive halfway, park and pedal from there.

• If you'll be commuting a short distance along busy city streets, buy a durable mountain bike. If you'll be riding longer distances on smooth back roads, but a faster road bike.

• Once or twice a week, drive to work as you normally would and take along fresh clothes and towels.

• If there's no shower at work, ask if you can use the facilities at a nearby health club, or mop off with a washcloth.

• If you don't have the time or energy to ride back and forth in one day, try this trick: Drive to work with your bike in the trunk, then pedal home. Next morning, do the opposite.

Go the Other Way

If you have a regular route that you cycle or run, but it's becoming increasingly tedious, reverse it. You'll be amazed at all the new things you'll see by doing it backward.

Pedal Farther with Less Effort

The cycling equivalent of a marathon is called a "century"—100 miles in one day. Here's how to survive it:

• Eat one energy bar (or banana) and drink 12 to 16 ounces of water 30 minutes before a bike ride. This will top off your fuel stores and postpone the fatiguing effects of dehydration.

• Once you're on the bike, stand and pedal for 15 seconds every 10 minutes. This relieves saddle pressure and stretches your muscles.

• Tell yourself to pedal *faster* instead of *harder*. Spinning an easier gear at 80 to 100 revolutions per minutes is the most efficient pedaling range.

• Drink one bottle of water per hour. Set your sports watch to beep every 15 minutes as a reminder to take a slug.

• Keep your elbows bent throughout the ride. This encourages a more aerodynamic, "flat-back" riding position, plus it prevents road shock from being transmitted up your arms into your shoulders.

Enter the Draft

By pedaling directly behind another bike rider, you conserve up to 30 percent of your energy. That's because you're letting him break through the air for you. Do this for a long ride and you'll have considerable energy left over by the end.

Bring the Mountain to You

Riding a mountain bike takes about a third more effort than riding a road bike, largely because of the increased rolling resistance from the fatter tires and the increased weight of the bike. So if your time is limited and you have a choice of bikes, it's always better to choose the mountain bike, even if you'll be riding it on the road. Riding 12 miles on fat tires is the equivalent of doing 15 on skinny rubber.

SAY SSSSO LONG

Next time you're sprinting to the finish line in a bike race, put your head down and softly hiss. It causes whomever you're riding with to look down and check if his tire's going flat. By the time he realizes it's not, you'll have a big jump on him.

FIX A FLAT BIKE TIRE WITH LEAVES

You've cycled miles into the outback and get a flat. Unfortunately, you forgot to pack a tube, patch kit, and pump. What now? Stuff the space between the tire and the rim with leaves, vines, ferns, dirty socks, trash, or anything else that will give the tire some semblance of shape, then ride back. Slowly.

Have a Happy Landing

You can bet it'll happen some day. You'll be cruising along on your bike and suddenly find yourself flying head over handlebar, a Superman in cycling tights. This is a very vulnerable position. Which is exactly why you should learn the Hail Mary pass of cycling, the tuck-and-roll. Practice it on a gym mat or grassy lawn until it becomes second nature.

1. While falling forward, instinct might force you to extend your arms to help break your fall. Don't lock your elbows or you might break your wrists or collarbone.

2. You now want to transform your fall into a shoulder roll. And, of course, you should be wearing a helmet whenever you're riding.

3. Stay loose and roll across one of your shoulders and your back. Control your lower body by keeping it bowed so it makes contact with the ground as softly as possible.

4. Depending on your speed, you'll come to a safe stop either sitting or back on your feet. Rolling onto your feet is always impressive, but don't stand straight right away. Do it slowly to avoid back strain.

5. Once standing, quickly move out of the path of traffic, check yourself for injuries, then wave to the cheering crowd.

Don't Stare at the Rock

When mountain biking look as far down the trail as possible, and think about where you

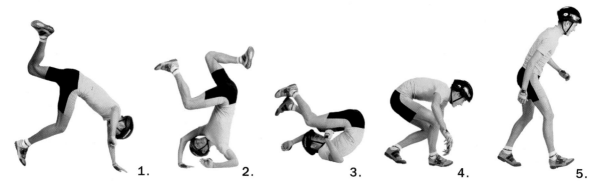

1.   2.   3.   4.   5.

want to go, not what you want to avoid. Generally speaking, your bike tends to go where you're looking, so if you focus on the obstacle, you're sure to hit it.

Climb Any Mountain

Most mountain bikers stand up on their pedals while climbing to generate more power on hills, but your best bet is to stay seated. When you stand, it takes weight off the back wheel, and you spin out. Also, gradually downshift before reaching the hill in order to maintain pedal speed from your seat. Sit back in the saddle and you'll use more of your powerful gluteal muscles.

Shake a Defender

To get open for a pass in football, run near enough to your defender that you can shake his hand. The closer you get, the easier it'll be to blow past him. As you close in on him, shorten your strides without slowing down—it'll help you cut faster.

Split the Uprights

The key to kicking a field goal is to have your holder angle the football slightly toward the goalposts and a touch toward himself. This will give you the best shot at hitting the sweet spot.

Make More Birdies

According to Jack Nicklaus, one of the most important elements of the golf swing is grip pressure. Squeeze that club too hard and you'll lose feeling and fluidity in your swing. The optimal grip pressure is the minimal amount required to prevent the club from flying out of your hands. (Imagine you're holding a bird.) If you feel any pressure on your left thumb, you're squeezing the club (and the bird) too hard.

Make Practice Perfect

Ben Hogan, the greatest golfer of his time, would practice his drive by hitting 50 balls in 2 hours. He'd think about each shot. He'd have a purpose for every one he hit. That's how you practice. The average guy gets a bucket of balls and shoots off 50 in 20 minutes. That's quantity, not quality. It just reinforces mistakes.

STEP BY STEP

KILL 'EM IN FOOSBALL

For a sizzling Foosball shot, perfect the "palm roll."

1. Cup your fingers beneath the rod handle.

2. Lower your arm, letting the handle roll up to your wrist.

3. When it's time to shoot, pull your arm swiftly upward, rolling the handle back into your cupped fingers.

FINAGLE YOUR WAY ONTO ANY COURSE

Find out if that swanky, private golf club is part of a real-estate community, then phone the marketing director and tell him you're considering purchasing a home but would like to play the course first to see if it suits you.

Drive More Carefully

Among beginning golfers, the driving range may be a more frequent source of injury than the golf course. In one hour of whacking balls, you swing more than you would in a month of weekend golf. And because the long shots in particular tend to work muscles that aren't used every day, there's a good chance of tiring, tightening, and even overstretching and tearing them. To lessen the chances of this, change clubs every 15 to 20 shots. Start with a midrange iron to warm up, then go to the driver, and follow with a short iron. Alternating clubs allow your muscles to rest, reducing the risk of injury.

Break a Hundred

Golfers always try to play the longest possible shot from the tee, hoping to smash a 280-yard drive and reduce the length of the next shot. But for duffers, this rarely works. Try this strategy instead: If the hole is more than 140 yards and less than 340 yards, divide the total yards by two. For example, let's say the hole is 320 yards. Divide by two and you have 160 yards. Can you consistently hit a straight shot 160 yards? If you can, play two 160-yard shots, and you'll be on or near the green. If you can't, play two shots of, say, 140 yards, and you'll be close enough to kick the next one on. If the hole is more than 340 yards, divide the total by three and use the same logic.

Read Any Green

If you're undecided about which way a putt will break, picture pouring water on the green. Imagine which way it will flow, and you'll have the line for your putt.

Sink Every Putt

As you stand over the ball to putt, use your throwing hand to determine how far you'd move that arm if you were rolling the ball toward the hole like a bowler. That's how long your stroke should be.

Get Out of a Bunker

To get out of a greenside sand trap, mentally glue a second ball to the back of your golf ball and swing at the second ball. That'll force you to hit just the right amount of sand so your ball will pop onto the green. Backswing should be slow; speed up as your club nears the ball.

Putt Cross-Handed

For putts shorter than 5 feet, try a reverse grip. Place your lead hand—the hand closest to the hole—below the hand farthest from the hole. This prevents your stronger hand from dominating the shot. The conventional putting technique is slightly more accurate on putts longer than 20 feet.

Spine-Tune Your Golf Muscles

As you age, the muscles closest to your spine become stiffer. This exercise can increase your spine's range of motion and lead to a full shoulder turn, and more yards for your drive. It's call the spine rotation stretch. To do it, stand with your back to a wall and your heels about 6 inches away from it. Keeping your feet flat, turn your body to the right so that your can place both hands on the wall. Ease your hips in toward the wall until you feel the stretch. Hold for 10 seconds. Push off the wall, and repeat the stretch on the left side. Continue stretching from one side to the other for 3 to 4 minutes, two or three times a day.

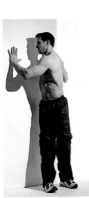

Find Your Way Home

If you're hiking in the woods and you find yourself slightly lost, make a compass with a razor blade and a piece of thread. Magnetize the blade by rubbing the dull end against the palm of your hand. Suspend it on the thread. The rubbed end will point north.

Start a Fire without Matches

On a hiking expedition with no lighter? No matches? No flint? Then lets hope you've got some steel wool and a battery. Roll the wool between your hands into a cigarette shape. Then pull the ends apart gently so there is only a fine mesh of steel wool in the center. Now touch one end to the battery's top, the other to the battery's bottom. Look at that! The current makes the wool in the center spark and burn. Get some tinder on it quick.

Put a Condom on Your Barrel

If you're packing a firearm into the wilderness, roll a condom over the barrel of the gun to keep debris and water out, as the Navy SEALs do. If you need to point and shoot quickly, the condom won't hinder the bullet.

MR. CLEAN

SCRUB YOUR ROD

The quickest way to clean a rod and reel: Take them into the shower and give them a gentle scrubbing with a big sponge or a car wash mitt.

Survive a Lightning Strike

If you feel the hair on the back of your neck stand up, you're about to be hit by lightning. Crouch on the balls of your feet, but don't put your hands on the ground. This will help keep the current from traveling through your body if lightning strikes the ground nearby.

Stay Cool on Hot Runs

Before exercising, dampen clothing, then wring it out. The evaporation will provide do-it-yourself air conditioning.

Keep Your Head Up

Researchers have found that runners who look down use more oxygen and run more slowly than runners who look straight ahead.

Listen to Your Feet

To be a better runner, you need quiet feet. If you hear them hitting the ground, you're not running well. Pounding is too hard on your joints. Keep your feet close to the ground with a quick, shuffling-type stride.

Warm Up on Cold Runs

After a winter run, gradually bring your heart rate back to normal with a 5-minute walk. Then head indoors for some stretching and calisthenics. This two-stage adjustment period is important because abrupt heating dilates blood vessels in the extremities. This steals blood from the heart and such sudden stress can prompt a coronary in susceptible individuals.

Become a Runner

Here's an easy-does-it running plan for absolute beginners. It requires no more than ½ hour per day, 2 to 4 days per week, and will get you gradually up to a 30-minute run in 12 weeks. It's intentionally easy at first and assumes a fitness level of zilch. If you are in okay shape, try beginning with Week 3.

Week	Run-Walk Schedule (to be done 2 to 4 times weekly)
1	Walk 20 minutes
2	Walk 30 minutes
3	Run 2 minutes; walk 4 minutes (repeat 5 times)
4	Run 3 minutes; walk 3 minutes (repeat 5 times)
5	Run 5 minutes; walk 2.5 minutes (repeat 4 times)
6	Run 7 minutes; walk 3 minutes (repeat 3 times)
7	Run 8 minutes; walk 2 minutes (repeat 3 times)
8	Run 9 minutes; walk 2 minutes (repeat 2 times, then run 8 minutes)
9	Run 9 minutes; walk 1 minute (repeat 3 times)
10	Run 13 minutes; walk 2 minutes (repeat 2 times)
11	Run 14 minutes, walk 1 minute (repeat 2 times)
12	Run 30 minutes

STEP BY STEP

BE A LORD OF THE FLIES

To learn how to put the fly where the fish are, put a Hula-Hoop on the ground in your backyard and follow these instructions:

1. *Start.* For practice purposes, tie a 1-inch piece of bright yarn to the end of your leader. Place the rod on the ground and pull about 25 feet of line straight out from the end of the rod. Now pick up the rod and grab the first foot of loose line coming off the reel. Hold it at waist level with your left hand between the reel and the lowest guide. With your feet positioned about shoulder-width apart, bend your knees slightly and square your shoulder to the rod. And relax; you can't cast if you're tense.

2. *Grip.* Hold the rod in your right hand with your thumb on top of the grip (your left hand if you're a lefty). The rod should be parallel with the ground.

3. *Backcast.* In one fluid motion, pull the rod up in an arc toward the front of your right shoulder, raising the tip. Start slowly and pick up speed as the reel approaches your shoulder. Keep a straight wrist. Stop the rod sharply when it's just behind your head. Don't begin the forward cast until the line has straightened out behind you.

4. *Cast.* Using your arm and not your wrist, bring the rod forward with a smooth, controlled motion. Accelerate your hand as it moves forward, but don't try to muscle the rod. Stop the rod firmly as soon as it passes a position parallel with the ground.

Keep Training on Track

If you run on a track, stick to the outermost lane. This way you'll turn more gradually, which eases the strain on ankles and knees. And every couple of laps, turn around and run in the opposite direction. Otherwise, you'll put undue stress on your inside foot and leg, which increases your risk of injury.

Run Stairs, Get Stares

Here's a nostalgic workout to do at your local high-school stadium: Run to the top row of the stands, touching every step; jog down; and immediately do 20 pushups. Repeat the stair-climbs three more times, doing a different one of these exercises after each: 20 squats (without weight), 20 close-grip pushups, 20 squats. It's a great workout.

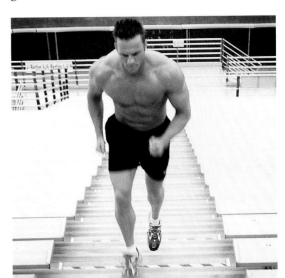

Keep Bugs Away

Don't wear red, blue, or black if you're going hiking in the woods. Those colors attract mosquitoes and bees. Also, try eating a garlic-heavy meal beforehand. When your pores release its odor, insects take cover. You'll be alone, but at least you won't be scratching.

Hold Two Potato Chips

When you run a long race, you can inadvertently build tension in your shoulders, arms, and fists, and this saps energy. To keep your fists relaxed, pretend you're holding a penny or potato chip between your thumb and index finger.

Run in Place with Dumbbells

Grab a pair of light dumbbells and stand with one foot about 24 inches in front of the other. Now do a smooth and controlled running motion with your arms, keeping your elbows bent 90 degrees and your feet stationary. Continue for 30 seconds, then reverse your stance and repeat. Arm movements are important in locomotion—if you doubt us, try running with your arms straight down at your sides. More powerful arm

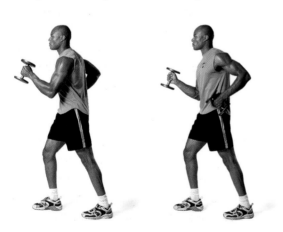

movements lead to more powerful locomotion. This is why sprinters do a lot of upper-body strength training, and why any runner can improve performance with this exercise.

Shorten Your Stride

It would seem logical that lengthening your stride would help you run faster. But taking longer steps actually slows you down by creating a braking action every time your foot meets the ground. Taking more steps, not longer ones, is the key to going faster. To monitor your progress, run around a track at race pace and count the number of times your right foot strikes the ground over a minute. The best rate for runners, weekend and elite alike, is about 90 strides per minute.

Run-Walk a Marathon

Running burns more calories than running/walking does, but the difference isn't as big as you might think. Running 3 miles burns about 400 calories; running/walking the same distance (with 1-minute walking breaks every 4 or 5 minutes) uses about 300 calories. But overall you'll use more calories running/walking because you'll be able to go farther. If you lower your exertion level by taking walking breaks, you'll be able to add mileage without burning out. You can even run/walk a marathon.

Here's the race plan: Run the first mile, walk 60 seconds, repeat 25 more times, then sprint like crazy.

WHEN ALL ELSE FAILS

CATCH FISH WITH YOUR HANDS

First, crash down the middle of the stream, scaring the fish into their hiding places under the banks. Then, once they're secure, like ostriches with heads in the sand, sneak toward the bank and slowly root around underneath. A fish in this position will actually let you touch it without moving. Once you feel it's belly, quickly spear its gills and tail between your fingers.

Master the Hills

The secret to hill running is maintaining a constant level of effort. When you're running uphill, slow to the point where you're not working much harder than you do on flat terrain—even if that means slowing your pace to nothing more than a crawl. On the downhill, run fast enough so it feels like work, even with the help of gravity.

Crank Yourself Up

Lots of guys look at their feet so they don't have to stare at the long stretch of upward-bound pavement ahead. Instead, imagine that a rope is attached to the middle of your chest, and it's being wound in from a point two stories above the top of the hill in front of you. Lifting your head opens your airways, so it's easier to breathe than when your upper body is hunching forward.

Start Doing Intervals

If you're regularly running 15 to 25 miles a week and don't feel like you're improving, add structured interval sessions to your training program. Once or twice a week, warm up for a mile, then alternate hard runs of 3 to 5 minutes each with a few minutes of jogging in between. Repeat three or four times.

Outrun Heart Trouble

Running faster has 13.3 times greater impact on lowering blood pressure than running at a leisurely pace. Conversely, running farther at a slower pace doesn't greatly affect blood pressure, but it has six times the effect on raising beneficial HDL cholesterol than short, quick runs. So if you want to lower blood pressure, increase your intensity. If you want to raise HDL, add duration.

Make the Grade 1 Percent

If you want to mimic road running on a treadmill, raise the incline to 1 percent before starting your run. Researchers found that's the degree of treadmill elevation that most closely approximates outdoor running.

Make Your Treadmill Last

Buy a new pair of running shoes and use them exclusively for your home treadmill workouts. Having a dedicated indoor pair will keep you from tracking dirt and grime onto the belt, which then takes it right into the engine.

Climb Stairs Backward

Leaning on the handles of a stairclimber can cut your caloric expenditure by 20 percent or more. For a better calorie burn, pump your arms as if you were walking or running briskly. Or you can just turn around. Facing away from the console burns even more calories than the traditional method.

Go Elliptical

Elliptical trainers provide the same cardiovascular benefits as treadmill running, without the impact on your joints. So they're a perfect solution if you're a runner who wants to stay in race shape without excessive pounding to your ankles, knees, and hips.

Don't Run on the Beach

The next time you're at the beach, stick to barefoot strolls. Because sand is loose, running on it puts unnatural strain on arches and the Achilles tendons. Also, most beaches slope, forcing you to run at a leg-stressing angle.

Predict Your Finish Time

Running a race at a distance you've never done before? You can predict your performance at that distance using your actual performance at another distance. Here are some examples:

5K	8K/5-mile	10K	Half Marathon	Marathon
16:00	26:30	33:00	1:13:00	2:33:00
16:30	27:00	34:00	1:15:00	2:38:00
17:00	28:00	35:00	1:18:00	2:43:00
17:30	29:00	36:00	1:20:00	2:48:00
18:00	30:00	37:00	1:22:00	2:52:00
18:30	30:30	38:00	1:24:00	2:56:00
19:00	31:30	39:00	1:26:00	3:01:00
19:30	32:00	40:00	1:29:00	3:06:00
20:00	33:00	41:00	1:31:00	3:11:00
20:30	34:00	42:00	1:33:00	3:15:00
21:00	34:30	43:00	1:35:00	3:20:00
21:30	35:30	44:00	1:37:00	3:24:00
22:00	36:00	45:00	1:40:00	3:29:00
22:30	37:00	46:00	1:42:00	3:34:00
23:00	38:00	47:00	1:44:00	3:38:00
23:30	39:00	48:00	1:46:00	3:42:00
24:00	39:30	49:00	1:49:00	3:48:00
24:30	40:30	50:00	1:51:00	3:53:00

Cut Back to Come Back

If an injury is causing you pain when you run, reduce your weekly mileage by half. If it still hurts, cut back by another half. If it *still* hurts, cut back again. Once you reach a level where you aren't feeling pain during your run or for several hours afterward, stick with it for a couple of weeks, then build back slowly. Apply ice before and after your workouts to minimize any swelling.

Get in Shape for Ski Season

If you're a skiier, we don't have to tell you that there's more to skiing than avoiding trees and women named Picabo. You need balance, endurance, and strength. These simple, at-home exercises, done with 1 minutes of rest in between, will give you all three.

Single-leg balance squat: Stand on a block or step (start with one that's 6 inches high) and move one foot off the edge. Bend the knee of the supporting leg so that the nonsupporting foot brushes the floor. Hold that position for 3 to 5 seconds; stand back up. When you can do 20 of these, increase the height of the block.

Single-leg ski squat: Stand on one leg; place the other leg in front of you with your heel about 6 inches above the floor. Squat down until the thigh of your back leg is almost parallel with the floor. Do 10 repetitions. Rest 15 seconds, then switch legs. Use two sturdy chairs only for balance (like ski poles).

Double-leg ski squat: Lean against a wall, with your feet about 2 feet away from it and shoulder-width apart. Bend your knees slightly

and hold that position for 5 to 10 seconds. Bend deeper and hold. Repeat until you've hit five different positions; go as low as you can. Work up to 30 seconds in each position.

Crush a Roach to Ski Better

To make your cross-country ski stride more powerful than a simple shuffle, imagine you're smashing a cockroach with the heel of your lead foot. Reach with that leg, plant the heel, then kick back to propel yourself forward on the other ski. To balance your weight, throw the opposite arm back. When you've glided as far as you can, repeat with the other leg. Eventually, you'll develop a steady rhythm.

Stretch before a Swim

To be a good swimmer, you need flexibility, but few guys ever stretch before jumping in the pool. You swim with your whole body, and you can't do that unless you're loose and supple. Do these three stretches before starting to do laps. Hold each for 30 to 40 seconds. Do the first and third stretches for both sides of your body.

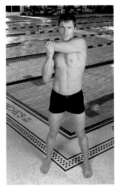 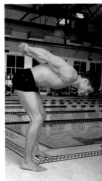 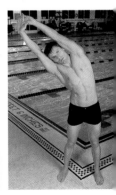

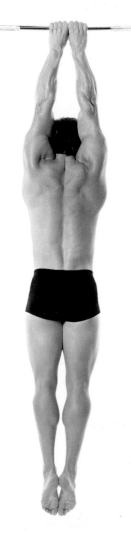

Become a Human Torpedo

Streamlining is the secret to swimming fast. It involves making your body as long and narrow as possible. It can trim as many as 10 strokes from a lap in an Olympic-size pool. To improve streamlining, competitive swimmers often hang from bars to stretch their shoulder and back muscles. Before your workout, simply grab a chin-up bar with both hands so your thumbs are touching each other and your palms are facing away from you. Let your body hang completely straight, with your toes pointing to the floor. Put your head between your arms, so your ears are in front of your biceps, and try to squeeze your shoulder blades together. Hang for 10 seconds, drop off the bar and take a 10-second breather, then hang for 10 seconds more. After a few ses-sions, increase your hang time to 20 seconds with a 15-second break.

Practice the Flutter-Kick

Using a kickboard would seem to be a good way to train your legs, since the foam board holds your body above water while your legs do all the work. In fact, a kickboard causes the hips and legs to drop lower, so they drag underwater. For a better workout, leave the kickboard on the pool deck and flutter-kick on your side. For proper freestyle form, extend your underwater arm in front of you and rest your surface arm against your side; every 10 to 12 kicks, take a stroke to switch sides. This drill keeps your legs in alignment with your torso, the perfect position for slicing through the water.

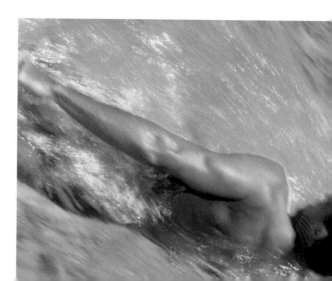

Do a Flip Turn

Swimming becomes an even more fluid workout when you master the flip turn.

1. Swim toward the wall. When you're about 15 feet out (you'll need to experiment with distances), give one or two strong pull 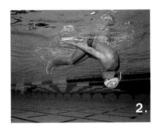 strokes and tuck your chin into your chest to start a forward somersault. Duck your head under, and push with your hands to plunge into a roll.

2. Quickly bend at the hips and begin to fold inward like a jackknife. Keep your chin tucked to your breastbone and your legs 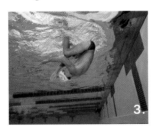 straight. Use your hands to maintain your momentum. Stay as shallow as possible while remaining completely submerged.

3. Tightly fold yourself like a book, nose to knees, hands to feet, keeping legs extended. Kick your heels toward 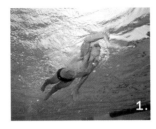 your butt as the rest of your body is rotating to achieve that streamlined egg shape. You'll have the urge to twist out of this position. Try to fight it.

4. After your legs whip over your head and you're upside down, stamp the soles of your feet against the wall 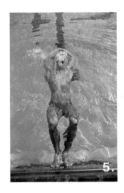 to initiate the rebound. Your feet should hit the wall about a foot or two below the water's surface. Your arms will automatically straighten behind your head.

5. Before you explode, nest your hands together to form a blade with your arms and squeeze your biceps to your ears. This is called "streamlining." Now push off the wall powerfully. Keep your feet and your hands together. You should torpedo straight off the wall, facing up.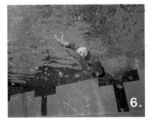

6. Cross your legs so that the water floating over your body rotates you to your side. When you're ready to resume your stroke, 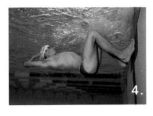 use the arm nearest to the bottom of the pool to propel you into your first stroke. If this is done right, you'll shoot more than 15 feet in 2 seconds before your hands break the surface. Then restart your stroke.

DO THE PERFECT BELLY FLOP

Everything is an art form. Done correctly, the classic belly flop can drench entire families—and more important, women in light summer dresses.

1. *Jump up and out as far as you can:* Put in some practice jumping off the side of the pool before you graduate to the diving board.

2. *Strike a "Superman" pose:* As you rocket forward, extend your arms and legs. Amateurs stay in this position, which is why they scream in pain when they hit the water.

3. *Arch your back:* Bend your body into the shape of a banana. This will maximize your splashing impact and prevent you from bashing your face or groin.

4. *Prepare for impact:* At the last moment, cock you head back to protect your face. For dramatic effect after the splash, bob on the surface like a dead man.

Give Her a Memorable Ride

To figure the proper boat speed for waterskiing, ask your girl her weight. Take the first two digits of her body weight, then add 20. (Example, 180 pounds = 18; 18 + 20 = 38 miles per hour.)

Prevent Swimmer's Ear

To keep bacteria in the water from causing the painful infection called "swimmer's ear," follow this quick routine after your workout:

1. Dry your ears with a hair dryer set on "low" for a minute or two.

2. Using a clean eyedropper, carefully put a few drops of a therapeutic solution in your ear— half white vinegar, half rubbing alcohol. This mixture dries your inner ear and prevents any bacterial growth.

Take a Dip

If you just finished some laps and want to squeeze in some resistance training, stay in the pool for a few dips. Just by swimming to the edge of the pool and raising your body in and out of the water (like you would with a dip machine) you'll exercise your triceps, chest, and back—and also get in some shoulder and forearm work.

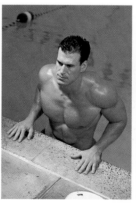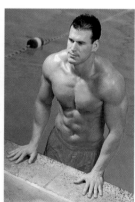

Drown-Proof Yourself

When you can't muster another 10 seconds of dog paddling, use an emergency move called "drown-proofing." While floating on your stomach, curl into a ball and wrap your arms around your knees. When you need air, gently lift your head and take a breath, then lower your head and rest again. This position conserves body heat and energy.

Make Your Serve Sizzle

If tennis is your game, to put more oomph in your serve, do this exercise: Hold a 3- or 4-pound medicine ball above and a little behind your head. Then bring it directly over your head and throw it forward with both hands. Do two or three sets of 15 repetitions every other day, throwing with a smooth motion and increasing your distance gradually over a period of weeks.

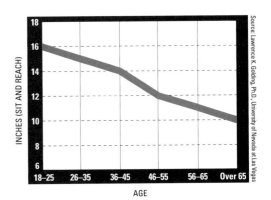

Watch the Ball

One of the most common tennis mistakes is to look at where you think you want your ball to go. Wrong. As it moves into your racket, look down, keeping your head still and your eyes fixed on the point of impact. Then look up. You should actually see your arm cross under your face on forehands and backhands.

Get It Together in 20 Seconds

Say you've just double-faulted for the third time in a row. You've got 20 seconds before you serve again. Use it. For the first 3 to 5 seconds, allow yourself to acknowledge the error, then let it go. During the next 6 to 10 seconds, breathe and relax. Take the final 3 to 5 seconds to visualize what you want to do. Then, do it.

Count Naturally

Instead of counting seconds while you stretch, which only adds to the tedium of it, try counting breaths. Ten breaths is all you need for any stretch. It will help your mind stay in better tune with your body.

Preserve Your Dignity

To maintain your flexibility well into old age, all you have to do is stretch your muscles for 30 minutes per week. That's 4 minutes per day. Still too daunting? Then think of the adjacent graph as a depiction of basic human dignity. Allow yourself to stiffen with age, and you'll eventually need help to leave bed, to walk, and even to use the bathroom. Regular stretching is your insurance against such embarrassment.

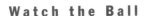

Source: Lawrence K. Golding, Ph.D., University of Nevada at Las Vegas

Don't Become a Bouncer

Bouncing during a stretch causes muscles to tighten in order to protect themselves, thereby defeating the purpose of the stretch. Muscles prefer to be coaxed rather than jolted, so as you begin a stretch, do so slowly and smoothly, working toward a position that starts to feel tight but never painful.

Stretch When You're Warm

A lot of guys confuse stretching and warming up. Warming up means 5 to 10 minutes of cardiovascular activity—enough to break a light sweat. It doesn't mean doing some twisting with a broomstick over your shoulders—that's actually stretching. The best time to stretch is after you've warmed up.

Stretch Your Entire Body with One Move

End every workout with this move: Sit on the floor with your right leg straight in front of you. Bend your left leg, and put the sole of your left foot on the inside of your right thigh. (Your legs will look like the number 4.) With your right hand, try to touch either your right ankle or your right big toe. This stretches your right calf, Achilles tendon, hamstring, hip, knee, glutes, lower back muscles, shoulder, arm, and wrist. Hold the position for 30 seconds to 1 minute, then switch and do the same for your left side.

Strike the Bow Pose

When time is short, the bow pose will stretch your entire body in one simple move. Lie on your stomach and draw your feet toward your butt. Bring your arms behind you and grab your ankles. Gently pull your feet close to your butt and hold. In time, you'll be ready for the next step: Continue to hold your ankles as you gently raise your upper body and legs off the floor. Hold for as long as is comfortable, then lower yourself.

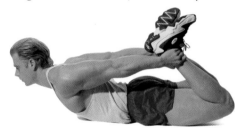

Don't Be a Working Stiff

If you sit at a desk all day, here's a stretching routine to do at the end of your shift.

Sit, straddle, reach: Do three times on each side. Hold each stretch for a maximum of 15 to 20 seconds. If you're just starting, do 5 to 10 seconds, no more. No rest between sets.

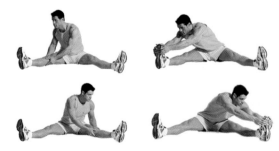

Shoulder-flexor stretch: Repeat the exercise two or three times. Hold for 15 to 20 seconds each time. Rest your arms for 10 seconds between stretches.

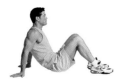 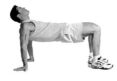

Hip-flexor stretch: Do two or three times with each leg. Hold for 15 to 20 seconds, then switch legs.

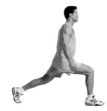

Don't Shock Yourself in the Shower

Take a lukewarm shower after a workout. Hot showers slow circulation and depress blood pressure. Cold showers tend to raise blood pressure and may overload the heart. A shower with water temperature around 98°F keeps you alert without any shocks.

Beat Calf Cramps with Tonic Water

If running gives you nighttime cramps in your calves, drink tonic water before you go to bed. It contains quinine, a plant extract that acts as a muscle relaxant. Add lemon to the tonic or mix it with orange juice to reduce its bitterness.

Strap on a Beer

Frozen or very cold cans of beer make great ice packs. Hold one against whatever is ailing you—a sore muscle, a sunburned neck, a pounding headache. With an Ace bandage, you can even wrap a frosty 16-ouncer against the back of your thigh. Or use a sweatband to strap a can near your elbow after a tennis match. A metal can transmits the cold very rapidly. Just make sure to put some thin fabric between the skin and can to avoid frostbite.

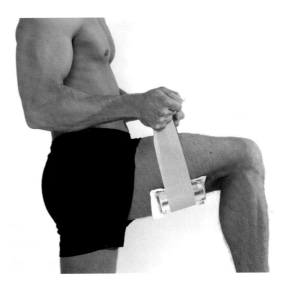

Escape a World of Hurt

No matter what your game, injuries can happen. If one's happened to you, don't wait till the morning after hard exercise to pop some ibuprofen. Taking it immediately after the game can help lessen the inflammation in your damaged muscles.

Tell If It's Broken

If you feel nauseous after injuring an arm or leg, you've probably fractured it.

PINCH AWAY A CRAMP
To get rid of a muscle cramp when all else fails, try pinching your upper lip. Experts don't understand why this acupressure point works, but it often does.

Chill Out for 25 Minutes
When you pull a muscle or wrench a knee, grab a bag of ice and a stopwatch. Doctors have concluded that icing an injury for exactly 25 minutes is the optimum time for quickest healing. The healing effect begins at 5 minutes and peaks at 25. Icing for longer than 30 minutes can damage the tissue and nerves.

Ice Yourself with a Tennis Ball
Slice a 1-inch opening in a tennis ball, fill it with water and stick it in the freezer. Then when you have a sore back, lie flat on your back, put the ice ball on the sore spot, and slowly roll your body over it. The ball will provide cold and pressure, both of which help heal sore muscles.

Heal Muscle Pulls Faster
The recipe for treating a minor muscle pull or strain is pretty simple—rest, ice, compression, and elevation—but a lot of guys screw up the elevation part. Resting your leg on the coffee table while you pop a couple of cold ones isn't enough. Unless you've got the injured area above the level of your heart—and preferably your head as well—you're not minimizing the swelling.

Also, within 24 to 48 hours, try to do some light aerobic exercise. This will deliver fresh blood to the injured site, blast out lactic-acid buildup, further reduce swelling, and significantly speed recovery time. Just make sure you don't stress the area. If you have tennis elbow, go for a run. A pulled hamstring? Ride the stationary bike.

Ride Out a Charley Horse
The next time you get one of these painful muscle spasms, try this remedy: Arch your toes back toward you while gently rubbing your calf. Start behind the knee and slide your hand down the muscle to the heel, then repeat. Rub along the length of the muscle, not across it.

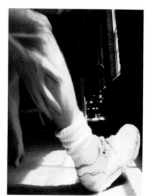

Get Rid of a Side Stitch
To get rid of a side stitch, push three fingers deep into your stomach just below your ribs on the side that hurts, purse your lips tightly, and blow out as hard as you can. Doing this should release the pressure on the diaphragm.

Stop a Sprain from Happening
If you have a tendency to twist or sprain your ankles, wear neoprene or elastic braces, not for the support they supply, which is negligible, but rather for the awareness they create of your gimpy ankles. You'll be better able to tell when your foot is turning in the wrong direction and stop a sprain before it happens.

Make Your Own Ice Pack

The ice-gel packs you can buy at sporting-goods stores are good for chilling sore muscles because they conform to a joint to cool it more thoroughly. But they can cost up to $20. To make a better and cheaper gel pack at home, mix 1½ cups of water with ½ cup of rubbing alcohol, seal it in a plastic bag, and throw it in your freezer for a few hours. Instead of freezing into a rock-solid brick, the alcohol forms a thick slush that will stay ice-cold for at least 60 minutes.

Apply the pack to your skin periodically.

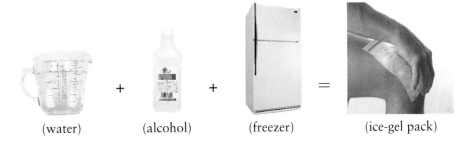

(water)   +   (alcohol)   +   (freezer)   =   (ice-gel pack)

Save Your Wind

If you start wheezing about 10 minutes into your workout regardless of how much aerobic exercise you do, there's a good chance you have exercise-induced asthma, a breathing disorder that affects an estimated 30 million Americans. It occurs when your airway constricts during exercise. Your doctor can prescribe an albuterol inhaler that will keep you from gasping. If chest pain accompanies your shortness of breath, that could be a sign of a heart problem, such as an arterial blockage. See a doctor.

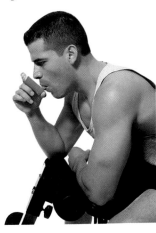

Avoid Finger Jams

If you have a finger that frequently gets jammed, try buddy-taping it to a neighboring digit. Two fingers are stronger than one, and less likely to bend at an odd angle.

Stuff a Sock In It

Remember that the penis is an appendage just as your fingers and toes are. When you're exercising in cold weather, the body draws blood away from these extremities to conserve heat in its core. Therefore, you have to take precautions to insulate it. One of the most indispensable pieces of winter clothing is a wind brief. This is nothing more than underwear with a nylon panel sewn across the front. Most sporting-goods stores carry them, and they are great protection for skiing, running, and mountain biking. If you're caught in the cold without one, stuff a handkerchief, sock, or even a plastic baggie down your pants.

SAVE YOUR CALVES

If your calves feel tight when you wake up in the morning, try sleeping on your stomach with your feet hanging off the bed. Gravity will take over, lightly stretching the calf muscles all night.

Soothe Your Aching Nuts

When you get hit in the balls, sit down and put your head between your legs. This will help stop that sick feeling in the pit of your stomach. Next, reach into your shorts and count your little buddies. If there's only one, his partner may have been knocked up into your abdomen. You'll need to see your doctor to coax it back down. You'll also need to see a doc if there's swelling, bruising, or prolonged pain. Ice the injured gonad on your way to the physician. The cold will be intense, so apply it over your underwear.

Let Your Back Uncrack

You may be able to ward off lower-back pain simply by waiting an hour after you wake up before starting vigorous exercise, such as running or weight lifting. When you're sleeping, fluid pools in your spinal disks, making your lower back tight. Simply walking around for about an hour heads off backaches by squeezing that fluid out and making your back more limber. If you're in a hurry to start your workout, you can try performing some other light exercises to help speed up the drainage process: Sit in a chair, feet flat on the floor, and gently bend forward. Or stand with your hands on your hips and lean slightly from side to side.

Stop a Nosebleed with a Tampon

Pinch your schnozz to stanch the flow of blood, and lean your head forward. Put a bag of ice on the bridge of your nose. The cold will help stop the bleeding even faster. Don't return to the game right away; ask one of the cheerleaders for a tampon, cut off a piece, and use it to plug your nostril. They are extra-absorbent, plus you'll feel "extra-fresh."

Insulate Your Knees

Cold air makes knee tissue less supple, which increases the risk of injury. Knees are especially vulnerable, because they have little fat insulation. The solution is to keep your knees warm while exercising. For temperatures in the 50° to 60°F range, wear basic LYCRA tights. For colder weather, try leg warmers or tights made of wool or polypropylene. For sub-20°F days, use pants made of warm breathable material such a Gore-Tex. Look for the kind with knee panels for wind protection.

Bust a Blister

Lancing a blister within the first 3 hours is much more effective than leaving it alone or removing it entirely. To lance a blister the right way, clean a needle with rubbing alcohol and make two punctures at opposite ends of the blister's perimeter. A single puncture is likely to clog and prevent all the fluid from draining. Check the blister about 8 hours later to make sure it has drained; if not, repeat the procedure.

To keep another blister from forming, apply a light coating of petroleum jelly or pieces of duct tape to other hot spots on your feet before exercising. Or spray your dogs with antiperspirant to minimize sweating and friction.

Put Your Socks on First

After you shower at the gym, always put on your socks before your underwear. Otherwise foot fungus can rub off onto your boxers or briefs and cause jock itch. By putting your socks on first, you keep your undies clean and yourself itch-free.

Likewise, always dry yourself from head to toe after showering—literally. That damp towel you dried your feet with can spread the fungus to your crotch.

Decide If You're Too Sick

It's usually safe to exercise when you have above-the-neck cold symptoms, such as a runny nose, sneezing, and scratchy throat. But intense workouts are not recommended if you have below-the-neck symptoms, such as muscle aches, loss of appetite, a hacking cough or other upper-respiratory ills, or when you have a fever.

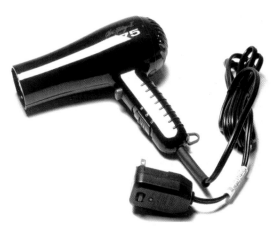

Blow-Dry Your Feet

To avoid athlete's foot, use a hair dryer to blow-dry your feet.

Rest 'em to Grow 'em

Actual gains in muscle size and strength occur not during the workouts, but in the time spent between them. Rest is when your body not only replaces the spent fuel in your muscles, but also adds protein filaments to repair the damage caused by heavy lifting. These tiny bits of protein are what eventually make muscles bigger. If you don't give them enough time to develop, your muscles will only be worn down, not built up. For a muscle to recover fully from a workout, you'll need to allow about 48 hours. But there's no hard-and-fast rule. If you find you're lifting less weight from one workout to the next, that's a pretty good sign you need more rest.

Take the Day Off

To see if you're overtraining, check your pulse first thing in the morning. If it's 10 beats per minute or more above normal, your body is still recovering.

Back Off, Mister

Every 4 to 6 weeks, take a week where your training volume and intensity are no more than half what they were in your toughest week. Without rest, you're training into oblivion.

Set Specific Goals

Research shows that people who set goals that are too general ("I want to get in shape") typically don't achieve them. Make sure your goals are specific and challenging, yet realistic, and have a deadline. ("Each week I'm going to run 10 minutes longer, and after a month I want to be able to run 5 miles without taking a break.")

Kill Your Excuse

If you think you're too busy to exercise, try this experiment: For one day, schedule a time to work out, and then stick to it—even if you can exercise for only 10 minutes. At the end of the day, ask yourself if you were any less productive than usual. The answer will probably be no—and your favorite excuse will be gone.

Save Your Best for Last

A big exercise mistake men make is doing their favorite exercise at the beginning of the workout routine and their least favorite at the end. The result: You either put little effort into these last few exercises or, if you're pressed for time, you skip them entirely. Doing what you hate first assures that you'll give these muscle groups the attention they deserve, and saving your favorites for last helps you recharge when your energy levels are on the decline.

5

HEALTH
and
WELLNESS

On average, American men die 7 years sooner than their female counterparts. If you're skeptical, just look around at all the widows drinking highballs and playing pinochle in retirement communities. If a guy can make it to his mid-70s and stay out of Depends, he suddenly becomes the Casanova he always was in his imagination. Don't let those canes fool you: They're not for balance; they're for fighting off horny blue-hairs. But all kidding aside, it's amazing that given the impressive list of medical advances in the last 2 decades men still lag so significantly behind women when it comes to lifespan. There are a number of reasons.

For one, research funding for male killers such as prostate cancer is still substantially less than for female diseases such as breast cancer. When it comes to lobbying for medical equality, men just aren't as vocal or as organized as women. As of 2003, there still wasn't even an office of men's health in our government (although one for women's health has existed since 1994).

Also, despite great gains by women in the workplace and society in general, men still continue to shoulder most of the burden for bread-winning. And with this ongoing responsibility comes great stress—the biggest of all health risks.

Plus, although pain is supposed to be a classic measure of manliness, most men are wusses when it comes to facing it. One theory holds that the reason women outlive men in such great numbers is because most women are toughened by the agony of childbirth. Therefore, when the pain of old age arrives—whether physical or emotional—they are better prepared to cope with it. Men, however, have no such yardstick and are often debilitated by it.

Our hunch, though, is that the real reason men die sooner is simply because we don't take care of ourselves as well as women do. Namely, we *hate* going to the doctor. While most women visit their gynecologist annually, most men only see a doc when they have a nasty flu or when they accidentally lop something off.

Are we stupid? Of course not. Anthropologists point out that the male in every species, from dogs to human beings, resists rolling over and being submissive. And when you think about it, that's exactly what doctors make men do every day in offices across America. We wait in

an endless succession of smaller and smaller rooms. We are forced to wear open-backed gowns. And when the time finally comes to meet the doctor, he is usually hurried and talks down to us. No wonder it's an experience we dread.

So here's an alternative. Here are the best 264 health and wellness tips from the editors of *Men's Health.* They will help you understand your woeful body a little better so the next time it does something funky and you wonder, "What the hell was that?" you'll at least have some semblance of an answer. Mind you, this isn't a substitute for professional medical care. Don't go reaching for this book instead of the phone if you feel any radiating chest pain. Rather, it's simply better than the traditional male alternative.

Now put on that open-backed gown and start reading.

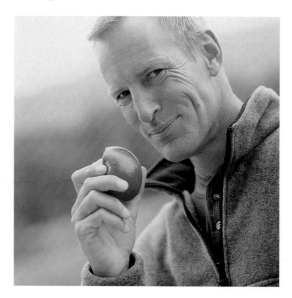

Tell Your True Age

You may not be as old as your driver's license says you are. Here's a quick way to measure your functional age, as opposed to your chronological one.

Skin elasticity: Pinch the skin on the back of your hand between thumb and forefinger for 5 seconds, then time how long it takes to flatten out completely. Up to 50 years of age, it requires only about 5 seconds; by 60, 10 to 15 seconds, and by 70, 35 to 55 seconds. Your initial measurement is less important than the rate of change over the years.

Reaction time: Ask a friend to suspend a thin 18-inch ruler vertically by holding it at the top. Keep the thumb and middle finger of your right hand 3½ inches apart, equidistant from the 18-inch mark on the ruler. As you friend drops the ruler without warning, catch it between your two fingers. Your score is whatever inch-mark you catch it at. Do this three times and take an average. The score usually decreases from the 11-inch mark at age 20 to the 6-inch mark at age 60.

Balance: Close your eyes and lift your dominant foot (right foot if you are right-handed) about 6 inches off the ground, bending your knee at about a 45-degree angle. Try this three times and average the number of seconds you can hold still before you have to open your eyes or move your foot to avoid falling. Typical scores: 28 seconds for ages 20 to 30, 18 seconds for ages 40 to 50, and 4 seconds for ages 60 to 70.

Give Yourself the Finger

Diagnose your health with these self-tests that you can do with just a finger or two.

• If you have a headache and want to know whether it's sinus-related (to better treat the symptoms), tap your face lightly above your eyebrows, between your eyes and nose, and on your cheeks. If you feel a sharp pain when you tap, you probably do have a sinus headache.

• To quickly assess whether you've been sun burned, use your finger to poke the area that has had the most sun exposure. If it blanches, the blood vessels have dilated—a sign of sun damage. If you find yourself believing that the blonde in the thong is checking you out, you're hallucinating—a more extreme indication that you've been in the sun too long.

• To take your pulse, place the first two fingers of one hand lightly on the inside of the opposite wrist, just below the thumb. Count the number of beats in 10 seconds and multiply that number by 6. The normal range while at rest is

HEED THESE 3 RULES

Humans die after 3 minutes without air, 3 hours without clothes (at 32°F), 3 days without water, 3 weeks without food, and 3 months without hope.

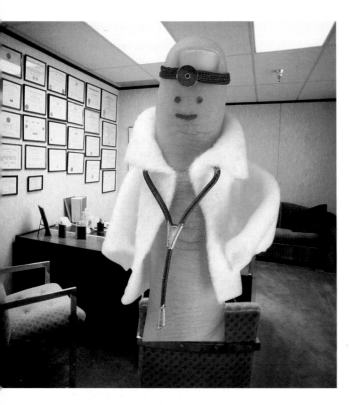

60 to 100 beats per minute, but highly trained athletes can have rates in the 40s.

• The length of your index finger compared with that of your ring finger may be a sign of fertility. In a test of 60 men at an infertility clinic, researchers found that men whose ring fingers are longer than their index fingers have higher testosterone levels.

Order the Perfect Physical

Following are the 20 components of a complete physical. (It's a good idea to have a baseline exam at about age 30, followed by a comprehensive exam every year after age 40.) Run down the list when you make the appointment. If your doctor balks or says you

don't need all these tests, either say your insurance company is "cash" or ask for a referral.

1. Blood work (as extensive as possible)
2. Body-fat test
3. Bone-density screening
4. Chest X-ray (if you're a smoker)
5. Colonoscopy (beginning at age 50, or earlier if you have a family history or other significant risk factors)
6. Comprehensive medical and family history
7. Head-to-toe physical exam
8. Hearing test and vision screening
9. HIV test
10. Kidney- and liver-function tests
11. Neurological exam
12. Prostate exam
13. Pulmonary-function test
14. Skin exam for melanoma and other possible malignancies
15. Stethoscope exam
16. Stool sample for occult blood (to test for colon cancer)
17. Stress test and resting electrocardiogram
18. Throat exam, including vocal cords
19. Thyroid-function test
20. Urinalysis

Save Your Marriage, Save Your Health

An unhappy marriage increases your chance of getting sick by 35 percent and shortens your life by 4 years. If fitness fanatics spent just 10 percent of their weekly exercise time working on their marriages instead of their bodies, they would get three times the health benefits.

Listen to Your Body Report

Does exercise make you feel stronger and more energetic? Do you feel better after a high-carbohydrate pasta-and-salad meal than you do after a high-fat prime-rib dinner? These are important news bulletins from your body. So are hangovers, overuse injuries, minor aches and pains, heartburn, constipation, headaches, and some types of impotence. A doctor can help you interpret these messages, but only you can detect them. Switch off the news once in a while and listen to your body's report.

TELL MOM SHE WAS WRONG

If you're like us, your mom probably threatened you with all kinds of medical mayhem when you were growing up. Finally, the truth:

Threat #1: *"You're gonna fall and crack your head open!"*

Truth: Your skull can split like an egg, but it would require a severe impact, such as falling into the corner of a coffee table. You're much more likely to fracture your skull.

Threat #2: *"Wear clean underwear in case you're in an accident!"*

Truth: When emergency-room personnel cut the clothes off trauma patients, it's done so quickly that they never pay attention to whether the underwear is stained, dirty, or full of holes.

Threat #3: *"Keep touching yourself, and it'll fall off!"*

Truth: There's no evidence that masturbation will causes your staff to revolt. Such exploration is a normal part of growing up.

Threat #4: *"Someday your face will freeze like that!"*

Truth: No matter how far you stretch the corners of your mouth or how deeply into your nostril you plunge your tongue, facial muscles will never become paralyzed as a result.

Threat #5: *"Don't go out without a coat or you'll get sick!"*

Truth: Colds and flu are not caused by catching a chill or by dejectedly walking home from your girlfriend's in the rain without your rubbers. This myth persists largely because most people get sick during winter, when these situations commonly occur. It may even be possible to think yourself ill. If you dread damp feet, your brain may depress your immune system when it happens.

Threat #6: *"You'll poke someone's eye out with that!"*

Truth: It's impossible to "poke out" an eyeball with a sharp instrument. What you'll probably do is pierce or rupture it. To actually pop an eyeball out, you have to get in there with your fingers and pull it out.

Threat #7: *"If you break a leg, don't come running to me!"*

Truth: It's unlikely that you'd be able to run with a broken leg, but you could still walk. There have been cases where people with broken legs walk into the ER. It hurts like crazy, but the muscles spasm and produce enough support to bear weight.

Decode Your Doctor

Typically an *intern* is a fresh grad, a *resident* has at least 1 year of experience, a *fellow* has at least 3, and *attending physicians* are the top dogs. All are fine for stitches. Tap the latter two for life-and-death matters.

Ditch This Doc

Don't go back to a doctor who prescribed medication for you without first asking about your diet, exercise program, and other drugs you're taking. He's either sloppy or ignorant.

Ask Your Doctor His Age

Find a doctor who's roughly your age—give or take 5 years. If your physician is facing the same health quirks you're facing, it'll help him anticipate what tests and treatments you really need. Plus, you'll feel that he understands you better.

Never Wait for a Doctor Again

A good doctor spends extra time with his patients. That means there will be times when he's running behind. To save yourself some grief, call ahead and ask the receptionist how the doctor is doing. If he's 20 minutes or so off schedule, bring some work with you or run an errand in the meantime. By calling ahead, you've also impressed upon the doctor's staff that you're a busy man. They're likely to do a little extra to get you in right away.

When scheduling your appointment, bear in mind that to get your doctor's undivided attention, being the day's first appointment is ideal. But being the last isn't bad, either. There's just not the same urgency as when he has 20 people in the waiting room.

Don't Sign Away Your Life

Researchers examined 42 pens from doctors' pockets and found them to be contaminated with multiple strains of disease-causing bacteria, including the types that cause impetigo, pinkeye, and urinary-tract infections. While doctors trash tongue depressors and rubber gloves faster than we dispose of paychecks, they probably tote the same pen for weeks, using them as pointers, probes, and drumsticks as they treat infectious patients. The chances you'll catch anything fatal from your doc's Bic are slim—but use your own to fill out those forms.

REAL-LIFE SURVIVAL

NEVER TRUST A NURSE WITH FAKE NAILS

Artificial fingernails harbor more bacteria than regular fingernails. Researchers studied 41 nurses and found that those wearing artificial nails were more than twice as likely to have bacteria on their hands after washing than those with natural nails. This increases the risk of transmitting infection.

WHEN ALL ELSE FAILS

STOCK UP ON VASELINE

It has many, many delightful uses:

Screw dipping. Dip screws in Vaseline before inserting. They'll be easy to remove, even years later.

Nipple protection. Yours, not hers. To prevent nipple and skin chafing while running, apply Vaseline to your nipples, armpits, and inner thighs.

Keeping Rover happy. Apply a little Vaseline to your dog's paws before he heads outside in snowy weather. Salt used on the roads can irritate canine feet if they aren't protected.

Nostril protection. If you're doing work in a dusty or smoky environment, a little Vaseline up your nose will prevent you from inhaling offensive particles.

Bait. Fake out those stupid fish by using small pieces of sponge coated with Vaseline to simulate fish-egg bait.

Tenderfoot tending. New shoes often rub, leaving sore heels. Dab a little Vaseline on the backs and heels of your feet to prevent blisters and soreness.

Unclogging the toilet. To increase suction on the rim of a plunger that won't grip, apply a film of Vaseline.

Stifling squeaks. Silence those annoying squeaks by applying a coating of Vaseline to hinges and other moving parts.

"Get That Thing Away from Me"

Next time your doctor pokes his stethoscope toward your chest, you might want to ask him to wash it first. Of 200 stethoscopes taken from four hospitals and clinics, 80 percent were contaminated, mostly with staph germs.

Carry Medical Data with You

Keeping important medical information in your wallet can speed your passage through an emergency room. Carry a list indicating drug sensitivities or allergies, prescription and non-prescription drugs you are taking, the name and phone number of your primary physician (and cardiologist, if you have one) and your doctor's backup physician, medical conditions you are being treated for, and a history of major medical problems experienced by your parents. Your doctor can help you prepare this information.

Also, have a baseline electrocardiogram (EKG) done and photocopy it reduced to wallet size. An EKG is a picture of your heart's electrical activity pattern. Emergency-room doctors will be able to compare that normal EKG with the one taken in the ambulance and decide on the best treatment.

Find a Great Doctor

Survey one of the following five people for the best doctor recommendation:

An operating-room nurse. If you're seeking a surgeon, pick the brain of an OR nurse. They see physicians in action.

A head nurse. Contact the vice-president of nursing and ask whom he or she would recommend. They've watched physicians come up through the ranks.

A chief resident at a teaching hospital. Chief residents (doctors in the last year of their residency) have spent the last few years observing their seasoned colleagues.

A health reporter for a large newspaper. These writers are usually very knowledgeable about the medical communities they cover.

A pathologist. These physicians perform autopsies regularly. They see the results of their colleague's handiwork—including the surgery mistakes and the missed diagnoses.

Ask Your Surgeon These Questions

Before surrendering your body, ask your doctor these key questions:

1. How many times have you done this particular procedure?

2. What are the outcomes of the procedure in terms of mortality and complication rates?

3. Are complications frequent?

4. Are you operating, or is a student?

5. Why do you want to use this particular operating technique?

6. What should I expect after the anesthesia wears off?

7. What potential problems could arise?

8. What is your philosophy about pain control?

9. How long is recovery?

Avoid Garlic Bread before Surgery

If you're planning to undergo surgery, stop using garlic, vitamin E, and fish-oil pills, which can thin your blood and cause excessive bleeding. Quit taking them about 2 weeks before your operation.

Play the Sedating Game

If you're heading for surgery, and a local anesthesia isn't an option, do these three things to ensure that you wake up.

1. *Cut the spuds.* Don't eat potatoes, tomatoes, or eggplant for at least a week before surgery. Researchers found that compounds in these foods can affect your body's ability to metabolize anesthetics.

2. *Bring your medications.* When you talk to the anesthesiologist before surgery, show her all the medications you take, including over-the-counter drugs. This will reduce the chance of unwanted interactions.

3. *Go intravenous.* Ask whether your anesthetic can be delivered intravenously rather than through a gas mask. Inhaled anesthetics can leave you groggy for a longer time after surgery.

Avoid 6 P.M. Surgery

It might not be a good idea to schedule an appointment with a dentist or doctor at 6 P.M. This is the time of day when your production of pain-blocking endorphins is low, as is your level of corticosteroids, your body's natural means of fighting inflammation. Most sufferers of chronic pain say it is worst in the late afternoon and evening.

Donate Some Blood to Yourself

Using your own donated blood during surgery could help you recover more quickly. In one study, patients who were given their own blood during operations had half the infection rate of patients who received blood from donors. Researchers think that receiving a transfusion of your own blood stimulates the immune system to fight infection.

Mark the Spot

Be certain that a nurse draws an "X" on the spot where the surgeon is supposed to cut you. We're not kidding. This is mandatory in many hospitals. It's intended to prevent the lamebrain surgical mistakes that make headlines a dozen times each year.

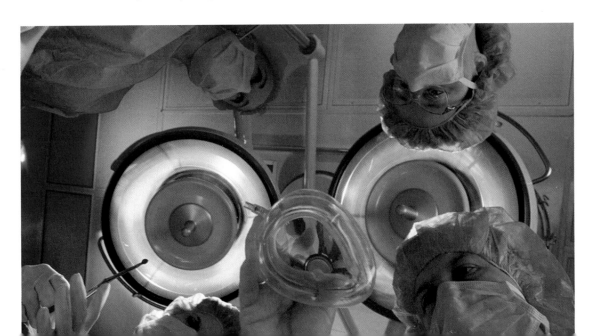

Take Your Best Shot

If you're just as queasy about getting a needle as you were when you were a kid, make sure to schedule it for early in the day. That's when your pain tolerance is highest. Also, take a deep breath during the injection. Your muscles are less tense when you're inhaling.

You can prevent the bruising that sometimes occurs after an injection by firmly pressing your palm or four fingers against the area for 5 minutes. Such gentle pressure forces your blood's clotting agents to seal the wound before the blood that causes the bruise can seep into your skin's upper layer.

WIN THE WAR ON BUGS

The single most effective way to sidestep the flu is to get vaccinated against it. Like many vaccines, a flu shot exposes you to parts of the virus that were killed and processed in a lab. Your body's immune system identifies and builds antibodies to the virus and is readied for combat if you are later exposed to a full-fledged viral attack. The vaccine is 70 to 90 percent effective in preventing flu in people up to age 65. And even if you do get the flu, the symptoms will be less severe. Get vaccinated in the late fall or very early winter, though. It takes about 2 weeks to become effective.

Forget This Myth

You can't catch the flu from a flu shot. Your arm might be a little sore for a day, but only one person in 100 will feel some fever and aches.

Watch Your Altitude

Here's another great reason to get a flu shot. If you plan to go skiing in altitudes much higher than you're accustomed to—say, 8,000 to 12,000 feet above sea level—ask your doctor about flu vaccination or antiviral medication first. Higher altitudes stress your body and make you extremely susceptible to influenza.

Buy Liquid-Gel Caps

It's not just the pain reliever you choose, but the form it comes in. Liquid-gel capsules of dissolved ibuprofen reach your bloodstream almost 60 percent faster than the solid form.

Move Your Medicine

If your medication is constantly exposed to light, heat, or humidity (which is exactly the climate in steamy bathrooms), it could degrade faster than it should. The worst place to store anything is in a bathroom. The refrigerator is a bad idea as well because it's humid inside, causing certain medicines to crystallize or crack. A linen closet is the best storage place.

Look for White Powder

Want your aspirin to beat back your headache? Check the bottle. If you see a white, powdery film on the inside surface, your Bayer is belly-up. This holds true even if the date it was supposed to expire hasn't arrived.

Grill Your Doctor about Your Drugs

Next time a doctor hands you a prescription, take a minute to ask some questions. You could save some money. Drug companies have perfected the art of modifying a best-selling drug just as the patent for it is about to expire and a cheaper generic substitute is ready to hit the market. The companies push the modified pills to doctors and patients and thus hang onto market share. A recent study showed that 65 percent of the drugs approved from 1989 to 2000 were simply modified versions of—or the same as—existing drugs. These medications can cost much more than a generic or an older version that does virtually the same thing. Ask your doc these questions:

• Is this a brand-name drug? Why am I getting it and not a generic?

• Is this a new drug with new active ingredients, or just a modified version of an older drug? Would the old one work?

• If it's new, what's the benefit: fewer side effects, longer lasting, more convenient?

Make the Medicine Go Down

A few moments before downing a brackish concoction, suck on some ice. It'll numb your tastebuds and make the medicine less nasty.

Swallow 'em Whole

Don't crush a pill into powder to make it easy to swallow. If it's a time-release medication, it was designed to enter the system slowly and steadily; taken in powdered form, the drug is absorbed at once and can cause an overdose. Also, crushing pills destroys coatings made to protect the lining of the throat and stomach. Instead of pulverizing your pills, see if the prescription comes in easier-to-swallow gel capsules.

Keep the Rib-Eye Out of Your Eye

If you have a black eye, resist the urge to slap a steak on it. It's an old wives' tale. Meat is full of bacteria that can give you conjunctivitis. A cold compress will relieve the pain and swelling more effectively. First, treat the injury for 15 minutes with an ice pack wrapped in a towel to constrict the blood vessels. Remove the pack for 10 minutes to let your skin warm, then repeat the treatment. Switch to heat the next day to dilate blood vessels and improve circulation (a warm, wet washcloth will work).

To get rid of the discoloration, eat a few papayas. An enzyme in this fruit makes it easier for the body to reabsorb the blood trapped under your skin.

While your skin is still bruised, avoid aspirin. Aspirin prevents blood from clotting, and it's the seepage of blood that leads to discoloration. If you need pain relief, try acetaminophen (Tylenol).

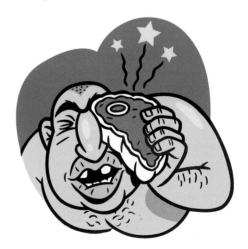

Yoplait It Again

Next time your doctor prescribes antibiotics, reach for the yogurt. Antibiotics kill the "good" stomach bacteria required for healthy digestion. Without it, you could develop diarrhea. A cup of yogurt can replenish these necessary germs. Yogurts labeled "live active culture" contain the beneficial bacteria.

Stop the Pilling

At least 20 percent of the antibiotic prescriptions written in the United States are unnecessary. Patients expect the antibiotics and the physician tries to keep his patients happy. Many doctors even prescribe them for viral infections, such as the flu, knowing full well they're useless. (They help with only bacterial infections.) Taking unnecessary antibiotics can help disease-causing bacteria develop a resistance to them, which could hurt you when you really need them. You only need antibiotics for sinus infections, strep throat, pneumonia, and serious skin infections. And always take every last pill the doctor gives, or you'll leave the strongest bugs alive to repopulate.

Skip the Antibacterial Soap

There's absolutely no reason to buy antibacterial soaps, according to the American Medical Association. While close to 50 percent of soaps sold in the States contain antimicrobial agents, the AMA claims that there's no solid scientific proof that these soaps are better at preventing infection than regular soap. In fact, the group argues that antibacterial soaps may be doing more harm than good—making bacteria stronger and more resistant to existing germ-killers.

Take 2 Gulps and Call Us in the Morning

Pills get stuck in your throat? Try taking them with two quick gulps of water without pausing rather than one larger gulp. The first swallow gets your epiglottis—the flap of tissue that covers the windpipe—to fold down, so pills don't get caught in it. The second gulp gets the pill past the epiglottis before it springs back.

KEEP A HEADACHE DIARY

If you suffer from frequent headaches, you can put your finger on what's triggering them. All you need to do is pick up a pen. By keeping a headache diary, a pattern could emerge that can help you identify the hidden causes of pain. When your headache comes, note what time it is, what you ate recently, and what you were doing just before you noticed the pain. This will point toward the troublemakers. Some commonly overlooked suspects include sex, flying, skipping meals, chewing gum, spicy foods, ice cream, and too much sleep.

Keep Your Head from Exploding

Migraines are highly individualized, but certain foods—especially those high in a compound called tyramine—are known to induce them in some people. Key suspects include organ meats such as kidneys, fermented products such as yeasts and soy sauces, wine and beer, monosodium glutamate (MSG), hot dogs, certain aged cheeses, chocolate, and caffeine.

Learn the ABCs of OTCs

It seems as if there are hundreds of over-the-counter pain relievers, but actually there are five main types: aspirin, acetaminophen, ibuprofen, naproxen sodium, and ketoprofen. The best one to take depends on why you're taking it. Aspirin, ibuprofen, naproxen sodium, and ketoprofen all have anti-inflammatory properties and work better than acetaminophen for muscular pain or sports injuries. For headaches, aspirin is the best all-around choice, unless it irritates your stomach. In that case, either buffered aspirin or acetaminophen (the active ingredient in Tylenol) is a good alternative.

Double-Team a Headache

Taking caffeine and ibuprofen relieves headaches more effectively than ibuprofen alone. Among 400 headache patients, 71 percent of those who took ibuprofen *and* the caffeine equivalent of two cups of coffee reported complete relief, compared to 58 percent of those who took ibuprofen *or* caffeine.

Take 2 Tennis Balls for a Nasty Headache

For a headache, stuff those two balls in a sock (preferably a clean one) and tie the end tightly so they won't move. Then lie on your back on the floor and place the socked balls right under the spot where your skull meets your neck. Lie there for a while. This kind of direct pressure on the nerves at the base of the neck may numb them, relieving pain.

Don't Blink the Water

Using tap water to clean or store contact lenses can cause a potentially blinding infection. Tap water contains microscopic organisms that, when trapped under lenses, can cause ulcers on the cornea.

Soothe Your Peepers

Brisky rub your hands together to generate heat. Then place them over your closed eyes. The gentle pressure and warmth will soothe your eyes.

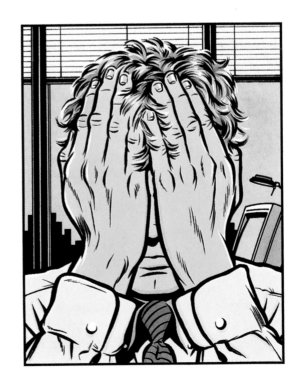

SOOTHE YOUR EYES BY CHANGING DEODORANT

If your eyes are constantly dry, try changing deodorants. Those that contain an antiperspirant can dry out eyes.

See If You're Ready for Bifocals

If you're over 40 and get headaches or eyestrain from reading, you may have presbyopia: loss of close focus. To tell if you do, open a telephone book and choose some numbers. (If you normally wear glasses, keep them on.) Move the book away until you can focus on the numbers. If you must fully extend your arms or bend them only slightly to see clearly, you're probably ready for bifocals. See an optometrist or ophthalmologist for a more precise test.

Poke Your Eyes

Here's a quick way to tell whether you're nearsighted: With a pencil, poke a hole in a piece of paper, hold the paper 2 to 4 inches from your face, and peer through the hole at an object that's at least 10 feet away. If you see the object more clearly through the hole, you might be myopic (nearsighted). If you're wearing corrective lenses for myopia, these results suggest it's time for a stronger prescription.

Test Your Hearing

In a quiet room, extend your arm straight out to the side and lightly rub your thumb and forefinger together. Slowly move the rubbing fingers toward one ear, taking note of how far away it is when the sound becomes audible. Repeat on the other side. Under age 60, a person with normal hearing should be able to make out the sound at 6 to 8 inches. If you're not able to hear at that range, you may not be catching everything people say to you—and that could put you out of the loop. If you can't hear beyond 4 inches, you have the hearing of a 70-year-old.

Plug Up the Stones

Here's where you draw the line on volume. When you turn off the stereo, do your ears ring or feel "full?" Are ordinary sounds muffled? If so, then the volume was too loud. At concerts, always wear foam earplugs; they'll not only protect your hearing, they'll also make the quality of sound better. In a lot of enclosed spaces, you're bombarded with reverberatory echo—plugs reduce the distortion.

Keep Your Window Up

Audiologists have noticed that the left ears of truck drivers tend to have significant hearing loss. That's the side of the head closer to the window—and the loss is probably caused by both wind and traffic noise. To protect yourself if you drive a lot, keep that window rolled up.

Shine a Bug Out of Your Ear

If an insect flies into your ear, shine a light in the canal. Chances are, the critter will crawl back toward the light.

Wax Eloquently

An aggressively applied Q-Tip can puncture your eardrum; the resulting scar tissue can give you hearing problems later. It's safer to clean your ears with a finger inside a washcloth. If wax tends to stop up your ears, have a doctor show you how to irrigate them with vinegar and water.

Thwart Cankers with Yogurt

If canker sores are a constant presence, your mouth may be screaming for more acidophilus. This beneficial bacterium can help regulate the natural flora in your mouth that can otherwise run amok and cause sores and gum problems. Eat a cup of yogurt as a mid-morning snack every day. And we don't mean the frozen TCBY kind. Look for yogurts that contain live active cultures.

Be a Sore Loser

Canker sores are like party crashers in your mouth—you don't know where they came from, and you just want them to go away before they ruin everything. These mouth ulcers are typically caused by trauma, an allergy, or stress, but a detergent called sodium lauryl sulfate (SLS) in most over-the-counter toothpastes may also be to blame. One theory is that SLS dries out the protective mucus in your mouth, making it more vulnerable to canker sores. If you have frequent sores, switch to an SLS-free paste such as Rembrandt Natural.

Put a Tea Bag on a Mouth Sore

Hold a wet tea bag on the canker sore; the tannin from the tea acts as an astringent.

Drink Less Beer to Avoid Cold Sores

The herpes simplex virus that causes cold sores needs the amino acid arginine to initiate its dirty work. Beer is rich in arginine, as are chocolate, cola, peas, peanuts, and cashews. Limiting your intake of these foods may help reduce outbreaks if you're prone to them.

Wipe Out Cold Sores with Aspirin

The herpes simplex virus can be fatal to your social life. Save it with aspirin. Researchers found that popping 125 milligrams of aspirin daily can cut the duration of a cold sore almost in half—from an average of 8 days down to just 5. Aspirin helps to reduce the inflammation that causes a cold sore, so the area heals faster.

Repair Your Roof

If you over-nuked your leftover pizza and scorched the roof of your mouth, use an over-the-counter cough lozenge with benzocaine to cut the pain. If you don't have any, try using sugar.

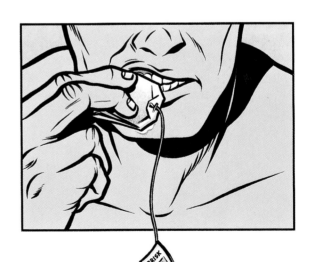

Replace a Lost Tooth

A tooth must be replaced within 30 to 60 minutes. Don't disinfect, scrape, or scrub the tooth, but if it's dirty, rinse it with water. Then push it back into its socket. Once in place, press it down with a finger or bite into a rolled handkerchief—then see a dentist. If you can't replace the tooth yourself, take it to your dentist in cool water or milk.

Handle a Toothache

Cut toothache pain in half by rubbing ice on the V-shaped area where the bones of your thumb and forefinger meet (not the web) for 5 to 7 minutes. This trick works with either hand, not just the one on the side with the toothache.

Stop Getting Cavities

Use a drinking straw. You may feel like your 4-year-old nephew, but a straw limits the amount of contact between your teeth and sugary sodas or fruit juices, so less dental damage occurs over time.

RINSE AFTER LUNCH

If you can't brush, rinse your mouth with water after lunch. Doing so reduces the bacteria in your mouth by 30 percent, which significantly cuts your risk of cavities. For a quick breath freshener, grab a handful of parsley sprigs and munch on the stems.

Store Your Toothbrush in Mouthwash

Store your toothbrush bristles-down in a glass of mouthwash (which you should replace every few days). This will minimize the germs you put in your mouth.

Give Germs the Brushoff

Changing toothbrushes more frequently when you're sick may help you get well faster. Well-worn brushes host bacteria and yeast associated with pneumonia, stomach ulcers, strep throat, sinus disease, upset stomach, and diarrhea.

Brush Your Tongue

Doing so reduces mouth odor by 75 percent, whereas brushing the teeth reduces it by only 25 percent. Combining the two methods is best. That approach reduces odor by 85 percent.

Be the Boss of Floss

Flossing is 10 times more important than brushing. The broad, flat surfaces of your teeth harbor few bacteria, but the unbrushable crevices between teeth are loaded with garbage. If you can't floss after every meal, at least do it once a day.

Knock Out Jaw Tension

Clenching the teeth can make muscles tight and provoke jaw pain. For quick relief, press a fist under your chin, then try to open your mouth, resisting the jaw movement with the fist. Hold for 10 seconds.

Put a Shoe on Your Pillow

In order to ward off neck pain, make sure your pillow supports your head and neck at a normal angle. To test, fold your pillow in half and put a shoe on top. If it springs back, it's okay. If not, it's incapable of providing proper support.

Handle a Smack in the Snout

If your nose is bleeding, lean forward. Leaning back can cause you to choke on your blood. Pinch your nostrils closed. The bleeding should stop within 5 minutes. Then test for a fracture. If the tip sounds squishy when you press it, it's broken.

Check for Thyroid Cancer

Pour a glass of water and hold a small mirror so you can see your Adam's apple. Watch the area below the Adam's apple for bumps and bulges as your drink. If you see any, have them checked, pronto.

Prevent an Allergy Attack

Ward off an allergic reaction to pollen by using a decongestant nasal spray or antihistamine *before* exercising or working outdoors in the summer. Warm-weather workouts can set you up for an allergy attack because the heavier you breathe, the more pollen you draw into your lungs. Anti-allergy medications work best if used before pollen exposure.

Shave Your 'Stache and Sneeze Less

If you're prone to allergies and have a mustache, wash it twice a day with liquid soap.

One study found that patients who did this used fewer antihistamines and decongestants. Reason: Cleaning got rid of stuck pollen grains.

Likewise, to minimize the effects of allergies, wash your hair before going to bed instead of in the morning. You'll rinse the pollen away instead of spending the night breathing it.

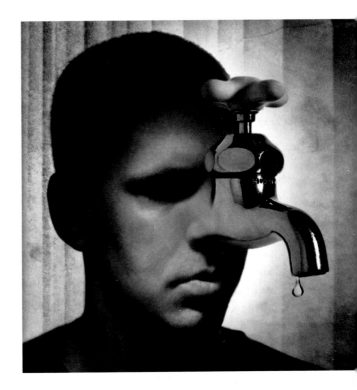

Dilute Your Decongestant

If you take a medicated nasal decongestant, like Afrin, don't overdo it. Using it for just 3 days in a row can irritate your nasal lining and make sinusitis worse. To prevent this, replace half of your decongestant spray with water that's been boiled for 10 minutes. This diluted solution should still relieve symptoms well, and you can use it for up to 6 days.

Avoid Swallowing a Sneeze

Feel a sneeze coming on? Don't hold your breath, seal your lips or pinch your nose to lessen the sound of your sneeze; the air pressure you build up can force infections deep into your sinuses or ears. First try pinching your nose when you feel the first tickle of a sneeze coming on. This usually makes the sensation subside. If not, lightly cover your nose and mouth with your cupped hand (preferably holding a handkerchief) and let 'er rip.

Never Catch a Cold

Cold viruses are transmitted through the air and by touch, so the best way to prevent a cold is to keep your distance from someone who has one. The most critical period to avoid contact is the first 2 to 3 days that the sufferer showcases symptoms.

By the way, you can't get a cold by catching a chill. On the contrary, the reason we get sick during winter is because we spend more time indoors in close contact with others.

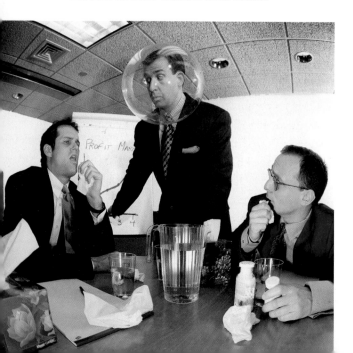

Hack It Up

When you have a bad cough, don't down tablespoonfuls of heavy-duty cough suppressants. The active ingredient you want to avoid is *dextromethorphan*. Suppressants short-circuit the brain signals that control the urge to cough. If you're coughing up matter, you need to let your body do its work. Stop this process and all the troublemakers stay in your lungs, where they can breed, prosper and set the stage for a nasty secondary infection. Instead, look for an over-the-counter remedy that says "expectorant"—the active ingredient will be *guaifenesin,* a chemical that liquefies the crud down there and makes it easier to cough up.

Follow This Hoarse Sense

Contrary to popular belief, if you have a hoarse throat you shouldn't whisper. Whispering is an abrasive way to use your voice, producing a tense, abnormal vocal-cord motion that may worsen the situation.

Blow Up Your Cold

Blowing your nose could make your cold last longer. Using X-rays, researchers discovered that nose blowing actually forces some mucus backward. You may propel bacteria and viruses directly into your sinuses, which may trigger reactions that could make your cold worse. Take antihistamines instead, as soon as symptoms appear.

Make All Symptoms Go

If you can't resist the urge to blow your nose, use a tissue to blow instead of a handkerchief.

You can actually re-infect yourself with a dirty handkerchief.

Thwart an Asthma Attack

If you're caught without your asthma medication, drink coffee. The caffeine in a cup or two of strong brew may open narrowed bronchial passages.

Test Your Lungs with a Candle

Hold a lit candle 6 inches from your face, open your mouth wide, and take a deep breath. Try to blow out the candle without pursing your lips. If you can extinguish the flame, your lungs are functioning well.

Stop Being a Heavy Breather

Guys who breathe through their mouths often are tired without knowing why. The reason: Mouth-breathing tends to be shallow and rapid, and your body works too hard for the oxygen it gets. Remedy this problem by making a conscious effort to breathe slowly and steadily through your nose.

Break a High Fever

Anything up to 100.9°F is mild and can be treated by drinking plenty of fluids. But to quickly bring down a reading above that, put an ice pack under your arm or near your groin. Icing either spot will cool your body's core. It's uncomfortable, but it works fast. Then see a doctor.

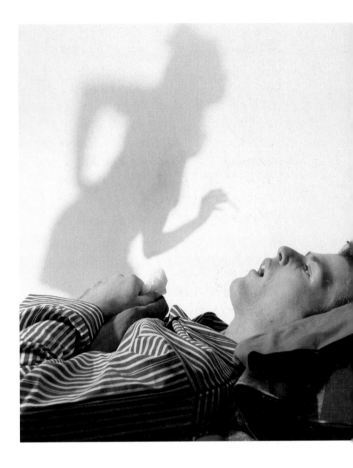

Take an Accurate Temperature

If you're sipping a hot or cold beverage to make yourself feel better, the liquid can throw off the temperature inside your mouth. Put the drink aside for 10 minutes before using a thermometer. That'll allow your mouth and core body temperatures to equalize. When the thermometer is in your mouth, keep your lips sealed. Breathing through your mouth while taking your temperature can throw off the reading by a significant amount.

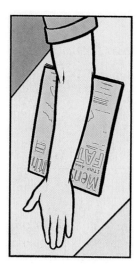 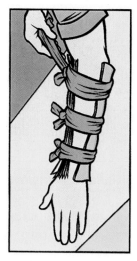

ice. Bad move. The tissue may freeze, making it impossible to reattach. Instead, wrap it in a clean, wet cloth, put the cloth in a plastic bag and *then* put it in the cooler.

& % * # % ! ! !

If you bash your finger with a hammer or slam it in a car door, plunge it in ice water for a minute. Then hold it over your head while pinching the wounded fingertip. After another minute, dunk it back into the ice water. Repeat this routine about 10 times. It will stop the throbbing pain and save your fingernail from blackening and falling off.

Splint a Broken Arm with a Magazine

To make an impromptu cast, place your wrist palm-down on top of a thick magazine. Roll the magazine into a U-shaped cradle, and secure it with tape, an Ace bandage, or long strips torn from a shirt.

Save a Severed Finger

If you happen to lop off a finger, your first inclination (after screaming and running around) may be to throw the digit into a cooler full of

Stop Biting Your Nails

If you're determined to stop chewing on yourself, have your hands manicured. It puts a different focus on the hands, which sometimes helps men stop biting their nails.

Fend Off Frosty Fingers

When your hands feel like they're going numb in freezing weather, swing your arms in a circle. This will bring blood rushing to your hands and warm them fast.

REAL-LIFE SURVIVAL

ATTACK A HEART ATTACK

Call 911 for help (better yet, have someone else do it). Then cough vigorously; you may be able to kick an irregular heartbeat back to normal. Grab an aspirin and chew it—the medicine will enter your bloodstream more quickly and may prevent the formation of a clot. Wait for the ambulance. If you try to drive yourself, you may black out behind the wheel.

Flip Through the Family Album

Worried about your heart disease risk? Many of the factors that lead to heart disease have a genetic link. Ask yourself what habits your parents might have had that lead to heart disease. Smoking, drinking, a regular diet of fine Slovakian cuisine—if you avoid their bad habits, you avoid much of their risk. By taking charge of your behavior, you can reduce your risk as much as 70 percent.

Build Your Heart Muscle

The heart responds to exercise the same way ordinary muscle does. Just as your chest expands with repeated bench presses, your heart grows with prolonged aerobic exercise. A well-trained heart can be about 30 to 40 percent larger than a normal one. And since it's so big, it can pump about 50 percent more blood with every beat.

Do a Gut Check

Studies show that "central obesity" (that's a potbelly to you) raises your heart-disease risk. This simple test will tell you how big a problem your belly is. With a measuring tape, get a reading on your waist at the midpoint between your bottom rib and hipbone. Then measure your hips at their widest point. Divide your waist size by your hip size, and you've got something called your waist-to-hip ratio. If that ratio is 0.95 or less, you've just eliminated one key risk factor for heart disease.

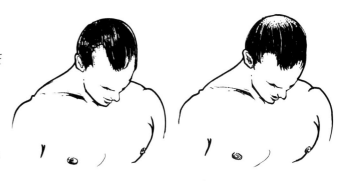

Lose Hair, Lose Heart

Baldness may indicate that you're at higher risk of heart disease. Men with frontal balding are 9 percent more likely to have coronary heart disease, while men with baldness originating from the spot on top of the head have a 23 to 36 percent greater risk than men with no hair loss. Researchers aren't sure how to explain the link. If you're balding, you might want to talk to your doctor about diagnostic tests that might give an early indication of possible heart trouble.

Read the Fine Print

Use this quick health test to rate your chances of developing high blood pressure. Take a look at the patterns on the fingertips of your right

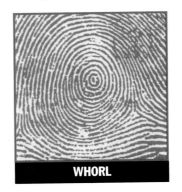

WHORL

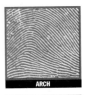

ARCH

LOOP

hand. Here's what you're looking for: whorl patterns and arching or looping patterns. How many of each? Men with three or more whorls tend to have significantly higher blood-pressure readings than those with fewer whorls. And whorls on the right hand were more strongly associated with increased blood pressure than were whorls on the left hand. If your prints are whorly, it might be a good idea to stop putting off plans to have your blood pressure checked.

Figure Your Heart-Disease Risk

Here's an easy equation that can determine your risk for heart disease: Subtract the diastolic number (the lower number) in your blood-pressure reading from the systolic number. If the result is greater than 60, you need to consult your doctor. As arteries stiffen, systolic blood pressure increases and diastolic pressure goes down.

Get Help Faster

Tell the 911 operator "chest pains," not "heart attack." If you say "heart attack," she'll likely waste time asking you to explain your symptoms more clearly.

Diagnose a Heart Skip

When your heart skips a beat, it's not always because there's a beautiful woman approaching. Every so often, the heart's sinus node screws up the electrical signals that keep it beating. Cardiologists call these disturbances arrhythmias. Although they may make you momentarily contemplate a Higher Being, they are generally harmless. Caffeine, alcohol, nicotine, cold and asthma medicines, even stress can cause the node to misfire. If arrhythmias occur several times a week, however, or if your heart rate fluctuates from below 40 beats per minute to more than 180, it's time to see a doctor.

Understand Your Blood Pressure

Here's the simple translation for those blood-pressure numbers that doctors and nurses rattle off: The first number (120) is the *systolic* pressure, which represents the pressure in the arteries at the moment your heart contracts and pumps blood. The second number (80) is the *diastolic* pressure, which represents the arterial pressure between beats, or the resting pressure. By the way, "120 over 80" is what you want to hear. That's a perfect reading for a healthy man. A cute nurse touching your arm can make your

---

REAL-LIFE SURVIVAL

DON'T WAIT ON CHEST PAIN

If you feel a persistent, uncomfortable pressure in your chest, don't waste time blaming those burritos. Head to the emergency room. A study of 2,404 heart-attack patients showed that 40 percent waited more than 6 hours before going to the hospital. That's too long. The longer you wait to seek treatment, the more heart muscle you'll lose.

STEP BY STEP

SAVE YOUR PET FROM CHOKING

It's not just for people anymore. Here's how to do the Heimlich Maneuver on your dog or cat:

1. Look in the monster's maw and determine whether the foreign object in his throat is visible. If possible, clear the airway by removing the object with pliers or tweezers.

2. If the object is lodged too deeply or if the pet collapses, place your hands on both sides of the animal's rib cage and apply firm, quick pressure.

3. As a last resort, place the animal on its side and strike the side of the rib cage firmly with the palm of your hand three or four times. Repeat this procedure until the object is dislodged or you arrive at the vet's office.

pressure surge, as can a morning cup of coffee, so don't be bashful about asking her—or someone else—to double-check a high reading. But if you hit 140/90 or better and don't edge down over a week or two, you've got high blood pressure, pal.

Take Your BP While Exercising

To find out how healthy your heart is, have your blood pressure measured while you're exercising, rather than at rest. Your levels will be higher, but according to one study, this reading may be a better indicator of your overall health. When you're exercising, a healthy BP can go above 120/80 but shouldn't top 200/80. Your doctor can measure your exercising BP during a cardiac stress test. Or, for a slightly less accurate reading, gauge your own BP using a battery-powered tester while riding a stationary bike.

Be a Sponge

Loma Linda University researchers found that drinking five or more 8-ounce glasses of water

a day could help lower your risk of heart disease by up to 60 percent—exactly the same drop you get from stopping smoking, lowering your LDL (bad) cholesterol numbers, exercising, or losing a little weight.

Pet Away High Blood Pressure

To lower your risk of heart attack and stroke, get a dog. Studies show that petting a dog lowers blood pressure almost immediately.

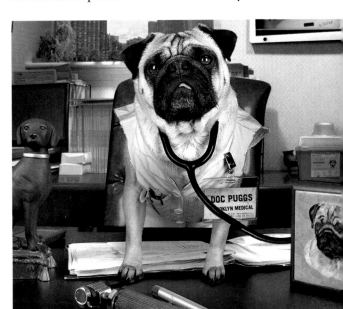

BEAT HYPERTENSION WITH BANANAS

Some people with high blood pressure are able to reduce their blood-pressure medications simply by raising their intake of potassium, which is plentiful in fresh fruits and vegetables, especially bananas. Guys with normal blood pressures can view this as an investment in the future.

Find Out If You're a Sensitive Guy

If you have a family history of high blood pressure, are hypertensive, or are just curious, you can do a simple at-home test to find out if you are salt-sensitive. All you need is a blood-pressure cuff and a food table that provides sodium values. Total your sodium and blood pressure for a week, getting a daily average for both. Then cut back on sodium and see what happens. Your blood pressure might inch down. Or it might plummet by 20 points.

Interrupt Heart Disease

A study showed that those who interrupt others had a 47 percent higher risk of coronary heart disease than those who let others finish talking. According to researchers, your body perceives the verbal competition as aggression—causing your heart rate to rise—which may eventually lead to heart disease.

Beware Loaded Gums

If you have a history of tooth and gum disease or an unusually high number of cavities, you might be at greater risk of heart disease. Researchers have identified a link between mouth and heart diseases. Certain people are predisposed to have more bacteria in their mouths. These bacteria not only cause more tooth and gum problems, but can also enter the bloodstream, causing blockages that may lead to heart disease.

Watch the Weather Channel

Heart attacks are more likely to occur on cold days and at extreme atmospheric pressures. Researchers found that each decrease of 18°F and each increase or decrease of 10 millibars of atmospheric pressure from sea level resulted in approximately 12 percent more heart attacks. Cold weather makes the heart work harder, increases its need for oxygen, and raises cholesterol concentrations. And differences in atmospheric pressure may cause fluctuations in blood pressure.

Survive the Next Snowstorm

Heed these hints to avoid having a heart attack while shoveling snow:

• Skip the morning coffee and avoid cigarettes and decongestants because, as stimulants, these constrict blood vessels and raise pulse rate, which puts additional strain on the heart.

• Warm up before you dig in.

• Dress in layers and remove them as you heat up to reduce heart stress.

• Pick a shovel with a smaller, lighter blade to limit the weight being lifted.

• Lift with your legs and not your back.

• Move your feet to dump the load rather than twisting at the waist.

• Take frequent breaks, pausing every so often to look imploringly at your neighbor and his Sno-Cat.

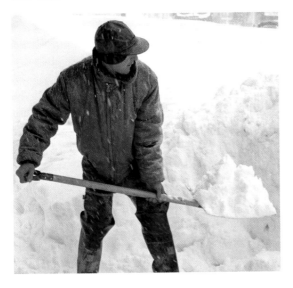

Toast Yourself

One or two alcoholic drinks per day can ward off heart disease in two ways: first, by modestly boosting blood levels of HDL, the cholesterol that clears arteries of fatty deposits; second, by making platelets or clot-forming cells less likely to stick together and obstruct blood flow. In fact, findings pooled from more than 30 long-term studies suggest that those who imbibe within this range reduce their risk of heart attack by 25 to 40 percent compared with non-drinkers. And just in case you were wondering, one drink means a 12-ounce beer, a 4- to 6-ounce glass of wine, or a shot (1.5 ounces) of anything stronger.

Laugh and Last

Half of a group of 48 heart-attack survivors watched a comedy video of their choice for 30 minutes a day for a year. The other half weren't allowed to watch anything funny. After 12 months, only two patients in the first group had suffered another heart attack, compared with 10 in the second group. Daily laughter seems to help restore the brain neurotransmitters that help us cope with stress.

Get a Flu Shot to Prevent a Heart Attack

Heart-attack survivors are one-third less likely to have a second heart attack if they get a flu vaccination before the flu season. The flu may contribute to inflammation that leads to rupturing of arterial plaques. It may also weaken your body in general, making you more susceptible to heart damage.

Toughen Your Ticker

Weights can make your biceps look good, but they're also good for your heart. Why? In addition to lowering cholesterol and blood-pressure levels, stronger muscles make physical exertion, especially lifting or carrying things, less taxing. Stronger muscles result in a significant reduction in heart rate and blood pressure while you're carrying a heavy object. This may help you avoid straining your heart during exertion, which can cause a heart attack.

Control Blood Pressure without Drugs

Exercise alone may be the most effective non-drug method for normalizing mild high blood pressure—although it can take 2 to 3 months to produce results. After a 3-month program of regular 20-minute, fast-paced workouts on a stationary bicycle, patients in one study saw their blood pressure drop by 10 to 50 points.

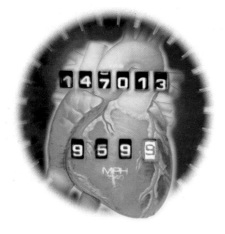

Lower Your Heart Rate

A lean, athletic man who maintains a resting heart rate (RHR) of 52 beats per minute will muster about 850 million heartbeats between the ages of 30 and 60—and that includes 3 hours per week at his peak exercise heart rate. An inactive guy with an RHR of 72 might clock 1.1 billion beats during those same 30 years—an extra 250 million beats, which could cut his life span by a decade. Over the long term, exercise can slow your RHR by as many as 20 beats per minute. To check your RHR, take your pulse in the morning, while you're still in bed. While looking at a watch, place two fingertips on the inner wrist of your nondominant hand. Apply pressure until you feel a pulse. Starting with the first pulse after the second hand reaches 12, count your pulses for 10 seconds. Multiply that number by 6. If it's more than 60, hit the treadmill.

Raise Your HDL

When looking over blood-test results, most men focus on their LDL cholesterol level and completely ignore the HDL cholesterol count. This is a huge mistake—a third of men at risk of dying of heart disease have perfectly normal levels of LDL. The fact is, if you don't have enough HDL scouring your arteries, even low amounts of LDL can form dangerous blockages. The higher the HDL, the better. Once you get over 60 mg/dl, it's a strong positive factor in avoiding heart disease. The best ways to boost HDL include drinking three glasses of orange juice per day, running at least 7 miles per week, and dropping 10 pounds if you're overweight.

Lower Cholesterol with Margarine

The stuff is called Benecol, and it contains stanol esters—a plant substance that inhibits cholesterol absorption. A study at the Mayo Clinic found that those eating 4½ tablespoons of Benecol daily lowered their LDL (bad) cholesterol by 14 percent in 8 weeks. When they stopped using it, their LDL returned to previous levels. Benecol can also be used for cooking.

Buy 6 Bottles of Aspirin

Aspirin can save your life. Chewing one can thin your blood enough to quell a heart attack. So buy six bottles and put one anywhere you may need it: in your glove box, in your desk at work, in your golf bag, your briefcase, your toolbox. Give one to the bartender down at the Regal Beagle. Then replace them every May—the same time you check the smoke detectors.

Avoid Extra Iron

If your multivitamin contains iron, you might want to put it back on the shelf. Men don't need extra iron; most of us get more than enough in our diets. Excess iron, some scientists believe, contributes to the formation of free radicals, harmful substances that damage the arteries, setting the stage for heart disease.

Double Dose Your Heart

Taking both vitamin E and aspirin every day may significantly lower your risk of heart disease—even if your cholesterol level is high. Researchers found that the antioxidant and blood-thinner combination helped to reduce levels of plaque in clogged arteries by more than 80 percent. The benefit of the two treatments together is so great it may help men prevent atherosclerosis even if they can't lower their cholesterol levels.

Have Some Fat with Your E

Take vitamin E with milk (but not skim). The nutrient, which helps protect against heart disease, is fat soluble, so you need to take it with a drink containing some fat—absorption won't be as effective if it's taken with water.

Take 2 Vitamin Cs

To get the maximum immune-boosting benefit from vitamin C, take two separate doses per day. The vitamin passes through your body within 12 hours of ingestion. So, for example, instead of taking one 1,000-milligram tablet per day, take two 500s—one in the morning and one with dinner. This practice may provide more protection from cancer and heart disease than a single large dose, experts say.

Go Fishing for Salmon

One serving of fish a week can halve your risk of a sudden fatal heart attack. And salmon has more heart-protecting omega-3 fatty acids than almost any other fish.

Don't Order the King Cut

Eating a single fatty meal may temporarily boost your risk of having a heart attack or stroke. Researchers found that some healthy men produced 60 percent more clotting agents after they ate meals with about 55 grams of fat.

Eat More Garlic

A diet rich in garlic makes your aorta more flexible and can increase circulation. In fact, a clove of fresh garlic every day can decrease your total cholesterol by almost 10 percent. Garlic also has powerful antiviral properties that fight infection. Just a couple of cloves of garlic, mixed into food, will jump-start your immune system and improve your chances of fighting off a cold or flu. To minimize the aromatic effects of a garlic-heavy diet, stick to tomatoey Italian foods, or drink a glass of tomato juice with each meal. Acids in the tomatoes will neutralize the odor-causing oils in the garlic, just as they do other scents—like skunk spray.

Assess Your Stroke Risk

We always though that strokes were an old man's problem, until we heard that roughly 25,000 men in their 30s and 40s suffer them every year. Here's how to tell if you're at risk:

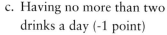

1. Your gut is. . . .
    a. Huge (4 points)
    b. Modest (2 points)
    c. Flat (0 points)
2. Your blood pressure . . .
    a. Consistently exceeds 140/90, and you don't take drugs or exercise (6 points)
    b. Was high, but you're making lifestyle changes and taking medication (4 points)
    c. Checks in at 120/80 or lower (0 points)
    d. Is, oh, who knows? (3 points)
3. Your diet includes . . . (count all that apply)
    a. Less than 30 percent of calories from fat and 10 percent from cholesterol (-1 point)
    b. Limited salt (-1 point)
    c. At least five servings of fruit and vegetables daily (-1 point)
    d. 25 grams of fiber daily; that's two big bowls of high-fiber bran cereal (-1 point)
    e. 400 micrograms of folate daily, which is found in kidney beans and OJ (-1 point)
4. Your vices include . . . (count all that apply)
    a. Binge drinking, which is five or more drinks in one sitting (6 points)
    b. Having more than two drinks a day, or more than 15 per week (4 points)
    c. Having no more than two drinks a day (-1 point)
    d. Smoking more than one pack of cigarettes a day (4 points)
    e. Smoking up to one pack a day (2 points)
5. Your exercise regimen is . . .
    a. Working out three times a week or more (-1 point)
    b. Off and on (0 points)
    c. Does reading this count? (4 points)
6. Your health history includes . . . (count all that apply)
    a. Atrial fibrillation, a specific kind of irregular heartbeat (6 points)
    b. Any kind of coronary heart disease (6 points)
    c. Blockages in your carotid arteries which deliver blood to the brain (3 points)
    d. Diabetes (3 points)
    e. Total cholesterol 240 or greater (1 point)
    f. Depression, if over 50 (1 point)
    g. Family history of stroke (3 points)

Scoring

18 points or more: High risk. See a doctor soon.

7 to 17 points: Medium risk. Make modifications in factors where you scored 3 points or more.

6 points or fewer: Low risk. Keep up the good work.

Judge Cholesterol with Contact Lenses

To tell if you have a cholesterol problem, examine your contact lenses. A diet full of fat, protein, or alcohol weakens your tears' ability to block lipids from adhering to the lenses. This results in cloudy deposits. If your lousy diet is destroying your contacts, just imagine what it's doing to your arteries.

Look Trouble in the Eye

If you see a white ring along the outer edge of your cornea, you may have high cholesterol. We all get this as we age, but younger men who see it should have a cholesterol test.

Use Honey, Not Sugar

The Irish have a lower incidence of diabetes than Americans, and some researchers think it's because they use honey instead of refined sugar in cooking and flavoring their food. Honey takes longer to digest than sugar, so it requires your pancreas to produce less insulin.

Inspect Your Mattress

Want to avoid a bad back? The fastest way we know to protect your back is to strip the sheets off your bed and inspect the surface of your mattress, searching for signs of worn fabric. The more you find, the worse your mattress springs are, and the greater your risk of back trouble.

See Your Tailor for Back Relief

If you have an aching back, it may be because one of your legs is shorter than the other. Even a slight imbalance can cause the spine to curve to the short side when you walk or run. Eventually, the bend puts painful pressure on disks. Most people can't tell if their legs are different lengths, but a tailor can. Ask one for a quick measurement. If he finds an imbalance, correct the problem with a therapeutic, Dr. Scholl's-type insert or see a podiatrist for a custom-made orthotic.

REAL-LIFE SURVIVAL

GET SOMEONE ELSE TO DO THIS

The money you'd save by doing these chores yourself just may not be worth it.

Activities most likely to lead to lower-back problems and hernia operations: Moving furniture, juggling a heavy suitcase into the car, carrying a TV or computer up stairs, and moving a refrigerator.

Activities most likely to break an arm, leg, or neck, or crack a skull: Climbing a tall ladder to paint the house, clean outside windows or venture into the attic and shoveling wet snow off the roof.

Activities most likely to trigger a heart attack: Shoveling snow, pushing a car that's out of fuel to the gas station, and playing tag, soccer, or basketball with the kids.

Rid Yourself of Hiccups

Rub an ice cube on your Adam's apple for a minute. The coldness interrupts the reflex arc from your brain to your diaphragm that causes hiccups.

Crunch Away Back Pain

Seventy-five percent of all lower-back problems can be prevented by building your abdominal muscles. Aim for 12 to 15 crunches a day.

Lose the Wallet, Beat Back Pain

If you're having low-back pain, try taking your wallet out of your back pocket. Sitting on your wallet can put pressure on your sciatic nerve, the major nerve running through the buttocks.

Get Out of Bed

The best way to get out of bed is to roll onto your side and gently push with your hands to lift your torso off the mattress. Why? At night, spinal disks fill with water and expand, and the surrounding muscles tend to stiffen. One sudden movement can damage your disks.

Fix Yourself with Tennis Balls

For a sore low back, lie on some tennis balls. Get two balls and lie down so they slide under the small of your back, one on each side of your spine. Take a deep breath, relax, and slowly work them up your back. You can vary the pressure by simply shifting your weight around.

Let Your Coffee Cool

Drinking coffee hotter than 157°F on a regular basis could increase your risk of esophageal cancer by a factor of four. (Restaurant coffee usually is served at between 170° and 190°F.)

Warm Up to Milk

If drinking milk twists your gut into knots, you may be able to train your stomach to tolerate it and other dairy products. Start by mixing regular milk with lactose-free milk in small but gradually increasing amounts. Your body will have a chance to adapt and may eventually be able to tolerate an 8-ounce glass of full-lactose milk.

WHEN ALL ELSE FAILS

DOUSE HEARTBURN

If, despite your best efforts, you get a nasty case of heartburn, try dousing the flames with a tall glass of water. Believe it or not, water works better than milk. Drinking a cool glass of water will wash the acid from the surface of the esophagus back into your stomach.

GIVE YOURSELF THE HEIMLICH

If you're choking, you don't have to rely on someone else to come to the rescue. Stand up and make a fist with one hand and place the thumb side on the abdomen just above your navel. Now grab your fist and press inward and upward with a quick, sharp thrust. If that doesn't dislodge the stuck food, try again, this time throwing your weight forward over the back of a chair, so your fist is driven up hard into your abdomen.

Chew Away Heartburn

Chewing a stick of sugarless gum for half an hour after meals can prevent or reduce heartburn. Chewing increases saliva flow, which neutralizes stomach acid and washes it away from your esophagus.

Give Spongebob a Bath

Run your kitchen sponge through the dishwasher every 2 days. It's the most common household hideout for *E. coli* and salmonella bacteria.

Mull This Over

A study showed that cinnamon kills *E. coli* bacteria. Researchers contaminated 64-ounce containers of apple cider with *E. coli*, then added cinnamon. After 24 hours, 1 teaspoon of cinnamon had reduced the *E. coli* to undetectable levels.

Avoid Seasickness

If you find yourself in a boat without any motion-sickness medication, limit your time below deck. The air is usually stale down there, and the sense of instability is more intense. Take note if you yawn—it's a warning sign of nausea when you're at sea. If you do feel queasy, eat Triscuits and drink Coke.

Cut Your Risk of Cancer

Only 5 to 10 percent of cancers are inherited. The rest are due to interactions with the environment. One of the most important things you can do to cut your risk is eat at least five servings a day of fruits and vegetables. A 14-year study found that men whose daily diets were highest in fruits and vegetables had a 70-percent lower risk of digestive tract cancers. Here's the easiest way to reach your quota: Never eat a snack or meal that doesn't contain a fruit or vegetable. Yes, it's that simple.

Chew Your Way to Recovery

Gum chewing can help speed your recovery after stomach or intestine surgery. In a study of men and women who'd had surgery, researchers found that the increase in saliva and other digestive juices from chewing gum significantly improved patients' recovery.

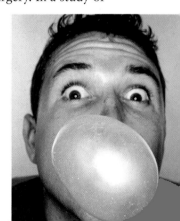

Calm an Upset Stomach

If the only time you drink sour-stomach standbys such as ginger ale or herbal tea is when you're ill, the mental association may actually make you feel worse. Instead, combine another old favorite, warm cola, with a teaspoon of baking soda to neutralize the acid.

Eat Less, Live Longer

The fewer calories you eat each day, the longer you can expect to live. Researchers found that mice on a low-calorie diet lived longer than those with a higher calorie intake. But more important, the researchers also discovered that switching a mouse from a higher-calorie diet to a lower-calorie one eliminated up to 70 percent of all genetic signs of aging that the animal had previously shown. This suggests that much of the damage of a high-calorie diet isn't permanent and can be rectified by a simple change in the amount you eat.

Protect Yourself against Ulcers

Men who are active are 30 to 50 percent less likely than nonexercisers to develop ulcers. Exercise may help to alter the way the body deals with anxiety and to modify the types and amounts of hormones released into the bloodstream—making it harder for ulcers to form. Even moderately intense physical activity like walking and jogging has been shown to protect against ulcers. Best of all, the results are cumulative, so the more a guy works out, the better protected he is.

Stand, Then Flush

You can catch intestinal bugs and hepatitis from toilet seats in restrooms. When toilets are flushed, a fine mist of water containing contagious bacteria lands on the seat. To protect yourself, stand before you flush. And always take the stall closest to the restroom door. After analyzing 51 public restrooms, experts found that this stall consistently had the lowest bacteria levels (and the most toilet paper). The first stall probably sees less traffic because it's near the door and people want privacy.

Stop Reading on the Can

Reading in the bathroom may be harmful to your health. Research shows that camping out on the bowl may damage nerves and muscles, possibly leading to hemorrhoids and other bad things.

ORDER THE CHILEAN RED

To reduce your risk of cancer, drink red wine from Chile. Chilean Cabernet Sauvignon is 38 percent higher than French wine in flavonols, antioxidants that plunder cancer-causing free radicals.

Cancel Your Runs

Prevent diarrhea by taking over-the-counter medications such as Pepto-Bismol *before* drinking questionable water. Pepto-Bismol kills germs and prevents infection as well as stopping diarrhea. Tablets are easier to pack than a bottle. Taking two tablets four times daily should do the trick.

Check Your Stool

If you're more than 40 years old, have your doctor test for hidden blood in your stool. It can be a sign of growths on the wall of the colon that may turn cancerous.

Cleanse Your Colon

Drinking more than four glass of water daily can lower your risk of colon cancer by 32 percent.

Prevent Kidney Stones

Drink at least 8 glasses of lemon water a day. Lemons contain citrate, a chemical that may stop kidney stones (like the ones below) from forming. Also, limit your salt intake and drink plenty of skim milk. The calcium binds with the stone-causing minerals and ushers them out of the body.

Here's an amazing finding: One study found that 76 percent of patients with recurring kidney

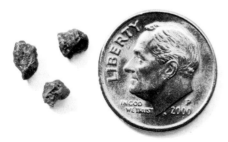

stones developed them only on the side they consistently slept on. Sleeping in the same position seems to alter the way bloodflow to the kidney is distributed, hurting its ability to stop stone formation. Every few nights, try to sack out on a different side to better distribute the flow of blood.

Tuna Creaky Joint

If your joints creak, try eating more omega-3 fatty acids. These can be found in fish such as salmon and tuna. It increases blood flow and reduces inflammation and pain around joints. Two portions per week should do it.

Repair Your Cartilage

If you're stiff and sore in the morning, spike your coffee with a scoop of NutraJoint Plus Glucosamine, a gelatin-based supplement you can find at your grocery store. Research shows that it relieves pain and may help repair cartilage; it contains nutrients your body turns into cartilage lubricant. But it doesn't work for everyone; if your body is going to respond, you should notice in about 2 months.

Roll Your Own

Testicular cancer is most likely to strike before age 40. Although more than 90 percent of men who get it survive, it must be discovered early. The best way to do this is with a monthly self-exam. Take a warm shower to relax the scrotum, then stand in front of a mirror. Look for any swelling of the scrotal skin. Examine each testicle with both hands, rolling it between thumbs and fingers. If you do find a lump, don't panic. This could be normal, but your doctor will have to confirm it.

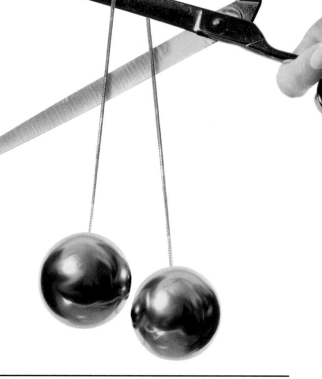

Take the Vasectomy Test

Is it time for you to get snipped? Answer the following questions to find out:

Are you married?	Yes	No
Do you have two or more kids?	Yes	No
Do you consider your marriage to be stable and happy?	Yes	No
Are you 35 or older?	Yes	No
Are you prepared for permanent contraception?	Yes	No

If you can answer yes to all of the above, you're a good candidate for a vasectomy. Even one no answer, however, and you should reconsider, especially if you're in a rocky or childless marriage. The majority of men who divorce remarry, often to women 10 to 20 years younger with no children of their own. These are the men who go back for a reversal.

Examine the Flow Chart

To see if you are experiencing signs of prostate trouble, answer the following questions. Over the past month, how often have you . . .

1. Had a sensation of not emptying your bladder completely after you finished urinating?	0 1 2 3 4 5
2. Had to urinate again less than 2 hours after urinating?	0 1 2 3 4 5
3. Found that the flow of urine stopped and started several times?	0 1 2 3 4 5
4. Found it difficult to postpone urination?	0 1 2 3 4 5
5. Had a weak urine stream?	0 1 2 3 4 5
6. Had to push or strain to begin urination?	0 1 2 3 4 5
7. Had to get up to urinate after going to bed on a typical night?	0 1 2 3 4 5

Add your score:_____

If you scored 10 or more, visit a urologist for an examination. (NOTE: This is not a test for prostate cancer. Ask your doctor about prostate exams and a screening for prostate cancer.)

Test Your Prostate

Regular screenings are the best way to diagnose prostate cancer early. The American Cancer Society and the American Urological Association recommend an annual digital-rectal exam for men 40 and over, and annual prostate-specific antigen (PSA) screenings beginning at age 50. (If you're African-American, or if you have a history of prostate cancer in your family, start this test at 40, too).

Avoid Sex before a PSA Test

If you're scheduled for a PSA test, don't have sex for a few days beforehand. Ejaculation within 48 hours of the test can cause your reading to be 60 percent higher than normal, which could lead your doctor to order unnecessary follow-up tests.

Give That Gland a Hand

Two to four servings of tomato sauce a week can cut your risk for prostate cancer by 34 percent.

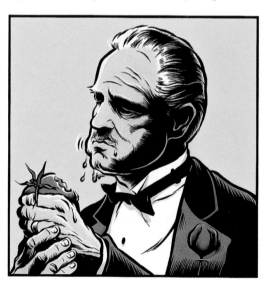

Eat More Watermelon

It may help you avoid prostate cancer. Watermelon is red for a reason. Like tomatoes, watermelon contains lycopene, a phytochemical that may reduce your prostate-cancer risk by as much as 40 percent. A single 1-inch slice has as much lycopene as four tomatoes.

Give Confidence to a Bashful Bladder

Up to one in 10 men has a disorder called paruresis, which is a fancy name for difficulty peeing in public. The best solution: Find a stall and lock the door. That'll give you enough privacy to relax and start things flowing (reading a paper helps). If there's no stall handy, take a deep breath and contract your pelvic muscles, then relax and exhale. Repeat until you hear a trickle. Or close your eyes and picture your ex-wife's face on the urinal cake.

Learn the Zip Code

You never realize what a tortuous device a zipper can be until it snags a sensitive piece of your penis. But since the skin there is loose most of the time, the very thing that makes it susceptible to zipping also protects it from serious damage. To free willy, gently back the zipper off, then wash the abrasion with soap and water and apply an antibiotic ointment such as Bacitracin. If you can't dislodge yourself and don't want to call the fire department, take a wire snipper and *carefully* cut the zipper's median bar. That's the little piece of metal that holds the front and back of the zipper clasp together. Once snipped, the zipper will easily come undone.

Bone Up

Osteoporosis is not just a woman's disease. Men get it, too. It takes very little to keep bones stocked with raw material. You need about 1,000 milligrams of calcium a day. Drinking just one 8-ounce glass of skim milk provides you with about 350 milligrams.

Men who toil at desks and are not active during a normal day should also exercise regularly by lifting weights. While bones also get stronger from walking and running, weight training is the best bone-building exercise. A full-body weight regimen has the potential to add bone, while aerobic exercise serves primarily to maintain existing bone.

Save Your Skeleton

Drinking soda may weaken your bones. The large amount of fructose that sodas contain changes how your body metabolizes the minerals responsible for healthy bones. Doctors discourage drinking more than two cans per day.

Never Pull Out

When a foreign object bigger than a splinter has entered your body, one rule sticks: Leave it in until you get to a doctor. The object is like a stopper. If you remove it, you might have massive bleeding and a much lower chance of surviving the injury.

Test Your Pain Tolerance

Fill a small cooler with one-third ice and two-thirds water, and maintain a water temperature of 32° to 35.6°F. Immerse one hand up to your wrist and start a stopwatch. Remove your hand and stop the watch the instant you can no longer tolerate the pain. Do not exceed 5 minutes, unless you like cryogenics.

Here's what your score means:

0-45 seconds: You have low pain tolerance. If you feel ex-

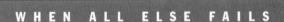

WHEN ALL ELSE FAILS

SOAK OUT A SPLINTER

Soak the invaded area in warm water for up to 15 minutes. This makes the wood swell, which often causes the splinter to pop out on its own. If that doesn't work, pour a thin layer of white glue over the spot. Let it dry, then peel it off. The splinter will usually come off with it.

WHEN ALL ELSE FAILS

CHASE AWAY MOSQUITOES

Lighted cattails put out a smoke that repels insects. If you recognize wild garlic or onion, they make an effective insect repellant when rubbed on the skin.

cruciating pain within 30 seconds, it's likely that aches and pains nag you constantly. Bumps and bruises that many people shrug off could send you scurrying for medical treatment.

46-90 seconds: You have average pain tolerance. Congratulations. You can suck it up when you're hurt, but you probably can't remove a bullet from your arm by using whisky and tweezers.

91+ seconds: You have a high pain tolerance. If you can last more than 2 minutes, you're probably unaware of pain. This can ultimately be unhealthy, though. You need to pay attention to injuries closely to determine whether you need a doctor.

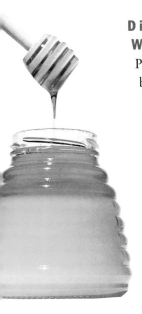

Disinfect a Wound with Honey

Pour a dab of honey on a cut before covering it with a bandage. Honey has powerful antibacterial properties. One study found that honey was capable of destroying almost all strains of the most common wound-infecting bacteria.

Vaccinate Yourself

If you play contact sports that can cause bloody injuries, ask your doctor about a hepatitis B vaccination to protect yourself. One player on an American football team accidentally infected 10 of his teammates with hepatitis B during practice.

Take the Bite Out of a Bite

Reduce the inflammation with ice. Then rub aspirin or meat tenderizer on the insect bite to break down the venom. Relieve the pain and itching by dabbing the bite with a pasty salve of water and baking soda. If you're in the wilderness, use a mud pack.

Scratch the Other Limb

For itchy skin under a cast, try scratching the same place on the other arm or foot. Your brain may think you're scratching the real itch.

Fix a Cut with Tea

The tannin in tea leaves promotes rapid blood clotting. Next time you have to treat a cut, press a cool, wet tea bag against it. You can cover the tea bag with a handkerchief, a towel or some gauze to soak up the excess liquid as you apply pressure.

Call Dr. Pepper

Next time you nick yourself in the kitchen, reach for the black pepper. Run cold water over the wound to clean it, using soap if you were handling meat. Then sprinkle on some pepper and apply pressure. In no time, the bleeding should stop. Turns out black pepper has analgesic, antibacterial, and antiseptic properties. Pepper doesn't sting, either—but don't tell that to your audience.

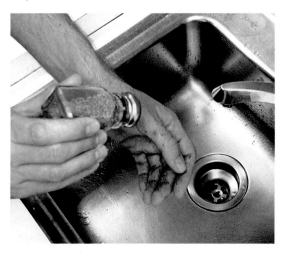

Patch a Cut with Super Glue

You can treat minor lacerations like paper cuts or cracked hands with Super Glue. Pull the edges of the wound together and put the glue on top in a thin film, making sure it doesn't penetrate the wound. Hold the cut together for about 30 seconds until the glue dries.

Put a Band-Aid on It

The idea that cuts need fresh air to heal is nonsense. Bandages aren't airtight, and studies show that wounds heal faster when they're covered.

Clean Strawberries

Road rash hurts bad enough. But it'll sting even worse if you try to disinfect the wound with hydrogen peroxide. Try rinsing the abrasion with the same stuff you use on contact lenses—saline solution. It'll wash away bacteria and keep the wound feeling cool. To help the area heal quickly, apply a mixture of Neosporin antibiotic ointment and zinc oxide two or three times a day. Keep it covered with nonstick gauze.

Stop Poison Ivy

If you know you've touched the stuff, you have 10 to 30 minutes to wash the area and prevent a skin reaction. Soap and water works fine.

Extinguish a Minor Burn

Submerge a superficial burn in cool water until it no longer hurts. You can also use shaving cream (it absorbs heat as it expands, halting the burning process) or a bag of frozen peas (you can mold it around your skin).

Cruise without These

Certain drugs and even some colognes can make your skin more sensitive to ultraviolet rays. Avoid using the following products on a sun-drenched vacation. If you must take them, be extra-liberal with the sunblock:

- Aftershaves with musk scents

- Diuretics such as Diuril and Hygroton

- Antibiotics such as sulfonamides and tetracycline

- Painkillers containing ibuprofen or naproxen

- Antihistamines such as Benadryl, Tavist-D, Actifed, and Chlor-Trimeton

TREAT AN ANKLE SPRAIN WITH CHEWING TOBACCO

If you twist an ankle and don't have any ice, grab some loose chewing tobacco. Moisten it slightly and pack it around the ankle. Secure it in place with a bandage or T-shirt. It's one of the quickest ways to reduce swelling. The nicotinic acid acts as an astringent, reducing swelling by drawing the fluid out of the injury site. Take care not to use the tobacco for more than 24 hours, however, because it can irritate the skin.

Scrape Off the Jelly

If you get too close to a stinging jellyfish, use a credit card to scrape the stinger off your skin. (Using your fingers only squeezes more venom into your body.) Then pour some diluted vinegar on your skin to soothe the pain.

Remove Warts with Duct Tape

The prescription calls for leaving the tape over the wart for 7 days, then uncovering it for 12 hours, and repeating the cycle until the wart falls off. Duct tape keeps the moisture in and helps soften and break down the tissue of the wart.

Take an Oatmeal Bath

To soothe a bad sunburn, wrap a cupful of oatmeal in sheeting or cheesecloth and hang it

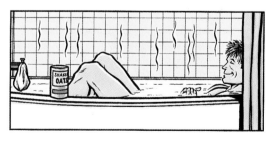

from your faucet, so that the bathwater runs directly over it as the tub is filling. No on knows exactly how the oatmeal works to soothe the pain, but you will feel better.

Peel Away Plantar Warts

Wash the offending foot and soak it in warm water for about 3 minutes. Next, eat a banana and cut out a square piece of peel that'll completely cover the wart. Put peel (fleshy side down) over wart and secure it to your foot with a couple of Band-Aids. Repeat for two consecutive nights, and then go ape when you see the wart fall off.

Diagnose an Ankle Injury

People try to judge ankle injuries by the swelling, but that's totally unreliable. Fractures may not swell at all, while sprains can be hugely swollen. Try this test: Grab your calf at its widest point with both hands and squeeze hard. (This puts pressure on the fibula and tibia, which are connected to the ankle joint.) If you feel a sharp pain in your ankle, it's probably broken. See a doctor to confirm.

Support a Crumbling Arch

To relieve plantar fasciitis, a painful strain in the ligaments that run the length of the foot, try rolling a can of frozen fruit juice back and forth under the arch. This applies ice therapy, while stretching your foot.

Rejuvenate Tired Dogs

Pour a handful of uncooked beans into your slippers and walk around for a few minutes. The rolling beans create an instant massage. Then hold your feet under the bathtub faucet. Run the water on hot one minute, cold the next. Alternate for 10 minutes, ending in a cold rinse. Ahhh.

Soothe Feet with a Golf Ball

For foot cramps and sore arches, roll a golf ball under the ball of your foot for 2 minutes to massage the tender area.

Reverse Lung Damage

If you smoke, quit. It may be the greatest thing you can do for your health. Stop smoking before age 40, and you'll add 5 years to your life. After 10 smoke-free years, you'll have cut your risk of dying of lung cancer in half. After 15 years, your risk of heart disease will be almost the same as that of people who've never lit up.

Count Down to Your Last Cigarette

Count the number of cigarettes you smoke in a day. That's your baseline. Let's say it's 24. Cut that by a third; you get 16. The key is to smoke those 16 at evenly spaced intervals—one for each of your waking hours. Smoke this way for a week; it will train you to suppress the urge to chainsmoke. The following week, smoke a third of your original number of daily cigarettes, in this case eight, or 1 every 2 hours. Final week: Day one, smoke one-third fewer cigarettes than you did in week one, or about 11 cigarettes in this case, and continue to cut a third of this number every other day until you are down to one or two. Then you're primed to quit for good. Twice as many people who use this method are smoke-free after one year than those who go cold turkey.

Sit on a Stool the Right Way

Laugh if you must, but sitting hunched over on a bar stool can hurt your lower back. Here's the right way to do it:

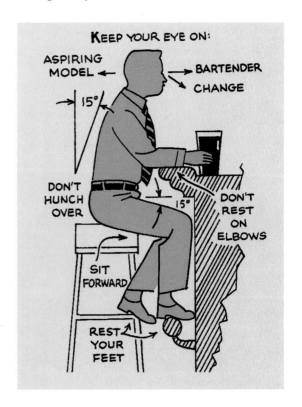

KEEP YOUR EYE ON:

ASPIRING MODEL ← → BARTENDER

CHANGE

15°

DON'T HUNCH OVER

15°

DON'T REST ON ELBOWS

SIT FORWARD

REST YOUR FEET

Try Sniffing Instead of Smoking

Researchers have found that sniffing strong odors reduces the urge to smoke. Evidently, the part of the brain that controls cravings also happens to be where you process odors. So if you're trying to quit, put something at your desk that gives off a pungent odor—vinegar, Vicks, coconut, peppermint—and take a whiff instead of reaching for a cigarette.

Drink Less Coffee, Smoke Fewer Butts

Taking fewer coffee breaks may increase your odds of quitting smoking. If a butt and a cup was your usual thing, you may have developed a "learned aspect" to your habit that makes you crave a cigarette whenever you sit down to sip. Less coffee, less chance you'll light up.

Massage Away Nicotine Cravings

If you're a smoker who's trying to quit, try this simple trick the next time a craving hits: Rub the skin between your index fingers and thumbs and the center of your palms. Researchers found that men using this technique smoked 25 percent fewer cigarettes in a month than 10 quitters who used traditional distraction methods such as chewing gum. The quick self-massage evidently calms you and keeps your hands busy.

Avoid Secondhand Smoke

Every hour you spend in a smoky bar is equivalent to smoking one or two cigarettes.

Smoke Stogies, Become a Fogie

Despite popular belief, cigars are not a healthful alternative to cigarettes. The tobacco content of a single cigar is five to 17 times greater than that of the average cigarette—and the nicotine content can be the equivalent of a whole pack. Provided you don't inhale, you're 11 times less likely to die of lung cancer if you puff three to four cigars a day than if you smoke a pack of cigarettes daily. Of course, you'll also be six times more likely to die of mouth and pharynx cancer (28 times more likely if you inhale your stogies), and your breath will smell like your cat's business end. If you really have to smoke something, try salmon.

Better the Buzz

The more alcohol you drink, the more tolerant (dulled) your body becomes to its effects. But if you drink less often and reduce the amount, you'll become more sensitive to alcohol. That means you'll be able to find greater enjoyment and stress relief in a lesser amount. Even a week of abstinence will increase your sensitivity.

Load Up before You Get Loaded

Drinking only on a full stomach is probably the single best thing you can do, besides drinking less, to reduce the severity of a hangover. Food slows the absorption of alcohol, and the slower you absorb it the less alcohol actually reaches your brain.

Don't Take Tylenol with Alcohol

If you drink alcohol frequently, even in moderation, stay away from medications that contain acetaminophen, including Tylenol. An alcohol/acetaminophen combination puts your liver at even greater risk than alcohol alone. The risk is most acute within 24 hours of drinking. So make sure your hangover cure doesn't include acetaminophen.

SIDESTEP A HANGOVER

For last call, order a double virgin screwdriver. Fructose, one of the sugars in orange juice, can speed up the metabolism of alcohol by as much as 25 percent. A couple of spoonfuls of honey immediately before or after drinking may also help prevent a hangover. Honey contains fructose, too, as does tomato juice—partially explaining why a Bloody Mary in the morning is sometimes considered a hangover remedy.

Avoid the Wrath of Grapes

It's not just drinking too much that did you in. The kinds of drinks you downed also played a part because of congeners, the compounds that give alcoholic beverages their distinctive flavors and colors. These are by-products of the raw materials of fermentation, distillation, even wood-cask conditioning, and there are many. A general rule is that the lighter alcohols (gin, vodka, and white wine) have fewer congeners and are less likely to cause a hangover than the darker ones (brandies, scotch, and red wine).

Don't Drive Drunk the Morning After

It's possible to be arrested for drunk driving the next day if you drank enough the night before. Let's say you're a 160-pound man and you drank 2 drinks per hour from 7 P.M. to 1 A.M. That's 12 drinks . . . a lot. At that point you may need help getting into a taxi. Or finding your pants. You sleep until 8 A.M., then drive to work. At 9 A.M.—8 hours after you stopped drinking—your blood-alcohol level will still be over 0.10 percent. Driving at that level would be illegal in most states.

Don't Make Us Repeat This

Memory wastes away if you don't use it. So start using yours. Go to the grocery store and shop without a list. Deprogram your speed dial and make yourself remember those important phone numbers. Try to get your kids' names right on the first try.

Stay Sharper Longer

To combat the dulling effects of age, go lefty. Use your nondominant hand for routine things such as brushing your teeth, answering the phone, and eating. This stimulates your brain into activating new pathways—and that means a more nimble mind.

Accuse Others of Taking Your Keys

Research suggests there's a marked difference between how younger and older people interpret misplacing their keys. A young guy usually blames it on someone else: "Who took my keys?" An old guy typically blames it on himself: "I must be getting old. I misplaced my keys again." Never use your age as an excuse—and see if you don't remain younger longer.

Take the 20-Second Stress Test

Lie on your back, place your left hand over your chest and your right hand over your belly button. If your right hand rises first and falls last with each breath, great. You're breathing with your diaphragm, which means you're a deep breather. If your left hand rises first or if it rises more than your right hand, you're a chest breather and your breathing is shallow—a sign of stress. Practice until you start breathing properly. You have until midnight tonight.

Get Happy Fast

More people than ever are taking antidepressants. But you don't necessarily need medication (or even a shrink) to lift your mood. Here are 10 alternatives:

1. Drive to a hardware store and buy a couple of gallons of light-blue latex paint, a roller, and a stepladder. Head home and quickly, vigorously, and without much care for cleanliness, paint the porch ceiling. Not only will the exercise lift your mood, but research also shows that staring at the color blue will relax you. (Bonus: According to Pennsylvania Dutch legend, a blue ceiling will keep flies away from your porch.)

2. Look in the yellow pages for the nearest Chinese restaurant that delivers. Call and order the ginger chicken with broccoli. Studies show that ginger and broccoli help relieve depression.

3. Call up an old friend and suggest a spur-of-the-moment road trip—to some weekend college basketball game, to the nearest warm-weather golf course, to Toledo, wherever. The point is to spend a lot of time in the car driving somewhere, throwing garbage into the backseat, and just being men.

4. Rent one of those giant metal Dumpsters. Tell 'em to park it in the backyard, within chucking distance of an upstairs window. Then methodically work your way through the house, throwing out all the accumulated crap in your life. In the end, you'll feel lighter, like you're starting over.

5. For the next few minutes, act happy. Grin, laugh, waggle your eyebrows, walk with a bounce in your step, whistle. People who are manipulated into smiling report feeling better instantly. Going through the motions can trigger the emotions.

6. Walk around the block or do 20 pushups. Aerobic exercise is just as effective as antidepressants in lifting mood.

7. Call your local community college and request a copy of its spring catalog. Pick a noncredit course you've always been interested in but never had time to pursue, then register for it. New challenges + new expertise = new enthusiasm.

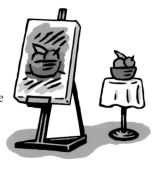

8. Go to the supermarket and buy the thickest, juiciest filet mignon you can find. Then take it home, dig out the charcoal grill and fire it up. (Never mind that it's the middle of January.) Let the aroma waft through the neighborhood. Sit on a lawn chair and drink a beer. You are now in touch with your primal self. Soon, you will find it easier to smile.

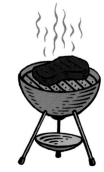

9. Make a list of five things you're going to accomplish before the end of today. Write them down; put them in your pocket. Get in the habit of doing this every day. One thing happy people have in common is that they feel in control of their lives.

10. Go to bed before 10 P.M. tonight and sleep until at least 6 A.M. tomorrow. Repeat for the next 7 days. Being happy is often as simple as being well-rested.

Spot Trouble Approaching

All men go through a midlife transition, but only some men go through a midlife crisis. Look for the following clues in your behavior.

If you recognize yourself, consider speaking with a good friend or therapist about it.

You feel cheated: After years of fighting your way to the top, you're sitting in your spacious corner office wondering, "I worked my butt off for *this*?"

Your wife suddenly looks old: We tend to see our own aging in other people first.

You take unusual money risks: You seriously begin considering pouring money into a startup company or entertaining career changes that involve travel and adventure.

You fantasize about sex: Plus, you flirt pointedly, chat up younger female co-workers, and try to engineer precarious situations with potential mates. You need to prove to yourself you still got it.

You become a happy-hour regular: You're using alcohol to numb the sense of depression that's stewing.

Your last kid just left home: The empty-nest syndrome is rarely about lost children—it's about who is left behind.

You change your look: Abrupt changes can give an esteem boost in the short term, but they won't cure the depression some men face as they try to come to terms with getting older.

You recently lost a parent: When you no longer have the solace of at least being somebody's kid, the rough, empty moments in life can become even darker and more isolated.

Relax in Seconds

Sit with your feet flat on the floor and your eyes closed. Pay attention to your breathing. As you breathe air into your body, imagine breathing in all the good things your body needs. As you let air out of your body, imagine letting things you don't need out of your body. Notice how you are feeling. Imagine the feelings you like growing stronger as you breathe inward. Imagine the feeling you don't like going out of your body as you let air out.

Sing along with Stress

Everyone needs some degree of stress in his life to be healthy and productive. It's very much like the tension on a violin string. If you don't have enough tension, the violin will play a dull, raspy note. If you have too much, there will be a shrill, shrieking sound or the string will snap. But just the right amount creates a beautiful tone. We all have to find the right amount of stress in our lives that allows us to make beautiful music.

Chill Out

Cold temperatures increase the level of serotonin in the brain, making you feel calmer. So after a tough day at work, put an ice pack wrapped in a towel on the back of your neck for 15 minutes.

Be Holy in New Ways

Any undivided attention is prayer. If we can stop the tumble in our heads and every day briefly devote our complete attention to something—a 10-foot putt, a 10-penny nail, or a 10-year-old child—we may acquire the serenity many find in formal faith.

Skip the Second Cup

The caffeine in two cups of coffee adds 16 beats a minute to your heart rate and makes you more irritable and anxious.

Declare an Info-Free Day

Stress is never listed as a cause of death, but it can usually be implicated as an accomplice. One fresh way to control it is to cut off all outside news 1 day a week. No television, no newspapers, no radio, no Internet, no magazines. Cut off the information, and you won't feel so overwhelmed.

Take the Wheel

A sense of control over some of the stressors in your life helps. If you blast a volunteer randomly with a noise, his stress hormones rise. But if you give him a button and tell him that pressing it will decrease the likelihood of the noise, there's a smaller stress response to the same sound. Getting organized, even in small ways, may help you feel more like the captain of your ship.

Solve All Your Problems

Check in with yourself for 5 minutes at the end of every day (just as you do with voice and e-mail). And during this respite, ask yourself two questions: 1) What have I done today that was meaningful? and 2) What meaningful change do I intend to make in my life tomorrow? If you practice this daily, you'll no longer find life so troublesome.

SWEAT TO RELAX

Exercising for 40 minutes can reduce stress for up to 3 hours. An equal period of rest and relaxation reduces stress for only 20 minutes.

GET CAUGHT NAPPING

If you can sneak one in, take a nap. It's perhaps the most underrated stress-reliever there is. One study found that men who napped at least 30 minutes a day had a 30 percent lower risk of heart attack than non-nappers. The ideal nap time is 2 to 3 P.M., if you get up at 6 to 7 A.M.

Get Past Tense

The neck is often the first place stress appears. To loosen it up, reach with your right hand over your head and behind your left ear, grasping your neck. Pull your head gently toward you right shoulder. Then use your left hand to pull your head toward your left shoulder. You'll feel instantly better.

Flush Away Trouble

Ever notice how satisfying it can be to flush a toilet, especially if it's one of those airport monsters that emit a roar and leave your tie fluttering in the vacuum? Well, you can use this joy to help clear your mind. Think of it as a stress laxative—a bit strange, but guaranteed to be gentle and effective. Before you go to bed put some small strips of flushable paper and a pencil in the bathroom. The following morning, take a seat and write down the names of all the people or situations in your life that are causing you angst. Then throw them in the bowl and flush. You'll be amazed at how great this feels and how well it works.

Be Mindful of This

The key to turning any day into a long, lazy August afternoon is to master a mental technique called mindfulness. It's the opposite of the "been there, done that" attitude. The idea is that each moment is a new moment we can be fully aware of. To bring a little mindfulness into your day, there's only one simple rule you have to obey: Don't focus on more than one thing at a time. In other words, don't eat while perusing the paper, don't wear headphones while exercising, and don't look in the mirror while having sex. By focusing your attention, you'll concentrate better on the task at hand and thereby enhance the experience. Food will taste better, exercise will be more enjoyable and sex, if you can believe it, will be more intense.

Give Yourself the Silent Treatment

What's the first thing you do when you walk into your house? Snap on the TV? Turn on the radio? Noise has become addictive for most of us. It distracts us from really knowing ourselves. While silence may not seem important, noise creates constant stress for our bodies. It weakens our immune systems, putting us at risk for all kinds of illnesses. To achieve a quieter life, first become aware to the noise level you routinely take for granted. Then turn down the volume in your house for several minutes every day. Create opportunities for silence.

Beat Depression

Eighty percent of people who are treated for depression, regardless of type, report substantial relief. The best treatment, studies show, is a mix of psychotherapy and antidepressants. But men require a different type of therapy than women—not the sappy, stereotypical, "tell-me-everything-you're-feeling" brand, but a more dynamic, opinionated style of coaching. To find a therapist like this, call around and ask two questions: Do you have experience helping men reconnect, and do you have an active or passive style? And demand progress. If you're in therapy for 6 months and you feel only 5 percent better, that's not good enough.

Answer This Question

Reply immediately without reflection: Are you winning? A positive answer probably means you feel up to the challenges you face and have a sense of control over your life. A negative answer may indicate that you feel you're in a losing situation and lack control over your life. In this case, you may be more vulnerable to stress. No answer at all indicates you have reservations about the direction your life is taking and you may also cope less effectively with stress.

Have Hope

People manage stress more effectively if they believe that things are improving. So make sure you always have something you're looking forward to. Help your wife understand why she should tease your saucily with a promise of the Lady of the Manor and the Gamekeeper on Friday night. Hope makes stress manageable.

Pop Some Bubbles

You know how much fun it is to pop those plastic bubbles used in packaging? Well, it

can actually be healthy, too. One study found that students were able to reduce their feelings of tension by popping two sheets of Bubble Wrap.

Call an Old Bud

Having friends is good for your health. Those people with the most friends typically respond better to medication, recover faster from personal loss or illness, and live longer. You need to do three things as you grow older: 1) create situations from which new friendships can grow, such as golf outings or poker nights; 2) make friends outside work, so you won't lose them if you change jobs; and 3) instead of talking about what's happening in the world, discuss what's happening in your life. Admit that you need a friend and don't be afraid to open up to him.

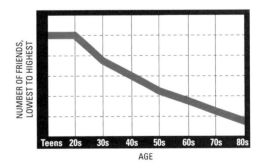

Start Collecting Friends

To live long and prosper, you need friends. In fact, one study estimates that being social can gain you nearly a decade. People with very poor social connections live 4.5 years less than expected, while those with very good connections live 4.5 years longer.

Give Her a Hand with That

Men who do volunteer work at least once a week have half the death rate of those who don't.

Live Relaxed, Live Long

If we had to give only one piece of health advice to men, it would be eliminate the stress in your life. Chronic stress in men has been linked to everything from allergies to heart disease. Experts say that up to 90 percent of physicians visits may be for stress-related disorders. For a few extra bucks, have the kid at the department store assemble the barbecue grill for you.

Have a Healthful Mid-Life Crisis

Men who have mid-life crises aren't neurotic. The desire to question and change your life comes from the healthiest part of you.

DON'T TRUST THE COFFEE

A few *New York Times* staffers checked decaffeinated coffee from 17 restaurants and found that five samples had more than the 60 milligrams of caffeine typically found in a cup of regular coffee. One even had 114 milligrams. It's a small test, but if it happens in New York eateries, it may happen at your joint. If you *really* need to avoid caffeine, bring your own packet of instant decaffeinated coffee and ask for hot water.

Keep the Willies at Bay

If you get claustrophobic in small spaces such as subways, elevators, and that closet of an office they stuck you in, visit your local fruit stand. A sniff of green apple may help relieve claustrophobic sensations. Carry one with you. Also, if you're selling your house, placing a basket of fresh green apples on the table may make potential buyers perceive the house as larger.

Stop a Panic Attack

Panicky people hyperventilate because they're breathing too fast—meaning their blood is losing carbon dioxide. To stay in control, breathe in while pinching one nostril shut. This forces you to breathe more slowly because you can't inhale as much air through one nostril as you can through two or through your mouth.

Stage a Hostile Takeover

Chronically angry men are five to seven times more likely to be dead by age 50 than their easygoing counterparts. Hostility weakens the immune system (by making your hormones overactive) and it puts the heart at risk (by clogging arteries). Here are two ways to control it:

Whack something: Beat a cardboard box with a stick, throw old plates into a Dumpster, or head for a slow-pitch batting cage and imagine your boss's face on each ball.

Exercise: Anger is a form of energy. Hitting a punching bag, lifting weights, or going for a run can help alleviate it.

Change Your Name

People with "positive" initials—they spell out things like J.O.Y. or W.O.W.—live nearly 4.5

years longer than people with neutral initials. D.U.D.'s and A.S.S.'s lived nearly 3 years less. Other initials that may shorter your life: I.L.L. and D.E.D.

Stay Challenged to Stay Happy

Men are not maintainers; we are builders. (That's why vacuuming holds no allure for us.) We are happiest when we're creating something—a career, a home, a family. Make sure there's always a project on your workbench, something new you're trying to accomplish.

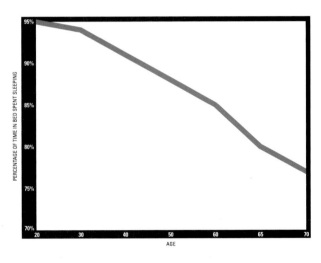

Increase Your Sleep Efficiency

Getting the right amount of sleep is critical to good health. The amount of sleep you need (typically 7 to 9 hours per day) remains constant throughout your life. Although older men may sleep less at night, they generally compen-

sate by napping during the day. Here are a few ways to increase your sleep efficiency:

• Avoid stimulants such as caffeine, nicotine, and alcohol in the later afternoon and evening.

• Don't exercise within 3 hours of bedtime.

• Establish a regular go-to-bed routine.

• Don't watch television, read, or eat in the sack. (Beds are for sleeping and sex.)

• If you don't fall asleep within 30 minutes, get up and do something relaxing until you do feel sleepy.

Trick Yourself into Sleeping Better

If the bags under your eyes are getting bigger, here are some ways to outwit insomnia:

• Tune your FM radio dial to a spot in between stations. This produces low-level "white noise."

• Face the alarm clock away from you. A digital-display light can wake a light sleeper.

• Choose restful colors for your bed linens. Try blues and greens. It's time to pack away your Bart Simpson sheets, friends.

• Have a couple bites of bagel, oatmeal, cereal, or pasta before bed. All these foods contain tryptophan, an amino acid that converts into serotonin, your brain's sleep agent.

Don't Take Peppermint Pattie to Bed

If you want to sleep soundly, don't eat Peppermint Patties, chew peppermint gum, or drink peppermint-flavored herbal teas before you go to bed. Just a whiff of peppermint may keep you

A C T   L I K E   A   M U T T

Here are 25 ways to live longer by imitating your dog:

Stretch: Every morning, immediately after waking up.

Visit the vet regularly: The best preventive medicine is an annual checkup.

Live in the present: It helps slow time and eases stress.

Sleep on the floor: An extra-firm mattress is best for your back.

Play: The opposite of work, it provides balance.

Nap: Even a few minutes is restorative.

Learn one trick to delight people: It works magic.

Run: No reason, whenever you feel like it.

Be good: Or at least try.

Yawn widely: It briefly lowers blood pressure and relieves anxiety.

Have a treat: Reward yourself, occasionally and guiltlessly.

Drink lots of water: The trick is keeping it handy.

Be loyal: Give every person a second chance.

Sleep like a dog: Feng shui masters say that sleeping with your head facing north (which some dogs do) increases circulation and improves metabolism.

Love unconditionally: Expect nothing in return.

Heed your instincts: Don't over-intellectualize your impulses.

Live simply: Shelter, food, love—is there really anything else?

Have a master: Find a mentor.

Get excited about going for a walk: It's still the simplest and safest exercise.

Bask in praise: Don't humbly deflect what you've earned.

Let yourself be petted: Periodically surrender to a massage therapist.

Be affectionate: It's unhealthy to hide your emotions.

Chew: A stick of gum after eating cleans teeth and aids digestion.

Wear a collar: Dress shirts get respect.

Keep yourself well groomed: But don't lick down there, please.

Woof!

up at night. On the other hand, if staying awake behind the wheel is your goal, sucking on a peppermint may be just what you need to do.

Hit Snoring with a Brick

To stop the nightly noise, elevate your head. This strategy helps keep the airway open. Place a brick or two under the bedposts at the head of the bed. Don't use extra pillows; they'll only kink your airway and make snoring worse.

Better Early Than Late

Getting an extra hour of sleep provides the energy equivalent of two cups of coffee. To get benefits from extra sleep, go to bed earlier. Sleeping later doesn't work. If you're used to getting up at 7 A.M., your body temperature and alerting hormones are all set to increase at about that time. When you sleep in, you disturb your circadian rhythms, and you'll feel somewhat groggy and out of sorts for the rest of the day.

Pop a Cherry

Drinking cherry juice or eating cherries before bed can help you fall asleep faster. Cherries provide a concentrated source of melatonin, a popular over-the-counter sleep aid.

Sniff This before Bed

Sniffing some lavender oil before bedtime is just as effective as sleep medication for some insomniacs.

Sit in Your Worry Chair

A lot of men bring their problems into bed with them. They lie in bed and think about their jobs, or they balance their checkbooks, or fight with their wives. If you find yourself falling into this pattern, set up a "worry chair." Ten minutes before bed just sit quietly in the same place and mull over the events of the day. You may not solve any pressing problems, but you'll at least be able to order them and set your priorities for the next day.

Sleep Around

If you're suffering from insomnia, you may want to try sleeping somewhere else for one night—a hotel, a relative's house, even a different room of your home. Many insomniacs come to associate their bedroom with their inability to sleep. By getting some solid shut-eye someplace else, you'll restore your confidence in your ability to sleep.

Find Your Ideal Bedtime

If you're not sure you're getting enough sleep, move your bedtime back a half-hour every night until you awaken when you want to without an alarm clock.

"Kur" Your Fatigue

If you wake unusually early, say 5 or 6 A.M., head for the bathroom and dampen a hand towel with cool water. Spend a few minutes lightly wiping your arms, legs, and torso, then go back to bed. The body is very warm when it comes out of REM sleep. Once it's cooled and you get back into bed, the body heats up even more, almost as if it has a slight fever. The result is a deep, restful sleep and more dreams. This technique is called a "kur," and it's standard treatment at many European spas.

Sleep with a Golf Ball

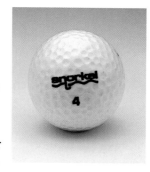

Many men are positional snorers—they only snore when they sleep sunny-side up and their tongues droop back over their airway. To cure yourself of this try wearing a pocket T-shirt backward to bed and put a golf ball in the pocket. Every time you roll onto your back, you'll land on the ball. It's tough to get cozy on top of a Titleist.

Avoid Your Last Gasp

If you're going to bed early enough but still feeling exhausted during the day, you could have sleep apnea. Ask you bedmate to listen to your snoring. Not all men who snore have this problem: The difference is in the sound of the snores. If it's a consistent, sawing-wood sound, up and down, you're fine. But if it's periods of silence followed by snorts or grunts, it's a reason to be concerned. You may not be getting enough oxygen. See your doctor.

Sweeten Your Dreams

If you're plagued by a recurrent nightmare, try consciously reworking it. When people in one study were told to change the content of a nightmare by writing down a new outcome and then rehearsing it, their bad dreams decreased dramatically.

Tinkle, Tinkle by the Stars

When nature calls in the middle of the night, don't turn on the overhead light. You may have trouble falling back to sleep. Light after midnight is extremely disrupting to your body clock. Instead, use a flashlight.

Answer the Alarm

Sleeping more than 10 hours nightly may shorten your life. A study of a million adults found that the mortality rate for long sleepers was 1½ to 2 times greater than the rate for people who slept 7 to 8 hours.

6

WORK

and

TRAVEL

If you average 8 hours of sleep per night and live to be 75, you'll have spent 25 years of your life in the sack. Even more sobering is the fact that if you're on the job an average of 10 hours per day, by the time you're ready for retirement you'll have logged an additional 13 years working. So 25 years snoring + 13 years slaving = 38 years, or more than half your life spent in either a complete or partial state of unconsciousness.

Lord help us.

Although there's not much we can do about the amount of sleep you need, there's quite a bit of advice we can lend on making those 13 years of work seem like less of a death sentence. The biggest cause of stress in most men's lives is their career. In their well-intentioned attempt to get ahead, a lot of guys end up dead. Strokes. Heart attacks. Depression. Obesity. Look around you. Or, even more sobering, look at yourself.

True story. We know a guy who used to be a reporter for a major newspaper. Young, talented, brimming with ambition just like his never-empty coffee mug. One night he returned to the office after covering an important city-council meeting. He had 30 minutes to write his story. It was a B1 piece, the lead to the local section, and his editor was all over him. But this guy was a pro. He pounded the story out, looking as calm as he always did, and beat his deadline by 5 full minutes. However, when his editor opened the electronic file, all the words were garbled. "Send it again!" the editor screamed. "There must be a transmission problem." But there wasn't. Our man had snapped, just like that. He was sitting at his desk, smiling, semi-catatonic—the sentences on his computer screen just as incomprehensible as this newsroom scene. Later, we learned he'd suffered a mild nervous breakdown. And although he's back to writing and reporting, he's not the same. A part of him left permanently that day.

The 157 tips in this section are designed to help you get the upper hand on this hairy, brute of a career you're wrestling. You'll learn amazing new ways to beat stress, build confidence, and even outsmart your boss. From money to management, business travel to office romance, it's all here. And because we realize that no matter how successful you are, there's always a part of you that'll be eyeing the door, we've also included tips on packing your bags and getting the hell out of here.

A career expert once told us that most men don't plan their careers, they let their careers plan them. It's a rudimentary mistake that steals satisfaction. Know where you're going, she advised, or at least be able to throw a dart in the general vicinity. Instead of waiting for "benevolent superiors" to decide what's best for you, decide it yourself. Instead of reacting to a supervisor's demands, make him react to you (with a counter-proposal or an entirely new way of doing things). This strategy is not as adversarial as it sounds. In fact, most bosses will admire and welcome your ambition. (After all, it's less work for them.) And you'll immediately begin to reap the benefits. Once you take control of your career, people will respect you more and stress will miraculously evaporate. Who knows? You may even need less sleep.

Let's get to work.

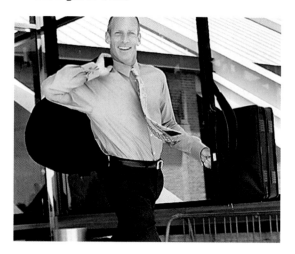

Get Started Right

People who wake up fully charged and ready to go often make a mistake by sitting down to read the paper or watch the news. That's like downshifting. Instead, do something creative, whether it's playing with the kids or working out a strategy for a business meeting. That way you'll keep your energy high and leave the house feeling like you've already done something constructive.

On the other hand, if you ooze off the mattress and into the shower, you're probably better off sticking to a dull morning routine.

Sip Yourself Sharp

Pay attention to the timing of your first cup of coffee. Several studies have found that introverted guys are generally sharper when they first wake up than are extroverts. As a result, an introvert performs better on morning mental tasks without coffee, while an extrovert does better with it. In the evening, the pattern flips. Introverts do better in tests when they've had caffeine, while extroverts do better without.

Set Your Alarm an Hour Earlier

Simply waking up 1 hour earlier each day during the work week will give you 5 extra hours per week, which works out to 32½ days in a year to accomplish whatever you "can't get done." Don't try staying up later at night, though. Time-management experts say most people find it easier to be more productive in the morning than late at night.

CATCH UP ON EXTRA WORK

One entrepreneur we know takes full advantage of his daily time on the hopper. He brings a hefty stack of work into the bathroom and spreads it out in front of him. Using what, you ask? The toilet tank, of course. He sits backward on the toilet and uses the tank as a temporary desk. (Talk about pushing paper.) Of course, this requires full removal of pants, as well as clearance room for the knees. And you really shouldn't stay on the can too long—no more than 5 minutes—or else you're inviting hemorrhoids. But still, it's strangely intriguing....

Make a Good First Impression

A person to whom you've just been introduced should get a clear impression that you're truly enthused to make his or her acquaintance. That requires more than a routine, "Nice to meet you" and a half-hearted extended hand. Consider switching to the slightly less common and more courtly, "I'm pleased to meet you," or even "It's a pleasure to meet you." The exact words are less important than deploying the happy-to-meet-you voice lilt. This subtle tone implies that you've heard wonderful things about this particular person and that you're glad, finally, to have met him.

Never Forget a Name

One of the easiest ways to remember someone's name is to look at the person you've been introduced to and imagine that her name is stamped on her forehead. No kidding, it works.

Maximize Your Message Machine

Your actual first impression is often on voice mail. So convince a woman to record your voice-mail greeting for you, as in "You've reached the office of Mr. Hot-Shot Who Has This Personal Assistant Who Is Clearly Both Competent and a Smokin' Babe." Now, you don't really have to have a personal assistant to do this, mind you. But this trick evokes an image of a man with a staff at his command, instead of a guy trying to jam a stack of paper into the fax machine.

Develop This Quality

Rudeness and incivility are disguises that the hideously insecure lurk behind. Confidence reveals the opposite, of course. No single characteristic carries such punch. Women deal with guys who lack confidence, but they don't swoon. Bosses delegate to men who lack confidence, but they don't trust them. It's confidence that shines your shoes and combs your hair. It's confidence that keeps you from being eager for approval. People will respect you more if you don't seem to give a damn whether they think you're worthy or not.

Plan Your Day This Way

You can pack more productivity into each day if you plan it around a few key guidelines.

Make major decisions between 7:00 and 11:00 A.M. You're most confident then and de-pression and anxiety are lowest. You grow less resolute between 2:00 and 8:00 P.M., when depression and anxiety can surge. One caveat: Avoid decisions on Mondays.

Push off big decisions until Tuesday. Making tough judgments after a weekend of relaxation is not only bad policy—Monday is the least productive day of the work-week—but it's also risky since Monday is when you're statistically most likely to have a heart attack. By waiting a day, your brain will be sharper and your body better able to cope with the stress.

Schedule meetings from 9:30 to 11:00 A.M. This gives people time to get organized, answer e-mail, and clear the decks, so they're ready to sit down and concentrate on the business at hand.

Plan deal meetings for lunch. People are most agreeable (so you sound most persuasive) over lunch. More business contracts are signed over lunch than at any other time.

Rather than arriving early, stay late. People will see your car in the lot when they leave, and that makes them feel guilty. Better, management will take notice and look the other way when you come in late for work wearing your bathrobe.

Add 20 Percent to Everything

Expect everything you do to take 20 percent longer than you think it will. Time constraints have a hold on all of us, so don't beat yourself up over them.

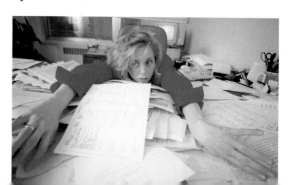

THWART BIKE THIEVES

Forced to leave your bike unattended while you pop into the mini-mart for a job application? These safeguards will slow thieves trying to steal your steed:

- Snap your helmet strap around the front wheel and the frame.
- Leave your bike in high gear (with the chain on the biggest ring in front and the smallest cog in back). This will help prevent fast getaways.
- If your front wheel is easily removable, take it with you. Ditto with your seat.

7 Signs of a Good Job

No matter what you do or where you do it, here are some signs of a job worth keeping:

1. You get regular feedback from your boss.

2. You respect your boss.

3. Teamwork is encouraged over competition.

4. Self-reliance is encouraged over conformity.

5. You have at least a certain measure of freedom and autonomy.

6. You're not held accountable for things you can't control.

7. There are no signs encouraging you to "Smile" anywhere on the premises.

Make a Stellar Speech

Here are a few hints to making a great presentation:

Exercise that morning. Hit the stair climber or treadmill. Aerobic exercise releases endorphins—literally "the morphine within"—which have a relaxing, calming effect.

Visualize first. Visualizing an upcoming speech improves your delivery. First relax, then picture how the day of your presentation will unfold. Imagine yourself waking up full of energy and confidence, getting dressed, looking sharp, and feeling prepared. Finally, imagine entering the room and seeing your peers and how they react to your well-organized, informative talk.

Eat an apple. Just before taking the podium, eat a Granny Smith apple. It's the tartest of the apple bunch. The acidity stimulates saliva production, which will help keep your talk crisp and fluid. If things still feel gummy, try a chaser of olive oil. Swish a spoonful in your mouth and spit it out; it will keep your lips from sticking to your teeth, eliminating that annoying lip smack when you're standing behind the microphone.

Keep it short. Once you start talking, keep speeches to 20 minutes to hold your audience's interest and no more than 40 minutes if you have a lot of information to convey. Figure that 170 words—three-quarters of a double-spaced, typed page—equal about 1 minute of talking.

Follow the three-point plan. If you want to win the respect of an audience, never make more than three major points. Anything more won't be remembered.

Sip away speaking anxiety. Room-temperature water with a touch of lemon is the best beverage for a nervous speaker with a dry throat. Avoid ice water; it'll constrict your throat. Tepid water will help your voice sound rich, and the lemon will clear any mucus buildup. You might want to put a small bottle of it in your briefcase, since the pitcher next to the podium is usually filled with ice.

Stand and Deliver

Getting up from your desk and standing can put you in a higher gear for decision-making. One study found that people under pressure make difficult decisions about 20 percent faster if they stand instead of sit. The researchers speculate that standing arouses your nervous system by increasing your heart rate 10 beats per minute.

IMPROVE YOUR MEMORY

Humans store information in chunks that are five to nine pieces long. We can remember a five-digit PIN number or a nine-item grocery list. When the memory tasks get longer, however, things get more difficult. To remedy this, divide the assignment. Instead of trying to remember 10 digits, split the numbers into two five-digit chunks.

Heed These Phone Hints

Talking on the phone all day can wear you down. Try these tricks to make it more bearable:

Hum a few bars. Before making a potentially stressful phone call, hum. That's right, hum. It'll help calm you down and make your voice sound richer.

Get off the phone. If you must call someone who's hard to get rid of, "accidentally" hang up on yourself in midsentence. He'll think you've been disconnected, and if he calls back and hears a busy signal, he'll just assume there's trouble on the line.

Let it ring. Instead of diving for the phone, let it ring two or three time before picking up. Use the ring as a signal to take a few breaths and relax. When you do answer, you'll feel more calm, confident, and in control.

Cut out interruptions. You'll accomplish more of your work on time if you don't interrupt your flow by periodically returning phone calls. Schedule your call-backs for one of those typically "unproductive" times of the day, like just before lunch or at 4 P.M.

Extend your vacation with voice mail. On your voice-mail message, say you'll be on vacation one day longer than you really will be. This will forestall the firestorm of phone calls, and give you time to come up with solutions to problems.

Use These E-Mail Tricks

Despite the state of your inbox, you're in control of your e-mail. Here are some ways to use it to your advantage:

• Want to e-mail your boss at 11:58 P.M. when you're actually sound asleep? Go to "File" and hunt for "Send options." You can program most e-mail to send the note hours, or years, later.

• The BCC (blind carbon copy) feature lets you forward a message to a group without revealing everyone's e-mail address. You see who's in the BCC box, but the recipients don't. Sneaky, but useful.

• Getting blown off? Hit "Read receipt" (look under "Options"), and you'll get an e-mail as soon as your note is read.

• To disable the pesky e-mail announcement feature in Outlook click on Tools/Options/E-mail Options/Advanced E-mail Options.

• Avoid smiley-face "emoticons"—they're a favorite of low-level employees yearning to be liked.

• Don't e-mail angry; e-mails live forever.

• Keep your e-mail fonts simple and the backgrounds clean. Anything elaborate makes people wonder what you're doing with all your time.

Become a Correspondent

In this e-mail era, the power of a handwritten follow-up letter is dramatic. A letter conveys professionalism and thoughtfulness. E-mail feels like a hasty attempt to cross something off a to-do list.

Jog Your Memory

To better remember what you're working on, do a couple of minutes of calisthenics for every hour of paperwork. Epinephrine and norepinephrine, two neurotransmitters that play a big role in converting short-term memory into long-term memory, are released whenever you subject yourself to physical or emotional stress. Scientists think this is why you can remember every detail of a car wreck, or why, if Cameron Diaz were to give you her phone number, you wouldn't need to write it down.

Fit Your Workout to Your Work

In order to best alleviate work stress, exercise in a mode opposite to your occupation. Here are some different job types, along with the style of workout that will best help you relax:

The Manager: This category includes executives, bosses, foremen—anyone who's got bottom-line responsibility. What you need is a change of scenery, at least 40 minutes of outdoor exercise. What you don't need are stationary bikes, treadmills, or anything that involves sitting still. A distraction-free environment will only let your mind wander back to your problems.

The Busy Body: These are guys who spend most of their time running around—whether it's as an executive assistant, an electrician, a cop, or a salesman. Stationary exercise machines let you stay put for a change. And they offer another advantage: They're solitary. Chances are, if you're running around a lot, you're running into people. You need a break from that.

The Number Cruncher: CPAs, stock analysts, researchers, and anybody else who deals with stats should forget about exercise logs, hard-and-fast workout rules, and whether they did 29 crunches or 30. Show up at the gym and do a variety of things on impulse.

The Creative Type: This group includes advertising executives, designers, promotion directors, and writers. Plan concrete, but achievable goals. Weight programs or aerobic activities such as bicycling or running, where you can compete with yourself and others and clearly chart how much faster and stronger you're getting, can give you the sense of day-to-day achievement that might be lacking at work.

The Assembly Liner: If you're engaged in any occupation where the routine is the same every day, be eclectic in your workouts. Try adding racquetball on Monday, swimming on Wednesday, and maybe yoga on Friday.

Take the Pulse of Your Workday

If you own a heart-rate monitor, you know how effective it can be for keeping your heart rate in your target zone while exercising. But you can also use it to beat stress at other times of day. If your job is highly stressful, wear it to work. Check your heart rate now and then. If it's high, you'll know it's time to take a break. A monitor provides a window to what's happening inside your body.

Loosen Up at the Office

It's 3 P.M. You haven't moved from your desk since lunch, and you're feeling as stiff as that plastic plant in the corner. Relief is as close as the door. Follow this 30-second stretching routine to loosen up:

1. Walk to the doorway and place your forearms up against each side of the frame. After positioning your arms, slide your left foot in front of your right and slowly lean forward. You'll feel the stretch in your arms, chest, and shoulders.

2. Keeping your forearms against the door frame, slide your left foot farther forward to focus the flex on your lower body. The farther forward you slide your foot, the more you stretch your calves and hamstrings and the muscles around your hips.

3. Now, twist your torso to one side while braced against the door frame and leaning forward. This will flex the muscles over the ribs. Hold for a count of three. Ease up and twist to the other side.

4. Repeat the three steps, this time with your right foot forward.

Avoid Pains in the Neck

Position your keyboard below your belly button, directly over your upper thighs, to avoid carpal tunnel syndrome. Resting your keyboard on your desk is a big mistake. It causes you to bend your wrists upward, which leaves your median nerve most vulnerable. It also forces your shoulders to stay tensed to elevate your arms, which causes back and neck pain.

Join a Focus Group

If you work on a computer all day, consider getting another pair of glasses designed for on-the-job wear. Most people need a different prescription strength for computer work. The screen is too far away for reading glasses, but too close for distance lenses. You can also have computer glasses made with built-in reading lenses.

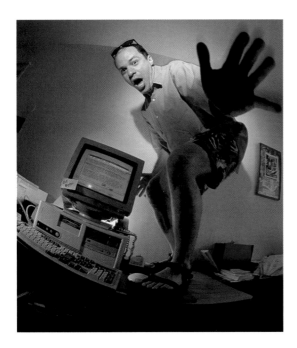

Be More Creative

To unleash your creative juices, force your brain out of its old grooves. Try things like re-arranging your clothes closet, wearing your watch on the other wrist, and brushing your teeth with your nondominant hand. Creativity means breaking habits and becoming more flexible. Even doing small things like this can jump-start you.

See Red

If you want a quick cure for fatigue, focus on something red. It's the color of bloodshed and fire. After eons of association, we are pro-grammed to respond to it.

Sniff Your Way Smart

Need a fast brain boost? Sniff a lemon. The scent stimulates your hippocampus, the part of your brain in charge of concentration and thinking skills.

Switch Off Headaches

One common cause of headaches is over your head—literally. Fluorescent lights flicker about 60 times per second. While this is unnoticeable to the naked eye, it can cause headaches and fatigue. If you work under fluorescent light, try to offset its effects with a table lamp or other incandescent lighting.

Order Up Some Bloom Service

Typical office ambiance, filled with paints, carpeting, vinyl furniture, and copying machines, gives off formaldehyde and ammonia fumes that can cause headaches and other health problems. The right potted plants in your office can filter them out. The most powerful air-conditioning plants are Boston fern, pot mum, dwarf date palm, dumb cane, dragon tree, and lady palm.

Polish a Paper Cut

To treat a paper cut, first make sure it's scrupulously clean. Then borrow a bottle of clear nail polish from somebody in the office and daub it on the cut to protect it from irritants such as air and soap.

Squeeze Your Balls

Keep a hand exerciser or a tennis ball at your desk and give it a few squeezes during tense times. When stress shoots adrenaline into the bloodstream, that calls for muscle action. Squeezing something provides a release that satisfies your body's fight-or-flight response.

Have Some Fun under Your Desk

For under-the-desk stress relief, try slipping off your shoes and rolling a golf ball under each foot.

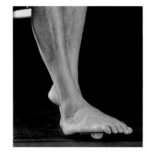

Nap on the Job

Thomas Edison got by on 3 hours of sleep a night by taking extremely short naps. The plan: Lean back in your chair, close your eyes (no need to lie down), and relax your body for a couple of minutes. Wait 5 or 6 minutes for dream images to appear in your brain; this is what's called "alpha sleep." When these images appear, open your eyes. You should feel refreshed. You'll also strengthen your attention to detail and improve your ability to make decisions—without the risk of unsightly drooling.

How to Cover Yourself

If you are self-employed, hiring an assistant may make you eligible for health insurance at group rates, which are generally much lower. Check out the regulations in your state.

Never Hire a Friend

There's an old adage: It's better to make friends of your employees than employees of your friends. Personnel directors we spoke with say that hiring a friend is often the quickest way to end a friendship. It's a very painful situation because both parties can easily feel some enormous breach of faith has occurred.

Take the Bullet, Then Scream

If you're the boss, take the heat. A good boss never lets the higher-ups know that his underling goofed up big-time. Are we clear? Patton never blamed his first looey. You can deliver as much heat to your staff as you want *after* you've taken it like a man from the guy above you.

Think Little to Think Big

It's important to separate "outcome goals" (the big stuff) into "process goals" (the little stuff) you can accomplish every day. Larger goals, like winning a championship or becoming the boss, can often seem abstract and distant, but when you break them into things you can do every day, your dreams gain power, and it gives you a sense of purpose and control. By doing it that way, you'll also learn to enjoy not just reaching the goal, but the daily pursuit of it.

Make Yourself Matter

It's so important to keep work in perspective. The cold, hard truth is that most of us just don't matter much at work. We're all pretty easily replaced at the office. But we matter a lot everywhere else we go. We matter to our fathers and brothers, to our neighbors, and to our women. We really matter to our children. The chance to matter is right there, in every other forum of our lives.

Retake Control of Your Life

If you're a successful guy who's constantly in demand and has trouble saying "no" at work, give yourself the 5-Year Test. Every time a possible commitment comes up—a meeting, fundraiser, dinner conference, speech—ask yourself if you're going to care about this event after 5 years. If so, accept. If not, decline. Learn to do this and you'll have a lot more time for the things you consider really important.

Spend Your Time

You don't really pay for things with money. You pay for them with time. "In 5 years, I'll have put enough away to buy that vacation house we want. Then I'll slow down or get out of this business altogether." Okay, that means the house will cost you 5 years. That's one twelfth of your adult life. Translate the dollar value of the car or the house or anything else into time, and then see if it's still worth it.

Die Broke

If you want to live a long and satisfying life, make it your goal to die broke. Although a sizable nest-egg relieves stress (which, in turn, enhances health), this is only true to a certain degree. After the mortgage is burned and the kids' college bills are paid, it's far better to spend than to save. The drive to accumulate money is Depression-era thinking. It's the old idea of leaving the farm to the kids so it will continue. But we don't live in that kind of society anymore. Instead of thinking of your legacy in terms of money, think of it as good memories generated by what you can do now by spending it.

Stop before It's Too Late

The failure to realize when enough's enough can leave a guy with a fat wallet but a life that's flat broke in every category that matters. One hundred percent in anything is unattainable. Settle for 80 or 90 percent and recognize that it's a pretty damned good accomplishment.

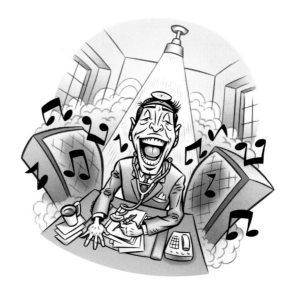

Shower Instead of Napping

Even better than napping, to stay productive when you're exhausted, take a shower. It's worth 2 hours of sleep. With any luck, your company has a gym with a locker room.

Be Wary of Workplace Romance

Don't sleep with anyone who you can fire or who can fire you and don't flirt at the office—especially with subordinates, and most particularly with lithesome young things fresh into the workplace. Even if you're only 25, you'll never be able to convince a jury you aren't a dirty old man. There are plenty of places for sexual conquests, but the office isn't one of them any longer. Any other attitude, and you're asking for trouble.

Wait to Date a Co-Worker

Wait 3 months after starting a new job before asking a co-worker for a date. When you're new, you're being judged. If you start dating too soon, you'll be in the spotlight even more.

Nobody needs that kind off pressure. Swing by her cube briefly on your way out the door. If it goes well, make it a habit. It opens up the evening and makes it easy to go from "I've had enough of those reports," to "Want to grab a beer?"

Don't Break Up on a Monday

If you're going to break up with a co-worker that you've been dating for a while, do it on a Friday night. You don't want to send a basket case back to work the next day.

Get Married to Further Your Career

If you want to further your career, get hitched. Numerous studies show that married men consistently get better employee evaluations and are more likely to be promoted than single men. Marrieds also make 10 to 50 percent more than their single counterparts. Employers seem to sympathize with family needs and view married men as more stable.

DON'T CATCH A DIVORCE AT WORK

Just like the flu, divorce is something you can catch on the job. Researchers in Sweden found that the risk of divorce is higher among men when they see colleagues move on to new partners. It evidently gives them the courage to take the same step. Women react differently, however. Seeing recent divorces makes them work harder at their marriages.

Imitate the Boss

Take cues from your boss and the people one level above you in deciding how to dress for work. You don't have to match them exactly, but at least be somewhat compatible.

Save Face after a Bad Joke

If you tell a tasteless joke at a meeting, and it doesn't go over well, say that it came from a respectable source. In other words, when your boss glares at you, wait a beat, and say: "Can you believe that was actually printed in *Time* magazine? I was appalled!"

Salvage a Screw-Up

So you bungled things badly at the office. After apologizing, ask your boss how he would have handled a similar situation. Suddenly you're showing good character, a desire to improve, and respect for his opinion. Who knows? Maybe he won't fire you.

Protect Your Interests

The next time your dingbat boss comes up with an idea that looks like a loser, politely outline your reservations in a memo. Send the memo. Keep a copy for yourself. Then if he rejects your advice and the project goes down in flames, keep quiet about whose fault it was and maybe he'll get the message. If he loses his job over it, you can start sucking up to the new boss by casually producing the memo and suggesting that things might have been different had he listened to you.

Win Every Argument

At the end of an argument, both participants usually declare themselves the winner, leaving the witnesses to make up their minds. Arguing is

Trick Your Boss into Giving You a Raise

Bring a cup of steaming cider with you the next time you ask your boss for a raise. Smells of cinnamon and cloves have been shown to entice people to spend money. Or better yet, rather than asking for a raise, ask for more responsibility. If you increase your value to the company, the money will follow.

If you find yourself in raise negotiations, try these helpful replies to your boss's excuses:

If the boss says. . . .	You say . . .
"Sorry, but you're already making the maximum for someone at your level."	"Then I deserve a promotion."
"I'd love to give you more money, but it would throw our salary structure out of whack."	"Then how about a one-time bonus? My productivity shows I've earned it."
"Our earnings are low this year. We need to watch payroll costs."	"Then how about paying my way to two industry conventions this year?"

If the answer is still no, then maybe you're not as valuable to this company as you thought and should start looking for a new job.

---

about overcoming the prejudices of onlookers. Here are three sneaky ways to do just that:

• Even people who used to know what "begging the question" means have probably forgotten, so it's a brilliant defense against almost any line of reasoning. No matter what your opponent says, answer by saying, "Now you're begging the question," or, "That begs the question, don't you think?"

• Continually restate your opponent's argument for him in grossly oversimplified terms. To prevent his case from seeming absurd, he will be forced to continually correct you and explain his position more fully, which will try the patience of any observers.

• An opponent who is demonstrably more intelligent than you is facing an uphill battle with your audience. He is dealing with the same

prejudices the BMW owner faces in a two-car accident with a Yugo. You can reinforce this bias if you occasionally answer your opponent's points by saying, "I'm sorry, I didn't quite follow that. Could you repeat it please?"

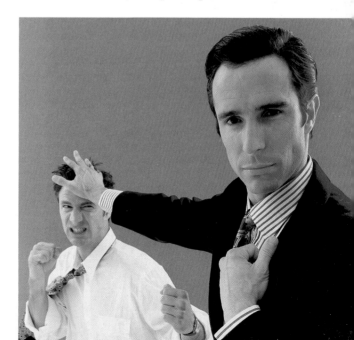

Be Prepared to Walk

Your single most powerful negotiating tool is the ability to leave the table. Deals seldom get worse when you walk away. The longer you sit on your hands, the better the terms are likely to become. An important *but:* Don't burn any bridges. The point is that you don't like the terms, not the person delivering them.

End a Meeting Right

Every meeting should end with a plan of action, and every attendee should have an assignment. Dan pulls the numbers from manufacturing. Judy drafts a preliminary letter of agreement. Fred works the shredder. Marching orders are vital—or you'll have the same meeting next week.

Run the Table

The seating arrangement at your weekly meeting can be more complicated than the one at a Jackson family reunion. Where do you sit? What does it mean? And why does that Website guy keep touching your thigh? Here are the best and worst spots to sit, (assuming your boss

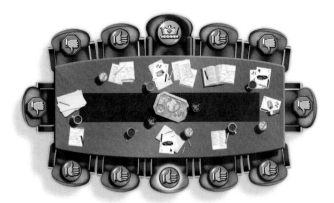

sits in the middle seat on one of the long sides of the table).

At either corner of the table on the same side as your boss: This is where unprepared guys go to hide. Bosses know this, and may single you out for the difficult questions. Like: "Who are you?"

Any seat on the side across from your boss: If you sit at any seat across from the boss (especially the one directly across), your boss will naturally make eye contact with you on important points.

The heads of the table: Sitting here—the old position of power—signals to everyone that

---

RIP A PHONE BOOK IN HALF

Taking out work frustrations by ripping a phone book in two isn't the feat of strength it seems. All you need to know is the trick to doing it. Start by placing the phone book on the edge of a table, with the pages facing you and the spine facing away. Grasp the phone book with your thumbs on bottom and fingers on top. Using the tops of your palms, slant the pages until their edges form a 45-degree angle. Now, slowly start ripping from the front of the book toward the spine. As long as you keep the same incline and have good wrist strength, you'll be ripping just a few pages at a time. After you've done it a while, you should be able to do it in no time.

Hint: If you want an unfair advantage, heat the book in an oven—on a low setting, please—for a few minutes beforehand. It'll make the pages brittle and easy to tear.

you could, or should, be in charge. The boss won't take kindly to that.

On either side of your boss: The boss is forced to turn to look at you when you talk, and that acknowledges your importance.

Outsmart Your Boss

Silently focus on some foible that blows his high-powered image: his bad grammar, his high-pitched voice, his nose-picking habit. Do a few of these negative visualizations before you talk to your boss to make him less of an intimidating ogre.

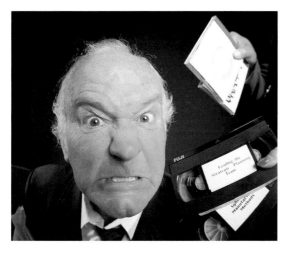

Get Your Boss a New Job

Let's say your worst-case scenario becomes a reality: That young climber, whom you can't stand, becomes your boss. You were here first, and you like it here or you would have left long ago. So what do you do? Call a headhunter—*for him*. Tell the recruiter all about your hotshot boss. If he is talented and ambitious, he'll jump at a better job. And who knows—maybe you'll get a promotion to fill that sudden vacancy.

Finish with Momentum

Ernest Hemingway would only stop working for the day when he knew exactly what he was going to write next. That way, it was easier for him to start the following day. Before you leave the office, write some notes on where you're headed. It'll be easier to regain the day's momentum tomorrow.

Also, before you go home, take some time to clean up your desk. There is a magical correlation between clutter and stress. Creating order out of chaos gives you a sense of closure on the day and fools people into believing you actually know what you're doing. Plus, this will make your evenings more relaxing. Reason: The human mind is a worry machine. At home, when you should be relaxing or asleep, it will scour your memory like a hungry shark looking for trouble. A to-do list and a clean desk help appease the beast.

Separate Work and Play

Taking work home is bad. The interesting thing is that many men take work home, poke at it a little, and then go do something else. They never actually get any substantial work done, but they don't enjoy their leisure because that work is sitting there tugging at their conscience. If you always have some work around, you'll never enjoy your time off and you'll resent your job. If you have a killer workload and simply can't avoid it, alternate evenings of intensive work and intensive leisure. On Monday, Wednesday, and Friday evenings (or whatever appeals to you), do your work and try not to get sidetracked. But on your leisure nights, don't even bother taking work home if you can help it. In fact, resist buying yourself a brief-case, because that's what they're designed for.

Think of Yourself As Autonomous

Instead of being a wage slave, picture yourself as an independent contractor with one major client—your employer. Then allocate your time so you not only meet the demands of your customer but also have room to develop certain aspects of your business that *you* (not the company) see as necessary for growth.

Change Jobs Often

Career-hopping extends life because it prevents men from making a common, fatal mistake: defining themselves by their jobs. Men's identities are often so wrapped up in their work that when they retire they lose their entire sense of self-worth. In fact, the highest suicide rate is among white men over age 65. Switching jobs and starting over teaches them to be more resilient, more flexible, and less afraid of making new beginnings.

Make a Mid-Life Shift

Around 45, you should consider changing your career—maybe not a new field completely, but a major change that will give you new perspectives and challenges and a renewed excitement about life.

WAIT OUT THE STORM

Never quit a job when you're angry. Give it time; think it through.

Turn a Pink Slip into Green

If you're about to be fired, here's what to do:

• Make a list of everyone you'd call if you got fired and call them now—while you have a job. Just calling to say, "Hi, how's the family?"

• If you don't have a 6-month money cushion, open a home-equity line of credit now. The banks won't help you once you've been cashiered.

Negotiate a Better Severance

Their severance package was the first offer. Get to work on your counterproposal:

• One month's severance pay for each year of employment.

• Another month for every dependent on your tax return.

• If you're fired in September, ask for an additional 3 months, since there's little hiring in the last quarter.

• If you weren't offered career counseling, ask for $5,000 to hire a counselor.

• Ask them to pay for your health insurance until you're covered by another employer.

• Insist on being paid in a lump sum so you immediately qualify for unemployment.

• If they won't negotiate, pack up your papers and say, "You'll be hearing from my attorney very soon." Even groundless lawsuits cost money, so it's in their interest to settle.

Keep Working after Being Fired

After being laid off, the most successful men operate as if they haven't been fired, just reassigned. They stick to their old work hours and start the day with a to-do list of contacts to make, letters to write, and job resource materials to plow through.

Start Planning Your Career

Some men don't realize that they're in the wrong line of work until they're out of work. Only then are they forced to reappraise their goals. When you think about it, very few people actually plan their careers. Most people just take what comes along, rather than finding the right fit for them.

Take This Job or Shove It

Before sending out your resume in response to a classified ad, learn to translate the jargon to make sure you know what you might be getting yourself into.

"*Good sense of humor required . . .*" Code for a tense environment. You'll have the door slammed in your face a lot, so you *must* have a sense of humor.

"*Self-motivated team player needed . . .*" The combination of the two traits means the company is looking for the impossible—a great performer who can work with a bunch of stooges.

"*Busy exec looking for . . .*" This job is going to be long on work and short on glory. This busy exec is looking for someone to do all his work so he can work on his golf game.

Be the Last One Interviewed

Don't rush to be the first guy interviewed for that new position. The last person interviewed gets the job the majority of the time. Worst times for job interviews are Mondays or just before quitting time.

Contain a Fire

If you were fired from your last job, here's how to handle it in your next interview. First, recruit a friend who works for a company in your field. Ask him to call your former boss and say he's thinking of hiring you. Your co-conspirator can then report back on what your old boss says about you, and how angrily he says it. Now you're ready to interview. Prospective employers don't mind hearing that you and your former boss disagreed. It happens all the time, but you should prepare them for the specific bad news. Speak highly of your old boss, too. Say there were some problems between you, and take responsibility for them.

Eat Chocolate Before an Interview

Immediately before a job interview, eat a piece of dark chocolate. It has the perfect mix of sugar and caffeine to help you do well under pressure. Caffeine makes you feel sharper and more aware of your surroundings. As for the sugar, researchers at Yale found that mental activity actually saps sugar from your bloodstream. By spiking blood-sugar levels with a bit of chocolate, you can think longer before feeling drained.

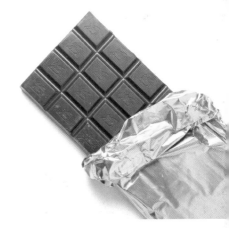

Interview the Interviewer

During the interview, you'll score major points not by talking about yourself, but by getting the interviewer to talk about himself. Don't wait until the end of the interview to ask about him and the company. Pepper him with questions throughout the interview so the session feels more like a conversation than a prosecution. As you're walking down the hall to his office, ask if he lives nearby or how long he's been with the organization. The more the interviewer talks, the more positive he'll feel about the interview and about you.

Consider This Clue

One factor you should consider when deciding to take a job is whether your prospective boss leaves the door open during your interview. If he does, the job may not be for you. Doing so is a clear indication of how much the company values trust and privacy. After all, how are you going to run you Amway business out of a cubicle?

Step Up, Commute Less

If you choose a new job that pays less but is 10 minutes from home over a current job that pays more but requires a 90-minute commute, you should not view that as a step down.

Take the Job That Sucks

If you have to choose between a good job in an industry in which you have no interest and a lousy job in an industry you find fascinating, take the lousy job. You may have to take a job in the mail room, but if you're smart, good, and work hard, it's not the job you'll have for long.

It's Your Move

When you're being wooed for a new job, you're in a strong position to negotiate. Ask your new employer to help sell your old house and find a new one, contribute to your living expenses, and even help your wife find a new job. Demand that the company pay for your moving expenses directly rather than reimbursing you; you'll have to pay taxes on the lump-sum check.

Wait 3 Months

After taking a new job, wait 90 days before making any dramatic changes. First impressions are important. Too many executives start off making big changes and turn people off permanently. Spend 3 months studying the situation.

Exhibit These Traits

If your goal is to be rich, start modeling yourself after those who are. According to the book *The Millionaire Next Door,* here are the typical traits that millionaires share:

Self-employed: Instead of laboring for someone else's success, they work for themselves.

Public-school product: They didn't attend pricey private schools (but they generally send their kids to them).

Working stiff: On average, they log 45 to 55 hours weekly.

Domestic brand: Married, three kids, and more than 50 years old when they made their first million.

Super saver: Their broker is on speed dial. Millionaires save and invest compulsively.

Humble abode: These guys don't live in palatial estates. The average cost of their homes is $320,000.

MEN'S WEALTH

RESIST A REFUND

After working way too hard for their money, far too many men feel good about receiving tax-refund checks. If you got one, you messed up. While Washington has held on to your money, you've lost months of compounding interest. Go to payroll and have them increase the number of dependents you claim on your W4 withholding form. For every $500 in refund you got, add one dependent. The number of dependents on your W4 doesn't have to match your actual number of dependents.

Modest duds: They rarely spend more than $400 for a suit or $235 for a watch.

Average wheels: Most drive Fords.

Relentless tracker: Millionaires know where their cash goes, from transportation to taxes to takeout. It's watching those pennies that helped them get rich in the first place.

Get Out of Credit-Card Debt

To slow the growth of credit-card debt, transfer the balances to the lowest-rate credit card you have. Then, right after you make a payment, call one of the credit-card companies you owe, and tell them you want to close the account because you've found a lower-rate card. They'll often negotiate a lower rate with you right on the phone.

Don't Work Late and Drive

After you've lived through another long day at work, avoid the terrible irony of getting yourself killed on the drive home. A late night at work can impair your senses as much as drinking a couple of shots. Researchers had one group of people stay awake for 28 hours and another group get drunk. After about 18 hours

of being awake, the subjects in the first group had mental and physical skills that were impaired as much as those who had drank two or three glasses of wine.

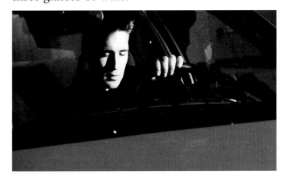

Drive Tall

If your lower back aches after your commute, it may be because you're slouching. Tilt your rearview mirror up a bit. That way, you make yourself sit up perfectly straight to see the cars behind you. You know if you can't see the cars, you're slumping.

Keep Your Headrest High

You can reduce the risk of whiplash and other neck injuries in an auto accident if you make sure your car's headrest is correctly positioned. Auto-safety experts say many are too low. In an accident, your body tends to slide up the seat; if your headrest isn't high enough, you may miss it entirely and suffer a whiplash injury. Check your headrest by sitting in the car and tilting your head back. The back of your head should touch the lower half of the headrest. If it touches the metal support post, the headrest is too high.

Talk Your Way Out of a Speeding Ticket

The longer an officer chats with you before writing a ticket, the better your chances of getting off with only a warning. To buy yourself as much time as possible, pull your car off the shoulder as far as you can so the officer can talk to you without fear of becoming roadkill.

Drink and Drive

Taking a long drive? Pretend someone poured a cold drink down your back—notice how your shoulders pull back and your spine curves? That's the position your back should be in when you drive.

Cool a Hot Engine with Heat

When coolant levels are low and there's no water to be added, crank up the heat and put the fan on high. The heater core will draw off some of the excess heat, making the job of cooling the engine a bit easier.

Adjust for Traction

If you're driving in bad weather, remember that tires lose a third of their grip in the rain. To compensate for that, generally cut a third off whatever speed you'd usually drive on a particular stretch of road.

Sharpen Your Blades

Instead of replacing "worn-out" wiper blades, soak a rag in rubbing alcohol and wipe them down. You'll be amazed how much better you drive when you can see.

Photograph the Accident

Keep a disposable camera in your glove box for that inevitable day when someone rams your car. Between "It wasn't my fault," insurance fraud, and civil litigation, the more evidence you have in your favor, the better. Snap pics of the damage, the intersection (with traffic signs

WHEN ALL ELSE FAILS

CLEAR A FROSTY WINDSHIELD

Crank up the defroster and turn down your sun visors. They'll help trap the warm air against the frozen glass and save you lots of scraping in the long-term lot.

BECOME A SCARECROW

If you're caught outside in a storm, keep hypothermia at bay by employing the "scarecrow technique." Take off your shoelaces and tie your cuffs around your ankles. Then start stuffing your pants and shirt with leaves or pine needles. You'll warm up almost immediately. If you're trapped in your car during a snowstorm, do the same thing using the stuffing from inside the seat cushions.

or lights), the other guy's license plate, and, just to be safe, the other guy (easy if he's pinned beneath the wreckage).

Pay a Toll Faster

Never take the exact-change lane. Few people ever have the exact change ready, so you'll end up waiting for them to find it. Instead, head for the manned booths and pick a lane with one or two trucks or busses as opposed to five or six cars. It may look longer, but it'll usually move faster.

Hammer Out an Exit Plan

Stash a hammer (or a hefty rock) under your driver's seat. If you need to get out of a mutilated car, your sneaker has zero chance of breaking ½-inch glass.

Keep Your Eyes on the Road

At 60 mph, you're traveling 90 feet per second. If you take your eyes off the road in front of you for just 3 seconds, you travel blind for 270 feet, nearly the length of a football field or a city block. Makes you think.

Take a Note with No Pen

Some guy on the radio offers a collection of Johnny Cash's greatest hits for only $10.95 and gives you an 800 number to call to order. But you're doing 90 mph on the Jersey Turnpike with 15 troopers in hot pursuit, plus you've got no pen. What do you do? Rub your finger on the side of your nose and write the number on the window. One wipe per number, please. You can read the number later by giving the window a blast of breath.

Count Yourself Out

To gauge if you're too drunk to drive, take this test: Stand with one foot in front of the other, arms at your sides, and tilt your head back to look at the ceiling. Now close your eyes and count backward from 30 by fours. If you flub it, call a cab.

Cure Carsickness

Does your stomach do flip-flops when you try to read in a car? You're suffering what's called *sensory mismatch*. To quell your belly, read brief sections, then glance out the front window. Also be sure to look out the front window whenever the vehicle changes direction and follow the turn until it straightens out. Not watching a turn is a sure way to make yourself nauseous.

Predict When Your Car Will Break Down

To diagnose a car's ills, examine the wet stuff underneath it. Coolant is bright green or orange, oil is brown, power-steering and transmission fluids are red, and brake fluid is clear or tan. Gasoline has an obvious odor. If you see a clear puddle in summer, it's condensation from the air conditioner.

Wait to Have Your Car Serviced

About to take a long car drive? Then forget about having your car serviced. Car trouble often occurs within the first several hundred miles after servicing. Get your vehicle to the shop 2 weeks before you're planning to leave.

Get Yourself out of a Fix

If the mechanic says your shocks or struts are shot, do the bounce test. Push down on each corner of your car until it starts to bounce on its own. Let go. If it settles after one full bounce, it's okay. If it bounces two or three times, he's probably not trying to rip you off.

Along the same lines, forget the 3,000-mile oil change. Most cars will do just fine if you wait until the manufacturer's specified interval in the owner's manual (usually every 7,500 miles).

Ask for Your Old Parts

Some less-than-scrupulous mechanics (a few do exist) substitute second-rate auto parts, while assuring you they've installed a premium brand. So before the mechanic does the job, ask him to stick the old parts in the new parts boxes when he's finished. You'll know what brand of parts you got and that your mechanic actually made the switch.

Measure Your Load

According to AAA, the most common cause of cold-weather auto breakdowns is a weak or dead battery. Unfortunately, this often happens without warning. Drivers in colder

---

WHEN ALL ELSE FAILS

PLUG A LEAKY RADIATOR WITH AN EGG

Should you happen to find yourself with an extra egg and a leaky radiator, as a stopgap measure to get you to the service station, break an egg into the radiator opening. Top off with water or coolant. Then close the radiator and start your engine. The egg will cook, and the particles will clog up the leak. Over time, the egg will break down, so it won't damage the cooling system.

MR. CLEAN

DE-STINK YOUR CAR

Pour pure vanilla extract on a cotton ball and place it in the ashtray. As the vanilla evaporates, so will the stench.

To get a fart out of the car, crack both front windows. The low-pressure zone outside the windows will suck out the gas. Key note: Keep the back windows closed. When all the windows are open, inside air doesn't exit, but is forced into the back.

climes with batteries that are more than 2 years old should get a "load test" at their local repair shop or auto-parts store. This gauges the battery's condition in minutes and is often done for free. Have one done every year as part of your car's regular pre-winter maintenance.

Drive on the Fumes

You're about to run out of gas, and there's no station in sight. Your best bet is to flip on the cruise control to maintain a constant speed of 55 mph—this will improve your gas mileage by 15 to 20 percent. Also, lose the AC—it burns 12 percent more gas.

Unlock Your Car, Dipstick

If you've locked your keys in your car, here's one way to possibly get back in. Pop the hood, grab the oil dipstick, wipe it clean, and insert the round end between the rubber door seal and the window. Move the dipstick around until you feel it catch the lock. Lift. There's a learning curve here, so give it a little time.

Change a Flat on a Sheet

Stow an old white bedsheet in your trunk. If you ever get a roadside flat, it'll make the change much easier. By spreading it on the ground you'll keep roadkill remains off your chinos and have an easier time keeping track of all those lug nuts.

Make the Bentley Gleam

A car's finish should sparkle like fine crystal. The secret to getting that chamois-dried look without the time-consuming buffing is in the rinsing. Working in the shade, hold the hose (without a spray attachment) an inch from the surface. The subsequent sheeting action will prevent the formation of those horrid water spots. Wrap the metal end of the hose with duct tape to prevent scratching.

Cover a Scratch with Crayon

You can temporarily repair unsightly scratches in your car's finish by coloring them with a wax crayon that matches your finish, then buffing the spot with a soft cloth.

Get Rid of Road Tar with Mayo

To remove road tar from your car's finish, put some mayonnaise on a cloth napkin, rub it on the offensive spot, let it set a few minutes, then wipe clean.

Break the Ice

Rock salt is good at what it does—destroying everything you dump it on, starting with ice and ending with asphalt. A better way to melt the ice is with magnesium chloride and water. Spray it on your driveway before a storm and it prevents ice buildup, and it's 70 percent less corrosive than salt. Colorado and Washington State highway plow guys swear by the stuff. It's sold in hardware stores as Reilly Freeze Fighter and runs about $9 a gallon, about what you would need to treat the average-size driveway.

Get Out of a Snowbank

The best way to maneuver your car out of a snowdrift is this:

1. Put something abrasive under the tires, such as sand, cat litter, a car mat, or your mother-in-law.

2. Start rocking the car back and forth, using the highest gear you can (the higher the gear, the better the traction).

3. Once you get the vehicle rocking significantly, apply the brakes when it reaches its highest point. (You want to perch atop the mini-snowbank you've created, not fall back into the hole.)

4. Now throw it into reverse and use the extra momentum to power out backward.

Pack Smart

If you're about to venture out on a trip, for work or for pleasure, here are six things you'd never think of bringing, but should:

Rubber door wedge: Jam the inside of hotel doors that have unreliable locks.

Antibacterial baby wipes: Clean off your hands or foreign toilets.

Racquetball: Use it as a sink plug so you can wash clothes in a hotel bathroom or as a stress-relief ball on long flights.

Safety pins: Seal your pockets when walking streets in cities where pickpockets have a higher annual income than you. Or, use a big pin to hold the curtains of your hotel room closed. They must be pinned unless you want a direct shaft of bright sunlight to fall across your eyes in the morning an hour and a half before it's time to get up.

Expired passport: It's collateral when foreign companies want to hold on to identification (never part with your real passport).

Extra meds: If you're traveling abroad and frequently take over-the-counter or prescription drugs, buy a spare bottle and toss it into your carry-on. A drug with the same name in a foreign country may be different from what's sold in the States. Standards for manufacturing differ, and the American Pharmaceutical Association warns that international versions of many drugs may include contaminants.

Know What to Pack Where

First, try to get your wife to pack for you. If that doesn't work, here are some hints:

• When flying, put toiletries in plastic bags and pack them in a carry-on bag. This guards against leaks caused by pressure changes and turbulence and will make life easier if the airline loses your luggage.

• Save dry-cleaning bags and put one over each item in your hanging wardrobe bag. This lets clothes slide against each other instead of bunching up and wrinkling. Or, slip some plastic Bubble Wrap into your suit sleeves to prevent crumpling.

• If you're bringing running shoes, store them in two 1-gallon zip-top freezer bags, so they don't stink up the rest of your clothes.

• To save precious luggage space, roll up belts and slip them in your shoes.

• On any trip longer than a couple of nights, bring two suits. One should be solid navy. That way, the jacket doubles as a navy blazer. The other should be a solid gray or a very subtle pattern that will allow you to wear the pants with your navy jacket.

Stuff In More Stuff

If you can't fit all your clothes in one suitcase, pack in what you can and then close it. Drop it on the floor a few times. This will help items settle and may give you more space.

Why You're Not There Yet

If that trip to Dayton with the kids seems to be taking longer than ever because you have to stop so often for gas, look at your roof. Boxy luggage on your car top can cut gas mileage by 10 percent. Use an aerodynamic roof rack instead.

Use Ethnic Travel Agents

If you're traveling by plane, here's a little-known way to save some cash. For discount fares, try travel agents in ethnic communities. Want a cheap flight to Korea from Los Angeles? Head to Koreatown and buy the ticket from just about any Korean travel agent. Even Japan becomes a discount destination if you go through an ethnic agent.

BOOK THE EARLY-BIRD SPECIAL

To reduce your risk of delayed flights, select departures early in the day. Later flights are far more likely to be delayed due to the ripple effect throughout the day.

Wing It When You Fly

If you're prone to motion sickness, request a seat over the wing on the right side of the aircraft. You'll feel less turbulence when sitting in the middle of the plane, plus most flight patterns turn left, so you won't be swung around so much.

Pop Two before Taking Off

Take two aspirin before a long flight. It'll thin your blood and reduce the risk of clots forming in your legs.

Avoid These Seats

On a recent fully booked 8-hour flight, we pressed the recline button on a coach seat and the damn thing wouldn't budge. The flight attendant explained that it wasn't broken; it was simply a "non-reclining seat." To skip this little infuriation, avoid booking a seat directly in front of an emergency row. These seats are almost always non-recliners.

Get Some Elbow Room

Aisle seats on planes allow the most freedom and leg room. But always choose one that is on the same side as your dominant hand. In other words, if you're right-handed, sit on the right side of the aisle, so when you're taking a drink or a forkful of dinner, your right elbow won't be the one bumped.

Pick the Best Seat on the Plane

When you make reservations, always ask what type of plane you'll be on. You can often find seat schematics either printed in the airlines' schedule books or on their websites. Then, when the airline reservation agent asks, "Window or aisle?" surprise her with a specific request for the best coach seat on the plane. This varies by airline and aircraft, but here are the seats to seek on some different carriers and planes:

• On a Delta 757, seat 19A has the extra legroom. On a United 757, ask for 8A. On a Northwest 757, score 16F or 15E. On a US Airway 737-400, 11A or 11F will let your stretch out. On an American Airlines 757, you want 10A or 10F. These are window seats, but you won't feel crammed in. Why? Because there are no seats 9A and 9F. You'll have lots of room in front of you. Kick back.

• On an American Airlines 767, if you're on a domestic flight, ask for seat 17H or 17J. They recline farther, have footrests, and give you more space in front because they have their own bulkhead. If you're going business class on a United 767 Model 200, claim 10A or 10F. They're both single seats with little desk areas on their sides. Very cool.

• If you're flying overseas on a British Airways 747, request seat J or B in row 52, 53 or 54. They're middle seats in the back, but because of the way the plane curves toward the rear, there are no window seats in these rows. So, you've got extra space between you and the window where you can actually stash a newspaper.

Beat Jet Lag

If you're flying west for an extended stay and the time difference is more than 5 hours, book your flight so you'll land at about 6 P.M. local time. Jet lag occurs when light hits you at the wrong time—your glandular watch says sundown, but the light outside says daytime. The combination throws off production of melatonin, a sleep inducer, and you may feel sleepy at midday and wide-awake at night. To put yourself in sync, you want to see light in the early evening. That will help reset your body clock.

If you don't have that much control over your arrival time, while you're on the plane, mimic what people are doing at your destination. If you board the plane and it's midnight at your destination, pass on the dinner the crew is serving and go to sleep. And when you arrive?

No matter where you're going and no matter what time you get there, stay up until at least 11 P.M. local time. If you can do that, you're well on your way to resetting your body clock.

Forget about Customer Service

Whether your flight has been canceled or delayed indefinitely, don't stand in line like a lemming. Pick up a phone and call the airline's 800 number. Whoever answers will probably have better info and more time for the task than the person on the scene.

REAL-LIFE SURVIVAL

WALK AWAY FROM A PLANE CRASH

In case the unthinkable happens, here are some ways to be prepared:

- Wear nonflammable clothing. Cotton is good; synthetics are deadly.

- Wear low-heeled, leather shoes such as loafers. These minimize tripping and don't burn as readily as sneakers.

- Empty your bladder regularly. Water weighs 8 pounds per gallon; full bladders burst on impact.

- Sit behind the wings, near an exit. These are generally the safest seats.

- Know whether your seat belt is a right- or left-hand release.

- Make your own air bag by putting pillows or seat cushions on your lap.

- Keep your feet flat on the floor. If your legs are stretched out, the metal bar beneath the seat in front of you could snap your ankles.

- Inflate your life jacket and snug it around your neck (even if you're not over water) to create a protective neck collar.

- Bend forward into a compact, fetal position.

- Pray.

STAY CALM OFF THE GROUND

Not eating before a flight may increase your anxiety when airborne. Here's how the bioscience goes: If your body is hungry, your blood-sugar level drops. When this happens, your body sends out a stress signal. Your adrenaline rises. So does your anxiety. To short-circuit this sequence, eat lots of preflight complex carbohydrates—some whole wheat bread, cereal, or a banana. They'll help keep your blood-sugar levels steady. On a day you're flying, don't go more than 3½ hours without having at least a snack. Also, stay away from coffee. Caffeine will ratchet up your tension level.

Ask for 3 Pillows

To avoid having a sore back when you deplane, ask the flight attendant for three pillows. Fold one in half and place it in the middle of your back, about 3 inches above the top of your buttocks. This will help you maintain the natural curve of your back and distribute weight evenly against your spine. Use another pillow on your lap to prop up your reading material. A lot of people lean over when they're reading on planes, which causes tremendous back strain. Use the third pillow—or a blanket or your briefcase—as a footrest. This will keep your knees higher than your hips, which forces you into a better sitting posture by ensuring that your back won't bow.

Snag a First-Class Meal

If the food is horrible in coach, tell your favorite crew member that you simply can't eat it. Or tell her you're allergic to orange cheese. Then say, "That poached salmon in first class wouldn't give me hives, though," and politely ask whether there are any first-class meals left over.

Sip This at 30,000 Feet

Every year, thousands of men are hospitalized after developing deep-vein thrombosis—a potentially fatal type of blood clotting caused by sitting in cramped seats and not moving around. To avoid this, the next time you have a long flight stick a sports drink in your carry-on. Drinks with a mixture of electrolytes and carbohydrates work better than water to prevent blood from pooling in your legs and clotting when you fly.

Take a Stand

If you get a leg or foot cramp from sitting too long in an uncomfortable airplane seat, don't rub the sore spot—that will only make things worse. For quick relief, stand firmly on the leg or foot, or just press it down on the floor as hard as you can.

Keep Your Ears Open

If you have trouble popping your ears on a plane, avoid cold drinks. The chill slows down the mucus-clearing movement of your cilia (hairlike structures in your nasal cavity). This causes your eustachian tubes to become blocked, so you can't equalize the pressure in your ear canals.

Grab the Right Bag

Before surrendering your luggage to the harried-looking attendant, tie pieces of green or red ribbon around the handles of your suitcases. You'll be able to find them on the luggage carousel immediately. Or apply some loud bumper stickers. Thieves will be less likely to steal your bag because it'll be easier to spot.

Bill 'em for Lost Clothes

If you land in Bermuda and your luggage goes to Budapest, the airline should bend over backward to make it up to you. Policies vary, but most airlines will cover the cost of replacing at least some of your stuff. Talk to the airline representative at the baggage claim and insist that the airline pay for replacement clothes. In most cases, they'll refund a percentage of your expenses—exactly how much is negotiable. If after hearing your tale of woe the rep offers you a smile and a new toothbrush, all is not lost. Go ahead and buy whatever you need to salvage your trip, but save your receipts. When you return home, send the airline an itemized list of the lost items, along with a copy of your frequent-flyer statement and a threatening letter. Often they'll make amends.

What to Eat When You Land

When you arrive at your destination, skip the local steak house and the hotel bar, especially if you arrive at night in preparation for a morning meeting. Fat and booze will make you sluggish. Instead, eat something small: salad, fruit, a baked potato, or a bowl of soup that isn't cream-based. If you're still groggy the next morning, wake yourself up with some lean protein—a glass of skim milk or some yogurt. Protein increases the supply of the brain chemical norepinephrine, which can make you more alert.

Have Grandma Unload

After you've survived the long drive, don't hurt yourself unpacking your car. Rather than rushing to unload the luggage from your trunk, take a breather. Ideally, wait about an hour to give your spine and back muscles time to loosen up. Then when you are lifting luggage out of the trunk, keep the weight as close to your body as possible. Don't lift with outstretched arms.

REAL-LIFE SURVIVAL

KNOW WHEN TO JUMP

It only takes a fall of 33 feet for a human body to reach terminal velocity. If you're higher than three stories, the lawn is just as likely to kill you as the flames devouring the word-processing department. No choice? Jump into a Dumpster. They're big, stinking safety nets.

Ask the Bellboy for a Loan

Let's say you're overseas and you need a little extra local currency. Your first thought is to go to an exchange bureau or ATM. Let us suggest a better alternative: your hotel. Ask for some local cash and have the hotel charge it to your room bill. It's called a "paid out" in hotelese. You'll pay for the cash on your credit card, thereby avoiding the often-hefty ATM and ex-change-bureau fees, and you get the best pos-sible exchange rate.

De-Stink a Hotel Room

If all the nonsmoking rooms at your destination are booked and the window doesn't even have a latch, you can quickly chase the smell of stale cigarettes by soaking a bath towel in cold water, wringing it out, and whirling it about the room. (Note: Please draw the blinds and keep your pants on.)

Let Pat Sajak Protect You

Whenever you leave your hotel room, make sure the television is on and the Do Not Dis-turb sign is hanging on the doorknob. An in-truder will think twice if he hears *Wheel of Fortune*. But it probably won't scare off maid services. Those ladies stop for no man.

When to Tip the Maid

Leaving a nice tip for the maid when you check out will earn you fond memories; leaving a tip each day of your stay will probably earn you better service while you're there.

Be the Perfect Houseguest

If you're staying with friends instead of at Motel 6, try to fall into the schedule and rhythm of your hosts. If they have their break-fast at 8:30 A.M. (an hour before you're usually awake), set a travel alarm and get up in time. If they go to bed at 10 P.M. (2 hours before you usually do) go to bed; if you can't sleep, read. Do not prowl the halls at night like a ghost.

Never Ask for Directions Again

If you're driving around an unfamiliar city and get hopelessly lost, get out of your car and flag a taxi. Tell him where you want to go and then jump in your car and follow the cab. Pay (and tip well) upon arrival.

Stay Safe in Perilous Places

When traveling in dangerous locales, carry a dummy wallet. Pad it with expired credit cards, foreign cash, and automatic teller receipts. If

---

REAL-LIFE SURVIVAL

BACKSTROKE OUT OF QUICKSAND

If your plane goes down in the jungle and you land in quicksand, don't panic. Just roll over onto your back and try to float. Then, with your arms and legs spread wide, slowly backstroke your way out. Don't be in a mad rush. Fast, jerky movements will only suck you in deeper.

Find a John Anywhere

When you gotta go, you gotta go.

To Find the Toilet In:	Say:	Or the International John Equivalent:
London	WC	John
Glasgow	loo	Ian
Sydney	dunny	John
Dublin	Jacks or loo	Sean
Berlin	toilette (*toy-LET-ta*)	Johannes or Johann
Paris	toilet (*twa-let*)	Jean
Bucharest	WC (*vee-cheeu*)	Ion
Rome	latrina (*la-TREE-na*)	Giovanni
Madrid	cervicio (*ser-VEE-see-o*)	Juan
Lisbon	banheiro (*ba-NEER-o*)	Joan
Moscow	toal-YET (phonetic)	Ivan
Tokyo	BEN-jo (phonetic)	John

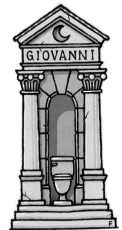

One exception: Never ask for a John in Amsterdam's red-light district.

---

you're held up, hand over the phony. Keep your real wallet in an inside coat pocket that buttons, and hope you don't get mugged twice on the same trip.

Also, before you go, photocopy all the important stuff in your wallet and give the copy to your secretary or a dependable coworker. He or she can fax it to you in case you lose your billfold.

Subdue an Alligator

Don't waste your time asking why you didn't take the family to Disney World, where all of the alligators are animatronics, instead of the Amazon, where you're outnumbered by the prehistoric beasts. Here's what you need to do:

1. Climb onto the back of the gator, facing its head.

2. Plant your feet *behind* the reptile's front legs. This keeps it immobilized. That way, if it turns its head to bite you, it'll bite off its own leg.

3. Come around the side of the gator's head and clasp its mouth shut with one quick motion of your hand. It's not as hard as it sounds because the muscles used to open the mouth are much smaller than those used to bite down.

4. Once the gator's mouth is closed, use your other hand to wrap it shut with duct tape or rope.

Survive a Shark Attack

If a shark attacks, punch it or poke it sharply in the snout, eye, or gills. Sharks, like many other animals, are sensitive around the schnozz, and a good punch in the nose makes you too much trouble to be dinner.

ESCAPE A COLLARING

If a mugger grabs your shirt collar with both hands, break his hold by powerfully windmilling your dominant arm (meaning right for righties) up, over, and down—crunching his wrists under your upper arm. Then run.

Or, if a big man attacks you from behind and locks his arms around you, use his weight against him. As he grabs you, you'll both stagger forward at least a step. Use that momentum: Let your legs collapse and rotate to one side. Your body will fall directly on his elbow, causing him to release his hold.

Plug Up a Hole in Your Tooth

You're on a trip and you lose a filling to a tough piece of steak. Now every sip of hot coffee or cold beer you take lets you know there's a gaping hole in your molar and a bunch of exposed nerve endings. What should you do until you can get to your dentist for a proper fix? Mold a piece of candle wax and plug up the hole with it. If you cover the exposed area, it won't be as sensitive to hot and cold. Don't have wax? Try sugarless chewing gym.

Get a Summer Flu Shot

It may seem out of season to get a flu shot, but if you're heading south of the equator in the summer, consider getting one before you leave. While it's summer where you live, it's winter in the southern hemisphere and, thus, flu season.

Think Nationally

If you travel often, consider joining a national health club, such as Gold's Gym, Bally's, or the YMCA. When the hotel gym is god-awful, you can exercise for free, or for a minimal fee, at the closest affiliated gym. If you move out of the area, transferring your membership to another branch will probably prove easier than wrangling a partial refund of your membership fee.

Return on Tuesday

Go back to work after a vacation on a Tuesday. It's less hectic than Monday. Plus, having a short week will keep that vacation-feeling alive a little longer.

PHOTO CREDITS

Achille: page 201 (tonic)

Jerome Albertini: page 271

Kelly Alder: pages 234, 242, 269

Roderick Angle: pages 11, 124

Paul Aresu: page 61

Guy Aroch: page 267

Daniel Arsenault/Image Bank: page 237

Michele Asselin: pages 73 (bottom), 277

Jerry Atnip: page 215

Ondrea Barbe: page 144

David Bartoloni: page 201 (man with ice pack)

David Bashaw: page 70 (man)

Al Bello/Allsport: page 195

Peter Berson: page 14

Candace Billman: page 51

Beth Bischoff: pages 58, 151, 161, 162, 163, 164, 165 (top 2), 167, 169 (Swiss ball), 171, 174 (bottom 2), 180, 181, 189, 192 (men), 200 (bottom 4), 201 (top 3), 202, 203 (man with ice pack)

Bob Blumer: pages 43, 45

Augustus Butera: page 92

Roger Cabello: page 176

Jonathan Carlson: pages 19 (bottle opener), 188

Coolife: pages 8 (McMuffin and bagel), 20, 178

Bill Cutter: page 227 (fingerprints)

Davies & Starr: pages 33, 233, 243

Lorraine Dey: pages 76, 90, 94

William Duke: page 223

Michael Edwards: pages 111 (bottom), 225

EyeWire: page 284

Ben Fink: page 40

Steven Freeman: page 258

Rafael Fuchs: page 224

A. J. Garces: page 192 (sign)

Philip Gatward/Dorling Kindersley: page 186

Robert Gerheart: pages 66, 129, 205

Girl Ray: pages 32, 54, 84 (top), 142, 210

Mitchel Gray: pages 168, 174 (top), 268

Lois Greenfield: page 74 (bottom)

Brad Guice: pages 170, 183

Brian Hagiwara: pages 8 (Dunkin' Donuts), 13, 18, 36, 106

Gary Hallgren: pages 100, 246

John P. Hamel: page 196 (swimmer)

Jeff Harris: pages 23, 39, 48, 81 (shoe)

Visko Hatfield: page 139 (top)

Tom Haynes: pages 111 (top), 200 (top)

Steven A. Heller: page 197

Hilmar: pages 208, 260

Anja Hinrichsen: page 99

John Hull: page 173

Courtesy of International Dairy Queen: page 16 (banana split)

Eric Jacobson: pages 2, 27

Laura Johansen: pages 24, 37, 41, 44, 113, 137

Johansson/Lodge Corbis Outline: page 102 (bottom)

Eric Anthony Johnson: page 84 (bottom)

Erik T. Johnson: pages 68, 71, 72, 80

Trevor Johnston: pages 247, 272

Robin Kachantones: page 165 (bottom)

John Kachik: page 81 (body types)

Jonathan Kantor: page 240

Ralph Kelliher: pages 138 (bottom 2), 232

John Kernick: page 88

Joshua Kessler: page 15

Andrew Kist: pages 112, 136

Michael Krasowitz/FPG: page 262

Michael Kraus: pages 21, 74 (top), 139 (bottom)

Dave Krieger: page 191

Dan Krovatin: pages 79, 102 (top 3), 135, 138 (top)

R. Krubner/Robertstock: page 231

Michael Lavine: page 19 (pretzels)

Allison Leach: page 52

Svend Lindbaek: pages 175 (bottom), 203 (man drinking)

Rod Little: page 175 (top)

Romilly Lockyer/Image Bank: page 101

Ian Logan: page 159

Brian Long: page 154

Mitch Mandel: pages 47, 152, 155, 196 (man hanging), 212, 275

John Manno: page 239

Gregory Nemec: pages 249, 250

Sylvia Otte: page 8 (muffin)

Particle 17/Mark S. Fisher: page 289

Bob Penn/MPTV: page 119

Mark Peterson: pages 35, 89

Maria Quiroga: pages 34, 203 (measuring cup and alcohol)

Victoria Rich: pages 16 (popcorn), 95, 244

John Ritter: page 140

Rodale Images: page 148

Dean Rohrer: pages 85, 127, 219, 221, 226, 241, 245

Danny Rothenberg: pages 65, 169 (top)

John Sterling Ruth: pages 31, 281

Roberto Sanchez: page 117

Chip Simons: page 273

Kevin Sprouls: page 115

Steven Stankiewicz: page 184

Robert Tardio: pages 70 (folding sweater), 73 (top)

Kenji Toma: page 97

Fabrice Trombert: page 172 (top 2)

Sally Ullman: page 57

Steven Wacksman: page 217

Sasha Waldman: page 229

Kurt W. C. Walters: page 227 (top 2)

John L. Wilkes: page 10

Kurt Wilson: pages 5, 166, 172 (bottom 2), 198, 199, 286

Steve Wisbauer: page 203 (refrigerator)

INDEX

Underscored page references indicate boxed text.

Conversion Chart

These equivalents have been slightly rounded to make measuring easier.

VOLUME MEASUREMENTS

U.S.	Imperial	Metric
¼ tsp	–	1 ml
½ tsp	–	2 ml
1 tsp	–	5 ml
1 Tbsp	–	15 ml
2 Tbsp (1 oz)	1 fl oz	30 ml
¼ cup (2 oz)	2 fl oz	60 ml
⅓ cup (3 oz)	3 fl oz	80 ml
½ cup (4 oz)	4 fl oz	120 ml
⅔ cup (5 oz)	5 fl oz	160 ml
¾ cup (6 oz)	6 fl oz	180 ml
1 cup (8 oz)	8 fl oz	240 ml

WEIGHT MEASUREMENTS

U.S.	Metric
1 oz	30 g
2 oz	60 g
4 oz (¼ lb)	115 g
5 oz (⅓ lb)	145 g
6 oz	170 g
7 oz	200 g
8 oz (½ lb)	230 g
10 oz	285 g
12 oz (¾ lb)	340 g
14 oz	400 g
16 oz (1 lb)	455 g
2.2 lb	1 kg

LENGTH MEASUREMENTS

U.S.	Metric
¼"	0.6 cm
½"	1.25 cm
1"	2.5 cm
2"	5 cm
4"	11 cm
6"	15 cm
8"	20 cm
10"	25 cm
12" (1')	30 cm

PAN SIZES

U.S.	Metric
8" cake pan	20 × 4 cm sandwich or cake tin
9" cake pan	23 × 3.5 cm sandwich or cake tin
11" × 7" baking pan	28 × 18 cm baking tin
13" × 9" baking pan	32.5 × 23 cm baking tin
15" × 10" baking pan	38 × 25.5 cm baking tin (Swiss roll tin)
1½ qt baking dish	1.5 liter baking dish
2 qt baking dish	2 liter baking dish
2 qt rectangular baking dish	30 × 19 cm baking dish
9" pie plate	22 × 4 or 23 × 4 cm pie plate
7" or 8' springform pan	18 or 20 cm springform or loose-bottom cake tin
9" × 5" loaf pan	23 × 13 cm or 2 lb narrow loaf tin or pâté tin

TEMPERATURES

Fahrenheit	Centigrade	Gas
140°	60°	–
160°	70°	–
180°	80°	–
225°	105°	¼
250°	120°	½
275°	135°	1
300°	150°	2
325°	160°	3
350°	180°	4
375°	190°	5
400°	200°	6
425°	220°	7
450°	230°	8
475°	245°	9
500°	260°	–